# BUILDING BETTER HEALTH

## A HANDBOOK OF BEHAVIORAL CHANGE

C. David Jenkins, Ph.D.

Professor of
Preventive Medicine and Community Health,
Epidemiology, and Psychiatry

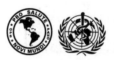

Scientific and Technical Publication No. 590

PAN AMERICAN HEALTH ORGANIZATION
Pan American Sanitary Bureau, Regional Office of the
WORLD HEALTH ORGANIZATION
525 Twenty-third Street, N.W.
Washington, D.C. 20037, U.S.A.

2003

**PAHO HQ Library Cataloguing-in-Publication Data**

Jenkins, C. David
    Building better health: a handbook for behavioral change
Washington D.C: PAHO, © 2003.
(Scientific and Technical Publication N° 590)

ISBN 92 75 11590 7

I. Title  II. (Series)
III. Pan American Health Organization

1. PRIMARY PREVENTION
2. HEALTH PROMOTION
3. EDUCATION, PUBLIC HEALTH PROFESSIONAL
4. BEHAVIORAL MEDICINE-education
5. MANUALS

NLM WA590.J52b 2003

# Table of Contents

# Prologue

At the beginning of the 21st century, our Region's health report card is mixed. On the plus side, the countries of the Americas have made clear gains in "Health for All" goals. Infant mortality rates are lower, for example, and this, in turn, has helped to add six years to life expectancy at birth in the last two decades. On the other hand, these gains have not been evenly attained throughout the Region, and some countries, as well as some areas and population groups within countries, have been deprived of these benefits. The fast pace of aging and urbanization has resulted in an exponential rise in chronic noncommunicable diseases, adding to the yet unsolved toll in death and disability wrought by communicable diseases, especially among the poor.

Already, noncommunicable diseases are the leading cause of disability and premature mortality in the vast majority of countries of the Americas. If projections hold, chronic degenerative diseases, lifestyle-related diseases, and violence will continue to take up an increasingly greater share of death and suffering, impairing the quality of life among the peoples of the Americas. They will also overtax health services and drive up health care costs. The good news is that many of these diseases and conditions can be prevented. At the very least, their development can be delayed or slowed, their severity mitigated. Because many of their determinants and risk factors respond to behavior change, health promotion holds the key in this battle.

Throughout its 100 years of work in and for health with the countries of the Americas, the Pan American Health Organization (PAHO) has championed the prevention of disease and the enhancement of health. Following the "Ottawa Charter for Health Promotion" issued by the First International Conference on Health Promotion in 1986, PAHO's health promotion efforts focused and gathered momentum. Since then, the Organization has worked with its Member States to fulfill the Charter's health promotion tenets, pursuing efforts that have included the fostering of healthy public policies, creation of supportive environments, strengthening of community actions, and development of personal skills. The book that you hold in your hands is PAHO's latest contribution to its overall health promotion effort.

The Handbook blends proven disease prevention practices and behavioral science principles into a one-of-a-kind, hands-on manual. Its pages spell out how to think about developing effective health promotion/disease prevention programs and how to carry them out so that they yield the best possible results. The book explores the causes of morbidity, disability, and premature mortality for each stage in the life cycle—from infancy to the elder years. The Handbook also looks at the protective and risk factors for each of the leading forms of death and disability, and recommends easily implemented, practical preventive interventions.

Health professionals battling to "add years to life and life to years" will find *Building Better Health: A Handbook of Behavioral Change* an invaluable tool in their work. In addition, national, provincial, and local health authorities will find it useful in planning health promotion programs. We hope that it also will become a popular textbook for teaching and training new generations of health workers.

We are grateful to the author, Dr. C. David Jenkins, a well-known professor of psychiatry, epidemiology, and preventive medicine and community health for partnering with PAHO to issue this important and useful work.

Dr. Mirta Roses Periago
Director

# Preface

Dear Reader:

Welcome to *Building Better Health: A Handbook of Behavioral Change.*

Today, the nations of the world devote huge sums of money to "health care." Sadly, about 98% of these budgets are actually spent on "disease care" and only about 1% or 2% on genuine care of health. In contrast, this Handbook devotes itself fully to health care, defined as improving and maintaining good health—which consists of feeling well and functioning well, physically, mentally and interpersonally; as well as having a high likelihood of continuing to live healthfully in the future.

The highway to "Health for All" for the 21st Century will be constructed by activating within communities already proven methods for advancing health and preventing disease and disability. The science is known, now its utilization must spread. Most of the programs we present are low technology, but people-intensive. Hence, they are sustainable even where financial resources are limited.

This book has been written by many people: those who have asked "What if?" and "Why not?"; those whose words and data I have read; and especially those in many parts of the world, in high and low places, to whom I have listened carefully over the years. Actually, these thoughtful people are much like you who read this Handbook. And I sincerely thank them. My task has been like that of a chef—to take these rich ingredients and blend them in a way that is appealing, nourishing, and energizing.

This Handbook was written for many kinds of persons, in many different countries, professions, and community niches. You may be a health worker in the countryside, a physician in a health clinic, a visiting nurse, a student in the health professions, someone updating their knowledge of community problems, a school teacher, a town council member, a dedicated parent, or someone else beyond my imagination. In any case, if you read this book, you are a student and a seeker. I am both of those, so we should get along well.

The Handbook covers many topics. I'm not an expert in most of them, but I've compared multiple resources and tried to select the better-validated and more practical wheat from acres and hectares of chaff. Expert reviewers have checked over each chapter, and I express my appreciation to all of them here. I am responsible for whatever errors may remain. You will find that reading the Handbook is different from reading a medical or public health textbook. I've tried to keep it fresh, personal, concrete, motivating, and sometimes even prodding. Comprehensive indexing makes the Handbook easier to use.

So, please—enjoy! Compare your ideas with those presented here, find new directions, see what actions can address the needs of the people around you. Be captured by a sense of urgency and an assurance that you can start this journey to a healthier world. Bring others with you to prevent disease and build health by means of behavioral and social changes.

*The sands of the Twenty-First Century await our footprints. . . .*

Respectfully yours,


C. David Jenkins, Ph.D.

# Acknowledgments

The author extends deep appreciation:

To stimulating and enabling mentors: John C. Cassel, MB, BCH; Irene Case Sherman, MD, Ph.D.; Stephen J. Zyzanski, Ph.D., Robert M. Rose, MD, Don W. Micks, Sc.D., and others at Universities and health agencies.

To everyday mentors in Chicago and Boston ghettos, in Suriname rainforests, in the South Yemen desert, and to patients in public health and medical clinics.

To the professors and practitioners who each reviewed parts of this Handbook: Seymour T. Barnes, B.J. Campbell, Neva T. Edens, Adam O. Goldstein, Berton H. Kaplan, George A. Kaplan, Ernest N. Kraybill, Robert Haggerty, William R. Harlan, Irving F. Hoffman, Barbara S. Hulka, David J. Lee, Itzhak Levav, Lewis Margolis, Kyriakos Markides, Cynthia Rosengard, Ross J. Simpson, Beat Steiner, T. Scott Stroup, and Stephen Zyzanski.

To Diane K. Godwin, for diligent work and solid advice on the many revisions of the manuscript.

And, especially to my wife, Perry, for her editorial help and for sustaining me during five years of work on this book.


C. David Jenkins, Ph.D.

# PART I.
# LAYING THE
# FOUNDATION

# 1. General Principles of Health Promotion and Disease Prevention

The scientific engines of the 20th century powered a revolution in biomedical sciences. These advances delivered deeper understanding of the dynamics of biological processes, amazing new pharmaceuticals, and space-age techniques for visualizing and treating problems deep inside the body. They have remedied many kinds of diseases and injuries for millions of people—but they have left the remaining billions with most of the same scourges their grandparents suffered 100 years ago.

The 21st century cries out for a new dimension of revolution, one that is not expressed mainly in organic chemistry, or in subcellular messengers, or in genomics. Rather, it will be expressed in the expectations, overriding goals, actions, and commitments of individuals, families, communities, and nations. No group of people, no matter how privileged and protected, can feel smugly safe and immune from the biopsychosocial epidemics of suffering that roam unchecked through the majority of the neighborhoods in this global village.

The new health revolution must carry the most potent advances in our scientific framework of knowledge to the people and places where they can make the difference between life and death. Only then can the possibility of "health for all" see its sunrise.

## HUMAN AND ECONOMIC VALUES OF PREVENTION

Health is the first and most important form of wealth. Health—the physical, mental, and social health of an *entire* population—is a nation's fundamental natural resource. If it is ignored or wasted, farms will wither, mines will close, factory engines will slow their production, families will break up, and children's laughter will no longer sing throughout the community. If health becomes only the province of the wealthy, that nation has an ominous future. The poor will struggle for equity, and even the wealthy, feeling isolated or disabled or in fear, will stop enjoying their riches.

Health is the essential foundation that supports and nurtures growth, learning, personal well being, social fulfillment, enrichment of others, economic production, and constructive citizenship. Cost-benefit research has become a popular

*Health is the essential foundation that supports and nurtures growth, learning, personal well being, social fulfillment, enrichment of others, economic production, and constructive citizenship.*

means to evaluate both medical treatment and preventive medicine, with the units of measurement usually being drawn from the monetary system. We should keep in mind, however, that successfully promoting good health has intrinsic values and enabling powers that reach far beyond a single year's budget.

With the world's national economies in transition from producing natural resources to adding value to resources through manufacturing, and now to the rise of the service economy and information management, the allocations for developing national infrastructures will increasingly shift to investing in the human infrastructure. Only by improving the health and learning opportunities of the next generation can the most valuable infrastructure for a nation's future be solidly built.

Since the 1950s, health care costs have skyrocketed in most nations. Advances in medical technology have made it possible to treat more and more illnesses and disabilities with increasingly sophisticated equipment, for both diagnostic and therapeutic purposes. Further, the miracles of medicine and surgery can now keep more patients with severe illnesses and injuries alive longer, often into older ages, at much greater cost to the community. As more of these patients survive, more and more persons need to be trained to provide rehabilitation and long-term care for this increasing percentage of the population. Thus, the proportion of the gross national product going into tertiary health care services is steadily increasing in most countries.

Successful health promotion and protection programs can be made available cost-effectively to the entire population. They have the potential to halt this expansion of preventable costs, or at least to slow its progress. Health-promoting prenatal care, for example, can deliver healthier babies, and preventive medicine in infancy and childhood will produce healthier children who can grow to their full potential and learn a full array of cognitive and motor skills. Effective programs to protect children and youth from injury and violence also will generate a healthier work force and lower the frequency of disabled persons needing health care. Introducing healthy lifestyle habits early in childhood, and reinforcing them through young adulthood, will prevent much of the current morbidity and mortality rates due to cardiovascular and respiratory diseases and cancers, which attack adults in their prime middle years. Clearly, keeping adults economically productive up to their retirement should be a goal both for health promotion and for economic development. Finally, as the elderly population in every nation grows, it becomes increasingly important to maximize the health and self-care abilities of retired citizens for as long as possible in their remaining years.

To reach all of these goals, an ounce of prevention is worth a pound of cure. This book will present, "ounce by ounce," specific preventive interventions that are beneficial, practical, inexpensive, and sustainable. They are currently the most visible signposts on the highway to improve health for all in the twenty-first century.

We know that it is always better to prevent a disease or an external trauma than to treat it after it happens—prevention saves individuals, *and* their families, from pain, suffering, loss of function, prolonged disability, or premature death.

*Keeping adults economically productive up to their retirement should be a goal both for health promotion and for economic development.*

Some prevention programs also save money, depending on the program, the population, the disease, and whether one is considering short-term or long-term community outcomes. For families and for nations, this is a most welcome message in these times of escalating costs of medical care, especially high technology care. The only time when prevention could be more expensive than treatment is when disease or injury is infrequent and moves quickly to death before major expenses are incurred—and this is even more painful for surviving family and friends.

But the argument for prevention cannot—and should not—be made primarily on economic grounds. Even though mortality from ischemic (coronary) heart disease has declined sharply since about 1970 (a 30% to 50% decline in some Westernized countries), the cost of treating each case has actually gone up because new technology has created new diagnostic tests and new therapeutic procedures. In addition, the fact that there is an ever-growing number of cardiologists, makes the overall economic benefit negligible.

And yet, we would not want to roll-back scientific advance or the achievement of a full complement of medical specialists. The justification for prevention is that it reduces suffering, makes disability and its diminishments less common, and keeps death off the family's doorstep until much later. As the wise professor Geoffrey Rose put it: "It is better to be healthy than ill or dead. That is the beginning and the end of the only real argument for preventive medicine. It is sufficient" (Rose, 1992).

Policymakers and the public alike also should consider that some diseases and disabilities, although preventable, are just not curable by any means—in the 20th century one immediately thinks of AIDS. Such issues as the damage caused by a cerebrovascular accident, an automobile crash that cripples a child, or the liver damage caused by excessive use of alcohol also must be weighed. Policymakers dealing in health issues and health professionals must recognize that prevention is the only "cure" available for such destructive maladies.

# DISEASE PREVENTION AND HEALTH PROMOTION

Promoting healthy lifestyles involves action on two fronts: disease prevention and health promotion. While there is much overlap between these efforts, disease prevention usually focuses more on specific kinds of illness and trauma and often relies more on the direct involvement of health professionals. There are a few biologically focused physicians who still claim that disease prevention programs cannot really succeed "because you cannot change people." This is obviously false: tens of millions of people change their health habits and other lifestyle aspects every year. The clear feasibility and success of prevention efforts have been demonstrated for many health problems in many nations. Consider the nearly 50% dramatic decline in cardiovascular mortality in North America and Western Europe since 1970.

In contrast, health promotion involves both individual and family behaviors—as well as healthy public policies in the community—that protect a person against numerous health threats and elicit a general sense of personal responsibility for maximizing one's safety, host resistance, vitality, and effective functioning. Health promotion, while often using guidance and motivation from health professionals, depends more heavily on individuals acting to change health behaviors in themselves, their families, and their community, as well as advocating preventive health priorities among policymakers, business, industry, and government. This Handbook lays out critical health problems and the social and behavioral changes needed to resolve them—both by means of health promotion and disease prevention.

## THREE LEVELS OF PREVENTION

Epidemiologists have identified three stages of the disease process at which preventive actions can be effective—primary prevention, secondary prevention, and tertiary prevention.

### PRIMARY PREVENTION

Primary prevention aims at keeping a disease from ever beginning or a trauma from ever occurring. Examples include immunization, reducing household hazards, motivating abstinence from illegal drugs, and reducing risk factors for heart disease. Primary prevention programs aim to reach the widest possible population group who is or might become at risk for a given health problem.

Health promotion programs are usually at the primary prevention level. Quite often a single behavioral habit will protect against a host of diseases. For example, helping children and youth never to start using tobacco (and adults to stop smoking) yields a 90% reduction in the risk of lung cancer, a 30% to 40% reduction (depending on the population) in the risk of heart attack, a 90% reduction in the risk of chronic lung disease, reductions in many sites of cancer, a reduction in auto accidents and injuries due to fire, and a reduction in the rates of acute respiratory diseases in young children in the home (Last, 1987).

Avoiding or limiting use of alcohol is another lifestyle choice that promotes health in many ways. Last (1987) lists 76 different biological, psychiatric, and behavioral problems caused or worsened by excessive alcohol use. These range all the way from acute intoxication to depression; suicide; cancers of the head, neck, stomach, large bowel, and liver; cirrhosis; cardiomyopathy; hypertension; depressed gonadal function; ethanol-drug interactions; traumatic injuries (especially when driving automobiles or boats); anemia; and many types of complications of pregnancy and birth defects.

> *The argument for prevention cannot—and should not—be made primarily on economic grounds. The justification for prevention—even when it does not save money—is that it reduces suffering, makes disability and its diminishments less common, and delays the arrival of death at the family's doorstep.*

Increasing regular, moderate physical exercise and maintaining proper appropriate eating patterns are other health promoting habits that also have a wide range of benefits, including preventing atherosclerosis, reducing high blood pressure, lowering LDL cholesterol, reducing the risk of adult onset diabetes, and strengthening the cardiorespiratory and musculoskeletal systems.

## SECONDARY PREVENTION

Secondary prevention involves the early detection and early intervention against disease before it develops fully. Screening programs are prime examples of secondary prevention efforts, providing that persons who screen positive for a disease or condition receive prompt and effective intervention. Conducting screening without full follow-up wastes money and creates anxiety and frustration in the community.

Some cancer screening seeks to identify malignancies while they are small. In contrast, cervical cancer screening (pap smears) seeks to identify pre-malignant cell changes. Screening for infectious diseases can identify sub-clinical cases needing treatment and also prevent spread to the community. This is especially important to healthy persons who otherwise would be exposed to "a carrier" of disease. Screening, at least at its first level, may not require expensive equipment or laboratory processing. Careful questioning and a focused brief observation can reveal many conditions, from nutritional problems to dyspnea to schizo-phrenia—and many more. This can be done by any trained health professional.

Such measures as wearing auto seat belts do not prevent accidents but clearly reduce the severity of human injury. The continuous use of appropriate anti-bacterials to treat Hanson's Disease (leprosy) and tuberculosis reduces the risk that the disease will spread to others and also halts the progression of pathology in the patient. Because these measures keep trauma and disease from becoming more severe after onset, they too are considered by some to constitute second-ary prevention.

## TERTIARY PREVENTION

Tertiary prevention takes place after a disease or injury has occurred. It seeks not only to prevent deterioration and complications from a disease or injury, but also to rehabilitate and return the patient to as full physical, mental, and social function as possible. This is primarily the work of health professionals, but the public needs to know the potential benefits of tertiary interventions and to ad-vocate giving them an appropriate priority in the light of a community's full spectrum of health care needs.

## THE ACTUAL CAUSES OF DEATH

When the public—and health professionals—think of the causes of death, they think of such things as heart disease, cancer, liver disease, or motor vehicle ac-cidents. These are just final diagnoses, however. What are the true causes that lead to these final outcomes? McGinnis and Foege (1993) have identified the non-genetic factors that increased total mortality in the United States and esti-mated their contributions to the ten leading mortality diagnoses.

---

### THE TEN "TRUE" LEADING CAUSES OF DEATH

- tobacco use
- inadequate or excessive nutrition (dietary habits)
- inadequate aerobic exercise
- excessive alcohol consumption
- lack of immunization against microbial agents
- exposure to poisons and toxins
- firearms
- risky sexual behaviors
- motor vehicle trauma
- use of illicit drugs

---

These same ten contributing causes are important risk factors throughout the world, but their relative impact will vary depending on local environments and cultures. Simple epidemiologic study should enable each country to set its own preventive priorities.

The McGinnis and Foege study was based on a wide literature review and consensus estimates of the prevalence of risk factors, proportional attributable risks, and 1990 numbers of deaths by cause in the United States. Of 1,238,000 deaths, approximately 400,000 were attributed to tobacco use; 300,000, to dietary and activity patterns; 100,000, to excess alcohol use; 90,000, to microbial agents; 60,000, to toxic exposures; 35,000, to firearms; 30,000, to sexual behavior; 25,000, to motor vehicles; and 20,000, to illicit-drug use. These proportional mortality rates by cause will differ by culture and geography. The good news is that all of these causes can be reduced by behavioral and social changes.

Low socioeconomic status and inadequate access to medical care also raise mortality, but usually in interaction with the ten social behavioral factors listed above. It is clear that these factors also contribute to long-term morbidity and impaired quality of life, and they also help to raise the costs for medical care astronomically before death closes each case.

## THE NEXT STEP NEEDED TO ADVANCE "HEALTH FOR ALL"

The causes and contributing risk factors for all the leading mortality and morbidity diagnoses in all nations are well established. Preventive measures to deal with them are also well enough known to be able to initiate programs. As the previous section demonstrates, the role of behavioral change in reducing every one of the above-mentioned major causes of disease and trauma is clear at both the individual and social levels. For the first time in the history of medical sciences, the first priority is not further discoveries in the basic physical and biological sciences, but rather the community-wide application of psychology and other social and behavioral sciences for the purpose of putting well-proven preventive health measures into wider daily use. Many of the discoveries in the behavioral sciences are already being successfully applied to clinical medical and public health problems. Technology dealing with behavior change must be applied to health promotion in many more nations and communities and it must be taught in every school for health professionals. **(Also see Chapters 2 and 12.)**

# 2. Principles of Community Health Intervention

Community health programs will be most effective and conserve more resources if they are built upon a foundation of solved puzzles. This chapter will discuss each of these puzzling questions in sequence, with the goal of providing local communities with a foundation upon which to build a dependable structure for local health interventions.

---

**PUZZLES TO SOLVE FOR BUILDING BETTER HEALTH**
- What factors contribute to the excess number of specified diseases, disabilities, or deaths?
- How can these factors be changed?
- What additional protective or health giving elements can reduce these health problems?
- With what subpopulations shall work be done, and in what sequence, to solve the problem?
- What overall intervention strategies will yield the greatest results?
- Precisely what needs to be done—and what can be omitted—to reach the goals?

---

## STRATEGIES FOR IDENTIFYING CAUSES

One of the early paradigms for explaining the spread of disease was the "epidemiological triangle":

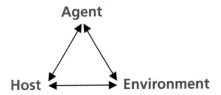

This section will examine how the concepts of agent, host, and environment have expanded in meaning since they were first used early in the fight against infectious diseases.

### AGENT

This term was first used to identify "the cause" of a disease, such as an infectious or parasitic agent. Today, agent also applies to excesses of heat, cold, dust, toxins, stressful events, instruments of injury, and even excessive amounts of calories or fats in the diet. Shortages or deficiencies of factors also may be considered as agents, as in hunger, thirst, iron or iodine deficiencies, lack of adequate mothering, lack of social contacts, lack of employment, poverty, and hopelessness.

In situations where no single element is a sufficient cause for disease, combinations of circumstances also can become agents. For example, among people without adequate protein, a serious lack of niacin will, in time, cause pellagra. This, however, occurs only among people who also lack tryptophan, such as those who eat maize, sorghum, or millet as the primary grain in their diet. Witness the fact that Southeast Asians, whose basic staple is rice, seldom get pellagra. Another example involves cancers that develop only after cells have been damaged in sequence by two separate chemical agents, then called co-carcinogens. Finally, patients taking certain psychiatric drugs can become severely sunburned and systemically sickened by only modest exposure to sunlight. What is the agent of this malady—the drug, the sunlight, both in combination?

### HOST

The host also must be considered from several aspects. It can be the target of disease, as originally conceived, and it also can be the disease's contributing cause and perpetuator, as it has come to be viewed later. Public health's goal is to make the host a preventor much more of the time, as well as an active participant in the healing process.

The host should not be viewed merely as a biological "hunk," however. Rather, the host is a complex set of systems, as is clearly seen when conducting a "review of systems" in making a diagnosis. The challenge of disease prevention and health promotion may require an evaluation and a change in the cognitive, emotional, behavioral, and social statuses of individuals, groups, and even communities. These efforts are in addition to such actions as raising host resistance by improving nutrition, providing immunizations, preventing immunodeficiency, and dealing with mood disorders, which can have many organic consequences.

Consider how the following conditions, all of which are parts of the host, might modify a disease prevention plan:

- Rural residents who fear or distrust doctors might not bring their children for immunizations or treatment.

- Families living in abject poverty will not be able to afford medicines nor follow the doctor's prescriptions.

- Urban subpopulations that live where violence is out of control may feel helpless and hopeless.

- People may be so depressed that they cannot function socially, staying at home and barely maintaining themselves.

- Among sexually promiscuous youth, antibiotics may treat the current infection, but they won't prevent the next one.

- Some factory managers may feel they will go broke if they have to add an effective chemical treatment system to the toxins they pour into the waterways.

- There may be proper citizens who see youth only as potential danger, and would just as soon see the homeless die of disease or violence rather than pay for kinder alternatives.

- There may be aged persons living alone with no one to help them in emergencies.

- People may know that cigarette smoking is damaging, but cannot get motivated to stop.

- Chronic alcoholics may be unable to stay in rehabilitation programs.

## ENVIRONMENT

In considering this term, we usually think first about what environmental scientists, engineers, and health inspectors have been dealing with for centuries—such physical factors as air and water pollution, and solid waste disposal. Then we might consider such issues as highway construction and product design, which also have come to concern environmental specialists. The biophysical pathogens against which environmental specialists have made great advances include reservoirs of infection, insect and animal disease vectors, food-borne diseases, organic allergens, toxic chemicals, radiation, and person-to-person transmission of disease in its various forms. All these remain very important, and public health programs in many nations have much work to do before all the plagues we know how to conquer have, in fact, been brought under control.

> *The challenge of disease prevention and health promotion may require an evaluation and a change in the cognitive, emotional, behavioral, and social statuses of individuals, groups, and even communities.*

At the same time, wise health professionals have for many years incorporated three more environmental levels into their work—the interpersonal, social/economic, and cultural/ideological levels of every person's environment. Unfortunately, this knowledge and practice is not yet widespread.

### Interpersonal Level

The elemental unit of the interpersonal environment is the dyad—the inter-relation between two persons. This begins with the bond between mother and child.

Even in lower mammals—from mice to dogs, to elephants, and up to primates—separation of the infant from its mother's feeding, nurturing, and protection usually means disease, deranged behavior, or death. This is even more striking in the human offspring, as many pediatric and psychiatric studies have shown.

There is powerful preventive therapy in having a "significant other" or several caring persons who are close physically, mentally, and emotionally. This protective effect actually begins before birth. A later section on pregnancy will describe several interpersonal factors during pregnancy that raise the risk for the baby to have low birthweight or fetal anomalies.

Similarly, loving and guiding family and friends can steer older children through the dangers and threats of adolescence and build a happy, caring personal adjustment and healthy habits that will last a lifetime. The quality of the relationship, the emotional connection, and the mentoring appear more important than the amount of contact itself.

In later childhood and teen years, the peer group becomes more important in shaping values, habits (including health habits), attitudes toward risk-taking, and whether expectations for the future are rewarding or punishing—or neither! ("Neither" here refers to the numbing fatalism of some inner city youth, for example, who have seen peers die suddenly.) Families, teachers, and health professionals need to become more active in steering youth to those peer groups whose thinking and behaviors are constructive and healthy.

The powerful therapy of a nurturing interpersonal environment continues throughout the adult years. In almost all nations, at all age strata over 25 years, married persons have lower death rates than persons the same age who are divorced, widowed, or never married. Longitudinal population studies of loneliness versus social supports have consistently shown that those with an adequate social network have lower death rates, even when controlled for other elements such as health status and economic status at the beginning of the years of follow-up. Studies of the elderly show the same effect, and some organizations and areas in Europe (Sweden, for example) are now providing elders who live alone with opportunities for socializing, to see if this extends the number of their healthy, functional years of life.

### Social/economic Level

Beyond direct, face-to-face interactions with family, neighbors, friends, coworkers, and members of one's religious or social group, lie the social structures of the community and nation. These include work groups, commercial enterprises, local governments, medical services, unemployment or disability assistance agencies, religious groups, civic betterment groups, professional associations, and many others, as well as the ways they are organized and function.

These social structures comprise far more than the sum of the people in them, and exert more power than separate individuals. They may cooperate and facilitate, or debate, or remain passive when decisions are made about a variety of issues. Some of these include water and sewage systems; electric and telephone utilities; road building; schools; clinics and hospitals; how industry treats its workers and the environment; how prisons will be run; who is responsible for public health, disease prevention, and health promotion; who will provide medical care and at what level of modernity, and who will pay for it; and even what the laws of the land will be. It is obvious that these societal forces have a tremendous impact on everyone's health—for better or for worse. From time to time, some of these social organizations will need to be targeted in order to enlist them in improving the health of their communities or region.

A population's low economic level is the strongest predictor of poor health and high mortality everywhere in the world. The next strongest predictor is low educational level. This is true when comparing from country to country and also when comparing districts within a country—even those countries that provide health care for all. These socioeconomic indicators are associated with a plethora of diseases and causes of injury that share little in their etiologies. They have been said to predict every malady, but to explain none. People who live in poverty have poorer diets, poorer housing, more environmental pollution, more exposure to pathogens, more dangerous occupations, less job security, more damaging life crises, less effective police and fire protection, more tobacco and alcohol use, and tend to follow lifestyles that raise risk factors. The poor have fewer physical, psychological, and social protective resources, and they are usually powerless to improve their lot. **(Also see Chapter 13)**.

> **A population's low economic level is the strongest predictor of poor health and high mortality everywhere in the world. The next strongest predictor is low educational level.**

The obvious solution is to eliminate poverty, but that has proven impossible to achieve and maintain in most eras and locations. The alternative is to identify the major "real" causes of death and disability in disadvantaged neighborhoods and enlist local government sectors and nongovernmental organizations to assist in reducing those environmental, individual, social, and cultural factors that perpetuate the real causes of death. **(See the section "The Actual Causes of Death" in Chapter 1)**.

### Cultural/ideological Level

Culture consists of a society's framework of knowledge and beliefs, the content of its books and mass media, its technology, the determination of how social roles are to be fulfilled, which behaviors are normal and which unacceptable, and which are its morals and value systems. It is culture that ranks the importance of families versus individuals, of industriousness versus leisure. It is culture that determines the relative value of competitiveness, equity among people, benevolence, valuation of health, and ultimate goals. A community's infrastructure—its roads, bridges, water, electricity, buildings, and medical technology—might be viewed as part of the physical environment, but it all has been created or borrowed by the culture.

Culture is the way of life of a people. Like health and disease, culture is transmitted from group to group, from generation to generation. Witness the power of television to transmit the culture of high-technology nations—both the useful and the destructive aspects—to every corner of the world. Raising the hopes for a healthier, happier life has been useful, but marketing materialism, consumerism, aggression, and violence has been harmful.

A community's ideology is part of its overall culture, and is often inferred, rather than seen. Ideology is the world of ideas, beliefs, and values in which the members of a society live. What people say is important to them is not always reflected in their behavior, however, and the written plan for many institutions is often not the "real" way they operate. In health planning, it is critical to understand this paradox.

Culture tells its possessor what is important. It may value fame, sports skills, or conforming to friends. Or, it may tell who is important and who can be left out—perhaps women, ethnic minorities, the poor, and the powerless, who are often neglected. The stream of illness generated in these subgroups by lack of resources, lack of knowledge and skills, and lack of "a way out," is forced under the surface in many communities. But illness filters upwards to and through the roots of the upper and powerful classes, and the garden at the top soon ceases to flourish.

Culture also tells us what is possible and what is not. For example, villagers in Suriname's interior had known malaria as far back as their spoken history could trace. And, they used the statistically powerful "persistency forecast"—the best predictor of the future is what has always happened in the past—to accept that malaria would always be a part of their lives. By developing trust in health workers, however, who themselves had seen malaria eradicated in their own communities, Surinamese villagers were able to change their perception of what "is possible," and so release hope and energy to eradicate the malaria scourge in their own communities (Barnes and Jenkins, 1972).

Millions of people scattered in smaller groups throughout cities and countryside do not believe it is possible—or, perhaps, not sufficiently rewarding—to always drive vehicles legally, to get along without street drugs, to get almost all of their children immunized, to prevent food poisoning, to stop family violence, to reduce heart attacks and strokes, and on and on and on. If they are to reach these people, health workers must enlist the help of behavioral scientists and communicators to use available channels to change culture and ideology; to help fill the environment with ideas, interactions, and communication about new beliefs about what is important; and to spread the idea that everyone is important and that far more is possible than current beliefs hold.

## USING THE EPIDEMIOLOGIC TRIANGLE IN PREVENTION PROGRAMS

High rates of disease could be reduced sharply by appropriate changes in one or more of the three components—host, agent, environment—or in selected inter-actions among them.

The triangle was first used to deal with infectious and parasitic diseases. Its application could go something like this:

- The infectious agent can be neutralized by disinfectants, heat, or radiation.

- The host's resistance can be raised passively or actively by immunization, exposure to a related but milder infectious agent, protective use of gamma globulin, and improved nutrition.

- The environment can be "treated," such as by eliminating reservoirs of the agent, proper disposal of toxic waste, chlorinating and fluoridating water sup-plies, and enforcing sanitary standards for food processors and restaurants.

- A toxic, infectious agent can be separated from the susceptible host by using barriers, protective devices on machines, protective clothing, the quarantine of infectious persons, or even the use of condoms.

- The spread of transmission of the agent can be halted. Some of the examples above also serve to block transmission, but to these must be added early case finding and treatment (such as for tuberculosis, typhoid, or head lice); chemoprophylaxis (such as for malaria); vector control (for insects, snails, infected animals); sanitary disposal of human wastes; providing pure water supplies; and putting in place aseptic techniques in medical facilities, day-care centers, and nursing homes for the elderly.

The five strategies shown in Table 2.1 also can be applied to different sorts of health problems. The table illustrates how strategies can be used to reduce such wide ranging conditions and injuries as trauma from automobile accidents, ischemic heart disease, or cigarette smoking.

17

**TABLE 2.1.** Applying the expanded epidemiologic triangle to preventive interventions.[a]

| Intervention | Auto accident | Ischemic heart disease | Tobacco-related diseases |
|---|---|---|---|
| Change the agent | • Make safer cars.<br>• Pad car interiors.<br>• Restrict speeds. | • Promote low-fat, low-salt foods.<br>• Reduce risk factors. | • Attempt (failed) to make safe cigarettes.<br>• All burning emits carbon monoxide. |
| Raise host resistance | • Train drivers in safety.<br>• Internalize belief that drivers do not drink alcohol. | • Increase exercise.<br>• Get commitment to "heart health." | • Teach smokers to quit and youth to refuse to start. |
| Modify the environment | • Enforce traffic laws.<br>• Make roads and intersections safer. | • Provide facilities for exercise fun.<br>• Have friends and family reinforce healthy habits.<br>• Make healthy foods more popular and accessible. | • Make tobacco harder to get.<br>• Increase taxes on tobacco products.<br>• Develop social norms against cigarettes as dirty, harmful. |
| Separate agent from host | • Wear seat belts.<br>• Install air bags. | • Keep fatty foods and cigarettes out of the home. | • Make the home, workplace, health facility smoke-free.<br>• Limit purchase places. |
| Interrupt transmission | • Move damage off-road.<br>• Set up flares to prevent additional automobile accidents.<br>• Issue penalties for recurring violations. | • Screen for risk factors.<br>• Teach youth about "heart health." | • Train school peers to teach classmates how to remain smoke-free. |

[a] For further discussion of these strategies, see Last JM. *Public Health and Human Ecology*. East Norwalk, CT: Appleton/Prentice Hall; 1987.

## MULTIPLE CONTRIBUTING CAUSES

Scientists in the 20th century have demonstrated that the causal matrix of disease and injury was much more complex than Koch's postulates could explain. Ischemic (coronary) heart disease, for example, has many possible contributing causes that can work cumulatively, interactively, or individually. And a single noxious agent (say, cigarettes) can cause or contribute to very different disorders (for example, emphysema, ischemic heart disease, or bladder cancer, to name just a few). So, the simple linear thinking of early germ theorists—the epidemiological triangle and, even, the five prevention strategies—must give way (for an increasing number of problems) to a conceptualization that includes both causation and remediation as a probabilistic, multidimensional matrix of interactions: a **web of etiology** and a **web of interventions**, if you will. This discussion is included here in the hope of stimulating the reader to study both the web of causation and the web of prevention imaginatively, and to find the most cost-effective ways to break the cycle of illness and injury in different cultures and communities.

The struggle to control diseases that have multiple contributing causes, such as ischemic heart disease and most cancers, gave birth to the concept of risk factors—those elements in host, agent, or environment that increase the incidence of specific health problems. The concept of protective factors soon followed, based on findings that physical exercise reduces atherosclerosis; that dietary folic acid reduces fetal anomalies; and that having a close, supportive, and encouraging family enhances child development.

Preventive programs for many diseases and sources of injury follow the risk factor strategy—reducing risks and increasing protective factors. This approach has dramatically reduced many endemic diseases, ranging from heart disease and stroke to automobile fatalities and oral cancer. The field of mental illness prevention has now also adopted the "risk factor-protective factor" strategy to intervene against the complex neurological, psychiatric, and social behavioral disorders in that field (Mrazek and Haggerty, 1994). **(Also see Chapter 7.)**

> *Preventive programs for many diseases and sources of injury follow the risk factor strategy—reducing risks and increasing protective factors.*

A review of the prevention strategies reveals that each involves changing behaviors. Some changes must come from community and government leaders, others must involve health professionals; many involve intersectoral cooperation and all require changing community priorities and personal and collective behavior of the public.

## SELECTING WHICH CONDITIONS TO PREVENT

Prevention is a contest that must be won. To mount a program and then to have it fail not only wastes money, it disillusions both the public and senior officials regarding the value of future public health proposals. So how can the playing field be set up so that prevention programs are sure to win?

The entire plan should be worked out in advance, starting from how to present the plan's advantages to officials and the public, to what baseline measures will be needed, what interventions will be done, how and with whom, how the outcome will be evaluated, and what budget and human resources will be needed.

Early on, it is critical to establish which condition is both of high priority to prevent and also has a high feasibility to be changed. The condition must be one that is costly to the community or nation—costly in terms of human suffering and economic impact. Ideally, the condition to be prevented should have a high prevalence; cause suffering, prolonged disability, or death; lead to loss of time from work or normal childhood activities; and be expensive in terms of medical care.

Respiratory infections, for example, have a high prevalence, but their severity is too low and they are self-remitting. They would not be an appropriate prevention target. And certain rare cancers, although severe and fatal, do not affect enough people to generate community support. A widespread preventive effort targeting these cancers would not be cost-effective. Back injuries in industrial workers, on the other hand, are very common in some jobs—such as those involving twisting the body or doing heavy lifting—are very costly to employers, create chronic pain in affected workers, and often force workers to leave their line of work. All of these costs are high. Furthermore, the population to be targeted for intervention is relatively small, which limits costs. Preventive measures targeting industrial back injuries have proven to be successful.

Mortality statistics are the most comprehensively gathered health data worldwide. Where ministries of health cannot obtain reliable data from their whole nation, they often focus on a reasonable sample of areas for death registration, so national estimates can be made to guide health policy. Information on non-fatal disease and disability is much more difficult to collect reliably. The World Health Organization (WHO), Harvard University, the World Bank, and others have set up a cooperative system of data collection, evaluation, and statistical adjustment of disability data. This project, called the Global Burden of Disease (GBD) Study, began publishing results in 1994, and has continued to do so at a rapid rate since (e.g., Murray and Lopez, 1996).

*An ideal intervention target has three conditions—it is a costly problem, it has moderate to high prevalence in a defined subpopulation, and effective interventions to address it are not unduly expensive.*

The concept of an overall statistic that combines deaths and disability in a single estimate of burden of disease has been under development and refinement since about 1980. WHO has approved the general concepts of Disability Adjusted Life Years (DALYs), Years Lived with Disability (YLDs), Years of Life Lost (YLLs), and related indicators. WHO has recommended more work on the equations and weightings of variables.

Future work with changed weights for specific diagnoses and more accurate assessment of numbers of cases, particularly from places where many conditions are incompletely recorded, may change rank order and final estimates of the leading causes of lost life and health. The GBD estimates, however, are widely

BUILDING BETTER HEALTH

accepted as the best available to date, and are dependable enough to serve as policy guidelines (Murray and Lopez, 1996). These indicators, especially DALYs, will be incorporated into this handbook to help identify priorities.

Another element that often enters into institutional or governmental decisions regarding which health problems receive high priority. For example, a medical university in a developing country gave its first priority to preventing ischemic heart disease. Although the condition was relatively rare in the area served by their medical facilities, two senior faculty members had had myocardial infarctions. And in the United States, the occurrence of an illness in the country's president is a good predictor of future appropriations for research on that topic. In contrast, diseases and injuries common in people living in poverty, among the homeless, or in groups who are criticized on moral grounds (such as illegal drug users or homosexuals) often are given a much lower priority than their prevalence, severity, and cost would warrant. Health professionals should be alert to these biases and work to correct them, but, for the sake of effectiveness, should always work in cooperation with formal and informal community leaders.

## SELECTING THE TARGET SUBPOPULATIONS TO RECEIVE HELP

Many readers probably already are saying, "Of course you help those who are sick." Or, "No, we're talking prevention here. You intervene with those who are at risk of becoming sick or injured." Well, the answers are getting closer, but no prizes need be awarded yet.

A community's health, as well as its continuing streams of ill health, is spread and sustained by a delicate, complex web of interactions among elements of the physical, biological, interpersonal, socioeconomic, and cultural environments. The persons whose health is of concern rest in the center where all the strands come together. Those persons are in constant interactive exchanges with different levels of their own functioning (biological, psychological, social, values, and lifestyle), as well as with the changing environments of their private worlds. Sometimes the easiest way to repair tears in the web, tears that bring illness and injury, is to deal with other persons or circumstances, rather than with the high-risk person or group.

The mechanisms of illness and injury are also interwoven, involving agents of disease, environmental circumstances, culture, socioeconomics, people and their behaviors. The task to be accomplished is simple to state, but difficult to achieve. Vaccination coverage rates need only be between 70% and 90% (depending on the pathogen) for "herd immunity" to be adequate to prevent epidemics, but that will not eliminate scattered individual cases. And cigarette smoking needs only to continue declining steadily. Once a society starts to perceive smoking as "out of style," dirty, and harmful to the smoker *and* to others, then the momentum of social change will make the ashtray as obsolete as the cuspidor.

*Once a society starts to perceive smoking as "out of style," dirty, and harmful to the smoker and to others, then the momentum of social change will make the ashtray as obsolete as the cuspidor.*

The task, then, is to study the strong and weak spots in the web of health and in the web of pathology to identify the very few linkages that must be broken—or those that must be strengthened—to reduce morbidity and promote health most efficiently, with the fewest side effects, and at the lowest possible cost.

Typically, such programs rely heavily on human interaction, and very little on advanced technology. In many cases, only limited groups need be targeted for interventions to help many people. The following are successful examples that may spark the imagination of those considering starting programs.

- To deal with an endemic level of neonatal tetanus in Haiti, Drs. W. and G. Berggen first studied the local mode of tetanus transmission. They then decided to work with traditional birth attendants to improve hygiene during delivery and to keep the newborn's navel free of infection after severing the umbilical cord. Neonatal tetanus dropped nearly to zero.

- To reduce the high level of infant and small child deaths in automobiles, many states in the United States have: (1) passed laws requiring that safety seats be used by all children riding in cars and trucks; (2) solved the distribution problem by enlisting hospitals and well-baby clinics to loan safety seats free of charge for several years, until the child is large enough to use regular safety belts; (3) solved the financial problem by having civic organizations, commercial enterprises, and others buy the seats and donate them for use; and (4) solved the compliance problem by requiring police to keep an eye out for violations in automobiles they observe, and to fine those in violation. The rates of child deaths in vehicles, as well as the extraordinarily larger rates of trauma, have declined dramatically. Yes, the public was educated about the problem and its solution, but the most critical interventions were with legislators, health professionals, government agencies, and nongovernmental and commercial resources.

- To reduce the rate of malaria transmission, anti-malarial medications are often distributed to populations. This is difficult where the population at risk is difficult to reach and compliance is poor. In PAHO's campaign against malaria in Suriname in the 1960s, the targets for intervention were storekeepers. They were given pink medicated salt to distribute free, in place of regular white salt, which was always sold. The pink color told the public that the product was "the real thing" and for free. Everyone needs salt, and free salt is, clearly, best. Acceptance was rapid and enthusiastic (Barnes and Jenkins, 1972).

- To cut the carnage wrought by motor vehicles, highway safety experts have successfully changed behaviors in four target groups: (1) highway engineers to get them to design safer roadways with better visibility, barriers where needed, and adequate signs; (2) vehicle designers and automobile company executives to construct safer cars equipped with seat belts, better cushioning, collapsible steering columns, anti-lock brakes, and many other safety provisions; (3) individual drivers (especially youth) to drive more safely through courses, driver licensing, and systems that take away driving privileges for repeated offenses; and (4) law enforcement personnel to enforce driving safety laws by providing clear legislation with non-trivial penalties and by enlarging the force to permit full enforcement of the laws.

- To improve dental health, an effective caries prevention involves providing a healthy level of fluoride in public water supplies (about 0.7 parts per million). The persons that receive the most intervention in this effort have been community leaders overseeing the water supply. In many communities in the past, this narrow approach created problems among some of the public, who felt they had lost control of their city and its services. To overcome those problems it may have been better to start with a public education program led by respected professionals such as dentists, physicians, teachers, and the clergy, thereby laying to rest fears and issues about loss of control. Currently, most organized public opposition to fluoridation has ended, based on the splendid results in so many communities. So, perhaps at this point a narrow intervention would be enough. It depends on the local culture.

Working with both formal and informal community leaders can help health workers decide which community group should receive the most information, motivation, and help for the plan of action. For a pleasantly and effectively implemented intervention for changing health, always work *within* and *with* as much of the community as possible. Never work *on* the community, *to* the community, or *for* the community.

Although most health promotion programs are directed at the general public, sometimes health promotion specialists enlist a target group to help them work with other target groups. The three following examples show some of these cases.

- When trained to identify the signs, schoolteachers can be the best case-finders for depressed, troubled, or neglected children.

- Health professionals may have the most influence in getting new mothers to breastfeed. However, they also may need to change the father's attitude to enlist his support, and they may need the young mother's mother to give encouragement.

- Health professionals may need to educate community and regional officials about the importance of establishing a district public health clinic, but the voting public and business leaders also may need to "motivate" officials to get the job done. In Chapter 12 you will find a discussion about which community segments are likely to accept new programs first and which last.

## WORKING WITH THE WHOLE COMMUNITY OR ONLY WITH THE HIGH-RISK GROUP

There are several convincing arguments for targeting a community risk-reduction intervention only at high-risk individuals. For example:

- It keeps the programs smaller.

- The target group is likely to be highly motivated. Its members have learned that doctors can fix what is, or may come to be, wrong with them.

- Persons in the high-risk group have, as individuals, the most to gain by reducing their higher probability of disease.

- Health professionals see this as what they have been trained to do, and so are well motivated.

- The general public remains unbothered.

There is, however, a convincing argument to the contrary for most widespread maladies. By targeting the intervention program at the whole community and getting the most community members to lower their risk factor by a small percentage, a much greater reduction in new cases and mortality will be achieved. This is the "population strategy" put forth by the late Professor Geoffrey Rose, Emeritus, from the London School of Hygiene (Rose, 1992) and others.

In his book, Professor Rose used epidemiologic data to put forward the following points:

- Most biologic, psychological, and social parameters associated with rates of disease are distributed in a roughly normal, or bell shaped, curve in the population. Blood pressure, IQ, and social participation are examples of such a distribution. It then follows that there are many more people that have moderate elevations of risk, compared to a few with extremely high risk.

- For many risk parameters, the chance of disease emergence is directly related (in some linear or nonlinear function) to the amount of deviancy (in either direction) from the levels of the healthiest subgroup. For example, the higher the blood pressure, the greater the risk of pathology; or, the lower the intake of protein in infants, the greater the risk of growth stunting.

- The percentage of people over any "high-risk cutoff point" (e.g., 160 mmHg/ 95 mmHg for blood pressure) is highly correlated with the population mean for that variable.

- The largest number of "cases" do not occur at the extreme "tail" of the risk factor distribution curve, but rather in the much larger group above the median, roughly from the 55th to the 90th percentile.

- By moving the entire population toward lower risk will lower the population mean modestly and lower the number of high-risk persons considerably.

Table 2.2 is taken from the screening phase of the United States Multiple Risk Factor Intervention Trial (MRFIT). The data are tabulated from Professor Rose's discussion of the original publication in *Lancet*.[1]

Row No. 1 in Table 2.2 shows the distribution of total serum cholesterol values observed in 361,000 United States men aged 35–57 years old who volunteered to participate in a study of men at higher risk of ischemic heart disease. This was not a representative sample. Based on earlier population studies (including the one conducted in Framingham, U.S.A., and others), the risk of ischemic heart disease attributable to total cholesterol was apportioned among the nine levels in percentages, as shown in row No. 2. The power of the total cholesterol risk factor (row No. 3) is shown by dividing the percentage of deaths attributable to total cholesterol by the percentage of the group that generated them. The potency keeps rising with level of total cholesterol, as past research has taught us to expect.

The message to take home from Table 2.2 is that intervening with the entire population enough to shift the whole population's distribution of total cholesterol lower by only 0.5 mmol—one category—would reduce ischemic heart disease mortality attributable to total cholesterol by about 34%. In contrast, a much larger reduction—three categories, or 1.5 mmol—applied to every high-risk person (≥6.0 mmol total cholesterol), but to no lower risk person, would achieve only an 18% reduction in ischemic heart disease mortality.

Table 2.2 illustrates more of Rose's arguments.

- When the common conditions are met—the risk factor has a bell-shaped distribution and the rates of disease keep increasing for each increment in the

---

[1] *Lancet* ii; 1986, pp. 933–936.

**TABLE 2.2.** Estimated association of total serum cholesterol to six year mortality with population data from the screened population of the United States Multiple Risk Factor Intervention Trial (MRFIT)[a], 1972–1973 (n = 361,622 men).

| | Total serum cholesterol (mmol/l) | | | | | | | | | Total cases (%) |
|---|---|---|---|---|---|---|---|---|---|---|
| | < 4 | 4–4.5 | 4.5–5 | 5–5.5 | 5.5–6 | 6–6.5 | 6.5–7 | 7–7.5 | > 7.5 | |
| 1. Population distribution by cholesterol level (%)[b] | 9 | 13 | 18 | 22 | 16 | 11 | 6 | 3 | 2 | |
| 2. Deaths attributable to high cholesterol effect | 0 | 4 | 8 | 17 | 22 | 19 | 13 | 9 | 8 | |
| 3. Potency of effect (L2)/(L1)[c] | 0 | .31 | .44 | .77 | 1.38 | 1.73 | 2.17 | 3.0 | 4.0 | |
| 4. Deaths after successful high-risk approach (%)[d] | 0 | 4 | 8 | 21.5 | 26.2 | 22.5 | — | — | — | |
| 5. Deaths after successful population approach (%)[e] | 0 | 5.6 | 9.7 | 12.3 | 15.2 | 10.4 | 6.5 | 6.0 | — | |

*Source:* United States Multiple Risk Factor Intervention Trial (MRFIT), as cited in Rose, 1992.
[a] MRFIT mortality data are the six year total for all causes, because total cholesterol affects several cardiovascular endpoints.
[b] Data from MRFIT screening.
[c] Ratio of percentage of deaths to percentage of persons at each total cholesterol level. This yields a relative risk ratio signifying the relative lethal potency of each level of total cholesterol. Ratios less than 1.0 indicate a protective effect.
[d] Percentage of the original (100%) deaths that would occur if the high-risk approach were applied to all persons having baseline total cholesterol of 6.5 mmol/l or greater and assumes that this intervention was successful in reducing all "high" cholesterols by 1.5 mmol/l—or three categories lower. The percent of deaths is then recalculated with every high-risk person experiencing the potency effect three categories below his original level. **There is now only 82.2% of the original burden of disease—about an 18% decline.**
[e] Percentage of the original (100%) deaths that would occur if the population approach were applied to the whole community, using mass media, group meetings, and all the other "total" approaches, and assumes that this intervention lowered the community's total cholesterol mean by only 0.5 mmol/l—just one category lower. The shape of the distribution curve remains the same, as is also assumed for row No. 4. **This results in the community experiencing only 65.7% of its earlier mortality—over a 34% decline.**

risk factor—then the population approach saves more lives and prevents more illness than the high-risk approach. This does not necessarily mean it is more cost-effective. The costs of each approach and the size of the targeted groups also must be considered.

- The population approach is more likely to be preferable in the following scenarios: (1) when the risk factors are widely diffused throughout the community; (2) when the gradient of disease risk continuously rises as the risk factor becomes more extreme; (3) when it is impossible or too expensive to separate the susceptible from the non-susceptible groups or persons; and (4) when the intervention is better achieved at a group or population level rather than at an individual level (for example, changing eating patterns of families or school groups; fluoridating the water supply, rather than hiring hundreds of dental aids to find and treat every child and adolescent).

- The high-risk approach will be more effective: (1) when the risk conditions are highly restricted (for example, exposure to fumes and solvents among furniture workers); (2) when susceptibility is limited and obvious (for example, persons with white, rather than tan or brown, skin for strict teaching about sun exposure and skin cancers); (3) when there is a "risk threshold" below which a risk factor confers no added danger *and* the low risk subpopulation can be easily identified; or (4) when the intervention causes enough inconvenience so that only high-risk, motivated persons will adhere to the hygienic program (for example, diabetics and pre-diabetics following needed strict dietary programs).

The population approach also reduces the size of the high-risk portion of the population. Rose (1992) estimates the reductions as follows:

- If high risk for systolic blood pressure begins at 140 mmHg, reducing a population's mean systolic blood pressure by 3% will decrease the number in the high-risk group by 25%.

- If excess body weight is judged to be more than 92 kg, reducing the population's mean weight by 1 kg (about 1%) will cut the number of excess weight persons by 25%.

- If heavy drinkers of alcohol are defined as persons drinking 300 ml of ethanol or more each week, reducing the drinking population's average ethanol intake by 10% will cut the number of heavy drinkers by 25%.

Comparisons of distributions of values of risk factors, such as those above in numerous populations, reveal that populations differ in means but not in the shape of the distribution. The above calculations are based on that assumption.

## THE PREVENTION PARADOX

The paradox goes something like this: preventive interventions often must involve many, many people in order to help just a few. This is an issue that dates back at least to the first immunization campaigns in the 1890s. And even in the early part of the 20th century, when diphtheria was epidemic, preventive programs had to immunize about 600 children to prevent one death. Of course, numerous non-fatal cases also were prevented. Similarly, today thousands of persons are wearing their automobile seatbelts for thousands of days each, for just one life to be saved.

These are examples of preventive measures—risk factor reductions—that bring large benefits to the population as a whole, but little or no benefit to most participating persons. Such high ratios of participants to persons benefiting must always be the case in situations where we know there will be many destructive events in a population but do not know who might become the victim.

The message for health promotion is to make preventive actions automatic and habitual, emphasizing their ease and simplicity, and also stressing that failure to do the preventive act may generate only a tiny risk but represents a huge penalty to anyone who becomes a victim. As Table 2.2 demonstrates, having many persons exposed to a modest risk of disease or injury costs a community far more damage than having a small number of persons exposed to a high risk.

Whether to choose the high-risk approach or the population approach hinges on several additional factors, including the inconvenience or possible side effects of the intervention program on persons at minimal risk and the shape of the gradient of potency of the risk factor. For example, a U-shaped effect—when both being too high and being too low are harmful—calls for the kind of program that encourages both extremes toward safe moderation. These decisions need to be worked out with the input of expert consultants. The purpose of this discussion is to alert all health workers to the issues and the options.

## SPECIFYING THE CHANGES IN BEHAVIORS AND ENVIRONMENTS REQUIRED TO REACH THE HEALTH GOALS

Once the type of health problem against which to intervene has been selected, as well as the population subsets whose changes in behavior will reduce the problem, those planning the program are ready to specify precisely what changes need to be made. A vague goal will doom public health leaders and workers to an enterprise akin to trying to catch a cloud in a butterfly net. A precise, operationally defined goal, on the other hand, will provide focus (thus eliminating unnecessary activities) and enable quantitative evaluation (both before the program begins and after it ends), both for the behavioral and environmental changes that the program aims to achieve and for the improved health outcomes the program is intended to produce.

Goals should be stated in terms of specific, measurable results. They should not be stated in terms of resources spent or activities conducted. For example, it is not recommended that a goal be set such as, "Use 25 nurses to do home visits to educate people about risk factors for cancer." Rather, state an outcome oriented goal, such as, "Raise public awareness of cancer risk factors so that 80% of adults know risk factors for cancer of the lung, head, neck, liver, and bowel." The following three examples of a third approach are more behaviorally oriented: "Decrease the proportion of adults (X%) who smoke cigarettes by 20%"; or "Decrease the X% who drink more than 7 alcoholic drinks per week by 20%"; or "Increase the X% who consume both three fruits or vegetables and two fiber-rich foods each day by 20%." Evaluation should be made in terms of measured changes. Since the cancers above may take 20 to 30 years to develop, early evaluation must be conducted in terms of risk factor changes. Don't look for changes in health statistics until the "incubation period" of the disease in question has elapsed. Simply to make people "more health conscious and knowledgeable" is not helpful, unless it spills over into measurable actions that really prevent disease.

Goals set for health interventions also should be attainable. Reducing the incidence of diarrhea in day care centers by 90% is not an attainable goal for the first intervention in most places. If a 20% reduction seems easy, set your goal at 30%, not at 50%. With some extra effort, you have a good chance of reaching 30% the first year, and then set another 30% reduction as the second year's goal. The prevention specialist should weigh the attitude of both health workers and the target population: Will they work harder the second year if they achieve their goal, if they fall somewhat short of it, or if they fail badly? Most behavior change specialists believe that a sequence of small or moderate successes is the best way to build morale, self-efficacy, and commitment for future goals—both among health workers and among the participating public.

Careful analysis of the etiology of a disease or class of trauma will usually reveal several risk factors in the people who later become victims. Certain places and times also confer greater risk. There are usually potential interventions to change the environment, to separate the agent from the host, or to activate any other of the five strategies for prevention (see Table 2.1).

> *Most behavior change specialists believe that a sequence of small or moderate successes is the best way to build morale, self-efficacy, and commitment for future goals—both among health workers and among the participating public.*

In general, combating a problem by launching two or more interventions simultaneously is often more effective than carrying out a single intervention, but it also can be more costly. The goal is to select cost-effective ways of intervening, and to combine them if indicated.

For example, some malaria control programs follow a probability model both to attack the vector (mosquitoes) and to raise human resistance with antimalarial medications. If the number of mosquitoes can be cut by half and the number of susceptible hosts can be cut by half (assuming equal and independent effects from each intervention and no changes in other factors), one would expect malaria transmission to fall to one-quarter of its previous rate. A similar multi-pronged approach also works well for highway safety and many other conditions.

In general, a program designed to change behavior and attitude will always be needed to gain public acceptance of environmental and health service programs. A highly successful polio immunization program conducted in the 1960s, when live-virus polio vaccine was new, was organized to include health professionals; elementary schools; churches; supermarkets; county offices; factories; recreational facilities; newspapers, radio, television, and billboards in two languages; community volunteers; and civic clubs. This enthusiastic, multi-faceted and many-channeled approach set records for community participation. The facilities, work hours, and media coverage were mostly free gifts to the health campaign. This "community saturation approach" is still being used with encouraging success.

The channels to be used to reach people, the nature of the message, and the times and places for providing services will differ greatly depending on the nature of the target disease and that of the target population. As an exercise, think how you would plan a program targeting measles in children, breast cancer in middle-aged women, AIDS among intravenous drug users, sexually transmitted diseases in teenagers, or reactive depression in recently widowed persons.

Before continuing, think about and write the nature and content of the program to be designed for each of these diseases and population subgroups, as well as where, how, and by what sorts of workers the services are to be rendered. Save the notes. You may want to review them after reading Chapter 12.

Chapter 12, on changing behavior, will provide further guidelines to use in planning for such programs. Before that, however, Chapters 3 through 6 in Part II will review the major health problems at each stage of life and will examine how they can be reduced.

# PART II.
# IMPROVING HEALTH THROUGHOUT THE LIFE CYCLE

# 3. Infants and Children up to 14 Years Old

## IN PREGNANCY

A healthy pregnancy and safe delivery are the essential foundation to a joyful and productive life. A damaged pregnancy, however, can result in mortality, malformation, and impaired functional status—both physically and mentally—that can last a lifetime.

Infant mortality (babies who die before their first birthday) is a traditional indicator of a population's overall health. As such, WHO has included it as a major indicator in its Global Strategy of Health for All (Rutter and Quine, 1990). Specific diagnoses for death during infancy may be assigned unreliably because often several contributing causes are present simultaneously and the assignment to primary cause is arbitrary or follows local custom.

Mortality data for 1993 in the United States suggests, however, that among live births who die before age 1, about 50% die from conditions that started during prenatal life. Their deaths are coded as being due to such conditions as congenital anomalies, disorders related to prematurity, low birthweight, respiratory distress of newborn, and maternal and perinatal complications (CDC, 1996). The risk factors for death, malformation, and disability, however, are more clearly defined and often preventable.

Poor nutrition, infections, and toxins are the three most frequent, yet preventable, causes of infant disability and mortality. Complications of pregnancy, often rooted in the first three causes, add their toll as well. The foundations for healthy babies come from educating and motivating youth well before their fertile years. Potential problems can be monitored and often prevented by alert prenatal care begun in the first trimester and continued throughout pregnancy.

Poor nutrition is more often due to a lack of protein, minerals (especially iodine and iron), and vitamins (especially folic acid), than to simple caloric deficits. However, women who are seriously deprived of food usually show all the deficiencies listed.

> **Poor nutrition, infections, and toxins are the three most frequent—and preventable—causes of infant disability and mortality.**

Infectious diseases can either interfere with the mother's body's ability to transmit adequate nutrients through the placenta, or the infectious agents themselves (or their toxins) can pass directly into the fetus. Rubella, dengue, HIV, hepatitis B, and other sexually transmitted diseases (e.g., gonorrhea, chlamydia, syphilis, herpes simplex, cytomegalovirus) are among those whose infectious agents can cross the placenta (Cates and Holmes, 1986:257–281; and Hutchinson and Sandall, 1995). Pregnant women at high risk for the above conditions should be screened for them at the first opportunity to protect the baby. All pregnant women should be screened as shown in the "Screening Checklist for Pregnant Women" later in this chapter. Diarrheal diseases and intestinal parasites reduce the nutrient stores in the mother, and, if severe enough, can malnourish the fetus (Perez-Escamilla and Pollitt, 1992; Last, 1986, pp. 1515–1531).

Research in recent decades has highlighted the damaging effects of "everyday toxins" such as those contained in cigarette smoke and alcohol. It has been well established that these are risk factors for low birthweight—which is a common intermediary for immature development—congenital anomalies, and infant mortality. Alcohol consumption can cause fetal alcohol syndrome, with its characteristic stigmata and disabilities. Even lesser amounts of maternal drinking are believed to cause non-specific damage, based on animal research. Many illegal drugs, and even some legitimate medications used inappropriately, can damage the fetus or create a state of acute narcotic withdrawal immediately after the baby is born. Cocaine is particularly damaging (Frank, Bresnahan, and Zuckerman, 1996).

*Poor family functioning* was found to be a predictor both of intrapartum complications and low birthweight in a study group of U.S. women of lower economic levels (Reeb et al., 1987). The study used three scales of family functioning. All of them asked about the woman's perception of her family's helpfulness and emotional support, her satisfaction with these circumstances, and her satisfaction with her family's performance in terms of taking care of the family's needs and getting along together without conflict. Discriminant function analysis showed poor family function, age over 35 years, and full-time employment outside the home to be the three strongest predictors of complications of pregnancy and delivery. Poor family functioning and more stressful life events were the strongest predictors of low birthweight. (See also Rutter and Quine (1990) for further documentation that life stresses and low socioeconomic status increase rates of low birthweight.) Ten biomedical variables were also evaluated, but they each had smaller predictive values. The relative strengths of risk factors vary by the stage of economic development and frequency of damaging diseases.

The main reason life stress may affect pregnancy outcome appears to be because it creates continuing anxiety and feelings of distress, which, in turn, change the levels of glucocorticoids, corticotrophin-releasing hormone, beta endorphins, and the interaction of the hypothalamic pituitary-adrenal system. A comprehensive review of the effects of stress and anxiety on pregnancy outcomes, the endocrinology involved, and possible treatment strategies has been presented by Lederman (1995, a and b).

**Low birthweight,** often caused by the factors above, has other less defined causes as well. Low birthweight, in turn, is a contributing cause to many physical and psychoneurological problems that emerge later in childhood. (See Chapter 7 for details.)

Excellent reviews of social inequalities in pregnancy outcome (Rutter and Quine, 1990), causes and consequences of intrauterine growth retardation (Perez-Escamilla and Pollitt, 1992), preventive perinatology for developing countries (Torres-Pereyra, 1988), and prevention of infant mortality by nurse-midwives (Willis and Fullerton, 1991) provide data and recommended actions for making pregnancy and infancy healthier.

WHO estimates that about 17% of the 122.3 million babies born worldwide each year have a low birthweight—under 2,500 g. The low birthweight rate was 18% in developing countries, but only 7% in industrialized countries (World Health Organization, 1980). Low birthweight babies have twice to four times the risk of dying in their first 3 days of life compared to normal weight babies, and the survivors are more likely to suffer impaired intelligence. Complications of pregnancy and delivery that involve fetal anoxia have been implicated as risk factors for schizophrenia emerging in the third decade of life (Mrazek and Haggerty, 1994). For babies whose pregnancies and deliveries leave residual physiologic dysfunctions involving the autonomic nervous system, the risks of conduct disorders later in childhood are raised fivefold (Mrazek and Haggerty, 1994). Low birthweight babies also have higher risks for many other abnormalities. (Also see Chapter 7.)

The material deprivation experienced by the poor, both in industrialized and developing countries, exacts a toll in the form of damaged pregnancies, fetal growth retardation, sick babies, and higher infant death. Clearly, impoverished areas are the places of greater need for preventive programs—but much of the fetal and infant damage is mediated by psychosocial, behavioral, and cultural correlates of poverty which can be modified by the determined efforts of health professionals and community resources (Rutter and Quine, 1990).

The two main strategies for improving infant health and development are: (1) reducing the frequency of low birthweight, and (2) increasing the delivery of prenatal care, both by starting care earlier in the pregnancy and by improving the rate of keeping subsequent appointments at the prenatal clinic.

*The material deprivation experienced by the poor, whether in industrialized or developing countries, exacts a toll in the form of damaged pregnancies, fetal growth retardation, sick babies, and higher rates of infant death.*

Much research has shown that early and comprehensive prenatal care can improve pregnancy outcomes. Such care provides early detection of correctable risk factors in the pregnant woman and provides her support to make the necessary arrangements for the latter portion of pregnancy, delivery, and early infant care.

Comprehensive descriptions of the recommended services and scheduling for prenatal care are published by national health authorities and can be found in textbooks of obstetrics. The list of prenatal risk factors, which follows in this section, should be used as a supplementary source. The first task of regional or community health authorities is to make prenatal services available, convenient, and culturally acceptable. The social groups at highest risk for prenatal and perinatal complications, low birthweight, and fetal anomalies, are people in low socioeconomic status and cultural minorities.

Low family income, unemployment, low education, poor housing, and lack of transportation each makes its independent—and interactive—impact to lower the utilization of prenatal care. If health care workers speak the same language the patients speak at home, the rate of women coming for initial care and keeping appointments is increased. Effective social networks in the community can be enlisted to encourage pregnant women to come for care (Willis and Fullerton, 1991). Health agencies must become proactive to enlist community participation.

The literature reviews have good agreement on the risk factors for low birthweight and fetal anomalies. The most detailed list appears in Willis and Fullerton (1991).

## RISK FACTORS FOR LOW BIRTHWEIGHT, FETAL ANOMALIES, AND INFANT DEATHS

### Social Risk Factors

- poverty and its correlates;

- low education of the mother (illiterate mothers experience three times the infant mortality rate in some areas compared to mothers who have finished high school (PAHO 1994, 1998, 2002);

- unmarried status (even after age and education are accounted for);

- poor family functioning, low emotional and practical helpfulness.

### Personal Biological Factors

- mother is too young (early teens);

- mother is too old (mid-40s or older);

- there are fewer than two years between pregnancies—a factor that can double infant mortality (PAHO, 1994, 1998, and 2002);

- the mother is obese;

- the mother is markedly underweight before pregnancy;

- the mother does not gain enough weight during pregnancy;

- the mother is undergoing her first pregnancy.

## Personal Behavioral Factors

- the mother smokes cigarettes;

- the mother consumes any alcohol;

- the mother uses illegal drugs;

- the mother misuses legal medications not approved as safe for use during pregnancy;

- the mother is exposed to workplace or farm toxins (chemicals, solvents, pesticides, some liquid fuels);

- the mother is exposed to infections (including sexually transmitted infections and poverty-related infections);

- the mother undergoes adverse life events without social support;

- the mother has inadequate nutrition before and during pregnancy **(population malnutrition is discussed in Chapter 13);**

- the mother receives insufficient professional prenatal care or it comes too late.

## Psychological Risk Factors[1]

- the mother experiences chronic elevated levels of anxiety or depression (Rutter and Quine, 1990);

- the mother undergoes a high frequency of stressful life events, especially in the absence of social supports (Lederman, 1995).

[1] This list is derived from Willis and Fullerton, 1991.

Note how these risk factors are heavily weighted with social conditions and behavioral habits. The steps to achieving the goal of reduced infant mortality and disability must follow the route of changing cultural norms and social expectations for women of childbearing age by educating and motivating each community and by supporting behavior change in individual women before their pregnancies begin. **(The general strategies of community intervention were presented in Chapter 2, and the technology for changing risk factors will be explained in Chapter 11.)**

### SCREENING PREGNANT WOMEN

Some localities may have many screening procedures, while others may have considerably fewer. The following checklist[2] includes those procedures best demon-

---

### SCREENING CHECKLIST FOR PREGNANT WOMEN

1. For iron deficiency anemia;
2. For pre-eclampsia via blood pressure measurement at each prenatal visit;
3. For weight: is mother clearly underweight or clearly obese; does she gain weight appropriately during pregnancy?
4. For tobacco use: urge and motivate stopping totally, at least during pregnancy and lactation;
5. For alcohol use: ask whether mother drinks and how much in a non-judgmental manner, then urge and motivate total cessation for the duration of pregnancy and lactation;
6. For mood altering drugs: ask about use in a non-threatening way, then urge cessation for duration of pregnancy, preferably permanently—drugs will damage fetus but not abort it;
7. For medications being taken, including over-the-counter compounds—urge discontinuance of all substances not known to be safe for the fetus;
8. For eating of non-food substances such as clay, starch, special folk-cure earths (ingesting such substances is sometimes called "pica of pregnancy")—some of these may contain traces of heavy metals (e.g., lead), other toxins, salts, or merely "empty calories." Urge stopping practice by substituting something safe to chew on or eat;
9. For asymptomatic bacteruria via urine test;
10. For rubella: ask about prior vaccination; if none, follow patient closely for infectious episodes during pregnancy, but *do not* immunize until after delivery;
11. For hepatitis B virus: based on community prevalence, do blood test to detect active (acute or chronic) infection;
12. For syphilis and for human immunodeficiency virus (HIV) in all pregnant women;
13. For gonorrhea and chlamydia: via sexual history and physical exam in all women; in higher risk women, by lab culture;
14. For Rh-incompatibility (now called D-blood typing and antibody screening).

---

[2] Various sources were used to compile the list, primarily the United States Preventive Services Task Force, 1996.

strated to be beneficial and efficient. As always, the availability and cost of certain technologies in the local setting will influence which procedure is selected.

Priorities for including or excluding items from all the screening checklists included in this Handbook should be based upon the local prevalence and seriousness of conditions and the local practicality and effectiveness of the proposed addition to program protocols. For example, investing in extending oral rehydration therapy may save more suffering than screening newborns for phenylketonuria abnormality.

The best "screening device" is a health professional who examines methodically, observes acutely, asks wisely, and listens intently to the mother and child. The health worker can then prioritize the more technical procedures based on the prevalence of conditions in the community and individual patient risk factors. Some of the screening items may not be feasible in underserved or under-equipped areas. Other items can be estimated clinically, such as iron-deficiency anemia by observing nail beds or eyelid mucosa, when laboratory tests are not cheaply available.

## FROM BIRTH THROUGH AGE 4 YEARS

This section deals with the major causes of death and disability in children through age 4.[3] The patterns of mortality differ, depending on whether a nation has an all-cause, age-specific mortality rate for ages 1–4 that is greater than about 150 deaths per 100,000 children of those ages or whether a nation's rates fall under about 120 per 100,000. Nations with rates between 120 and 150 can follow either pattern.

For nations with higher rates of early childhood deaths, the leading cause (using the International Classification of Diseases (ICD-9)) is infectious and parasitic diseases, followed by intestinal diseases and respiratory diseases. External causes usually rank fourth, but sometimes are higher.

For nations with lower early childhood mortality, external causes (including accidents, neglectful or intentional trauma) usually are the leading cause of death, with drowning common especially for boys. Congenital anomalies or infectious and parasitic diseases usually run second in frequency.

---

[3] Mortality figures are drawn from selected nations that have reported their age- and sex-specific mortality to the *World Health Statistics Annual* in recent years and from the Global Burden of Disease Study (Murray and Lopez (eds.), 1996). The impact of disability from non-fatal conditions and their responsible risk factors is drawn from estimates by the Global Burden of Disease Study (Murray and Lopez, 1997, a–d) and from José L. Bobadilla and colleagues (1994).

In nations that have warm climates year round, the many "tropical diseases" exact a heavy toll, especially among young children, resulting in impaired development, risk of recurrent disease, or, all too often, death. The world's most prevalent communicable diseases include malaria, schistosomiasis, amebiasis, insect-borne viral and parasitic diseases, tick-borne diseases, oral-fecal transmitted parasitic worms, and diseases associated with poor sanitation. These diseases often arrive as epidemics in communities and remain endemic thereafter. As recently as 1990, malaria alone caused an estimated 31 million healthy life years lost (QALYs) in the world's children. This figure includes both deaths and the disability among survivors.

Control of these diseases may involve separating flying insects from people by screening, insecticide spraying, chemoprophylaxis, using "clean" water and food, improving sanitation, separation from or pharmacologic treatment of human carriers, and changing various environmental aspects. Malaria, schistosomiasis, and other diseases involving living vectors can be prevented successfully only by large-scale community and regional programs. Much useful guidance in this regard can be obtained from recent editions of *Control of Communicable Diseases in Man* (Chin, 2000). The role of local health professionals and the public is to advocate specific community preventive interventions as needed and to assist in their successful completion.

An underlying determinant of the severity—the risk of permanent disability or death—of all these children's diseases is the children's nutritional state. Protein-energy malnutrition and iron-deficiency anemias are estimated to be responsible for a total loss of more than 45 million life years of healthy function—Disability Adjusted Life Years (DALYs) (Murray and Lopez, 1997, a–d). Vitamin A deficiency adds to these losses by causing eye lesions, which can lead to blindness. This deficiency also affects the skin and reduces resistance to infections. Malnutrition is seldom coded as the primary cause of death, but it aggravates respiratory disorders, diarrheas, and the immunizable diseases, and they, in turn, drain out what limited nutritional reserves remain in the body. Nutritional diseases are common in developing countries and among poor families everywhere, especially in urban settings. Even in wealthier nations, malnutrition can be found in children, adults, and the elderly in impoverished areas. **(Malnutrition as a community and regional problem is discussed in the section on malnutrition in Chapter 13.)**

*Breastfeeding* provides the best nutritional start in a baby's life. A well-nourished mother provides better nourishment for her baby, as well as essential immunologic protection. Breast milk can be fed exclusively until such time as the baby's rate of growth falters (slows down from local averages). This usually occurs between 4 to 6 months of age (Hijazi et al., 1989). In some places, a child's partial breastfeeding may continue for as long as 24 months of age.[4]

---

[4] See Jakobsen et al. (1993) for methods of promoting breastfeeding.

Extended breastfeeding delays the return of regular menses in most women. It also reduces the frequency and severity of diarrheas and respiratory infections in infants and tends to protect against obesity developing when the babies reach childhood and adolescence. In a study in New Zealand that followed more than 1,000 children for 18 years, longer duration of breastfeeding was associated with measurable advantages in cognitive ability at ages 8 to 13 years and higher scores on school-leaving examinations (Horwood and Fergusson, 1998).

The United States Government initiative "Healthy People 2010" urges that breastfeeding be continued until at least age 6 months. Studies show that giving new mothers promotional material from manufacturers of infant formula encourages many of them to give up breastfeeding as early as two weeks after the baby's birth. For most this is an unhealthy choice.

The solution to these nutritional problems is adequate food—enough calories; protein sources; green, yellow, and other vegetables and fruits. Iodine deficiency can be remedied by area-wide distribution of iodized salt. Vitamin A deficiency can be dealt with by fortifying a staple food or by large oral doses twice yearly. Both Vitamin A supplementation (included in WHO's "EPI-plus" program) and iodine supplementation (where required) are extremely cost effective in terms of healthy life years gained for the money spent (Bobadilla, 1994). Textbooks on public health nutrition also will be useful in this regard.

The probability that a child born live will live to his fifth birthday depends largely on where that child lives. The World Bank has

**Breastfeeding provides the best nutritional start in a baby's life.**

utilized mortality statistics for the latter 1980s from 169 nations and reporting areas to project the estimated percentages of live-born children who will die before turning 5 years old. The estimates are available from the original source for each reporting nation (Feacham et al. (eds.), 1992). Table 3.1 summarizes these data by six geographic/economic regions and shows both median percentages and ranges of percent mortality in the 1980s and 1990s.

Mortality medians differ substantially across regions: 12-fold differences for males, and nearly 17-fold differences for females. The ranking for regional mortality before age 5 follows that for economic development. In all nations, boys have higher rates than girls. Even more important for health policy-makers are the wide ranges of child mortality within each region. Within Latin America and the Caribbean, for example, the range is 10-fold for males and 12-fold for females. Other transitional and developing regions show similar disparities. This table can be read as a score card on child health for regions and nations, but it can far more productively be used as a searchlight of opportunity, to guide nations and districts to the subpopulations in greatest need and to the nature of those health needs. The remainder of this chapter will review major ways to save children's lives and health.

**TABLE 3.1.** Median percentages of live births projected to die before their fifth birthday by gender, region, and economic development (for 1990s).

| National Groupings | Males | Females |
|---|---|---|
| Asia and Pacific (36 nations and areas) | 5.2[a] (0.8 – 22.7)[b] | 4.5[a] (0.7 – 22.0)[b] |
| Latin America and the Caribbean (40 nations and areas) | 3.5[a] (1.3 – 12.8)[b] | 3.1[a] (0.9 – 10.6)[b] |
| Middle East and North Africa (25 nations and areas) | 9.5[a] (1.6 – 30.3)[b] | 8.0[a] (1.1 – 27.5)[b] |
| Sub-Saharan Africa (31 nations and areas) | 16.2[a] (1.9 – 26.1)[b] | 15.1[a] (1.3 – 23.5)[b] |
| Industrialized socialist and Eastern Europe (9 nations) | 2.2[a] (1.1 – 5.0)[b] | 1.7[a] (0.7 – 4.0)[b] |
| Industrialized free-market (28 nations and areas) | 1.3[a] (0.6 – 4.1)[b] | 0.9[a] (0.5 – 3.0)[b] |

*Source:* Data abstracted and summarized from Feachem, Kjellstrom, Murray, et al., 1992.

[a] Median of group.
[b] Range of group.

Mortality projections are based on World Bank model estimates calculated from data from 1985 or later (157 areas) or 1980–1984 (12 areas).

## PREVENTION AND EARLY DETECTION OF DEVELOPMENTAL PROBLEMS

The path of choice is primary prevention—keeping the risk factors from ever arriving. The section on pregnancy reviews the steps to take. **(Protection for the central nervous system is further discussed in Chapter 7.)**

As for secondary prevention, some developmental problems can be prevented by early detection of risk; others can be reversed, or at least have their damage minimized, if treated early. Detection without treatment not only is useless, it actually may cause harm by creating anxiety and guilt in parents who feel helpless in facing their child's problem without any solution. Treatment may be curative or it may help the children learn ways to keep their disabilities from impairing their functioning too seriously. Human beings possess a great force for life and growth, and this force is strongest in children. Caring health professionals and a loving family can help remove some barriers to children's growth and development.

### Screening Checklist for Newborns

1. For congenital hypothyroidism;

2. For phenylketonuria (PKU);

3. For sickle cell disease where parents are at elevated risk;

4. Perform ocular antibiotic prophylaxis to prevent gonococcal or chlamydial infection of the eyes;

5. Have a health professional perform a full pediatric examination;

6. Urge breastfeeding for the first year of life, supplemented by soft foods as needed.

## PREVENTING POSTNATAL DISABILITIES

A healthy pregnancy can prevent many congenital defects, but a considerable number of permanent limitations and disabilities develop after birth. Among these (depending on the nation) are malnutrition and growth stunting evolving from inadequate calories and proteins in the baby's diet. These are aggravated by diarrhea, sequelae of childhood infections, parasitic diseases, and trauma (both accidental and inflicted). All these causes can be diminished by social and behavioral changes.

In a review of the epidemiology of developmental disabilities (including both those of prenatal and postnatal origin), Lipkin (1991) concludes that developmental disabilities overall appear about as frequently as the most common of serious pediatric diseases. Hence, their prevention is vitally important to improve child health.

In the United States, a 1987 survey estimated that almost 1% of children under age 18 years had some kind of physical impairment. Psychological and neurological impairments were counted separately. The most frequent impairments were orthopedic (0.35%), two-thirds of which affected the lower limbs. Speech and hearing impairments were next in frequency (0.18% and 0.16%, respectively). Scandinavian surveys cited by Lipkin (1991) combine childhood disabilities with chronic diseases, and generally from 6% to 12% of children are affected (according to the definitions used). Gortmaker and Sappenfield (1984) included psychological and neurological as well as physical disabilities in their survey. Much higher estimated prevalences were found. Their listing is led by attention deficit disorders (15%), followed by learning disabilities (7.5%), speech and language disabilities (7%), mental retardation (2%), and moderate to severe asthma (1%).

Determining the causes of these disorders is a major concern. Current thinking estimates that genetic factors contribute to many disabilities, but that the following external factors are primary causes for many other cases and contribute to multifactor etiology in still others: intra-uterine toxins, such as alcohol, to-

43

bacco, and cocaine; intra-uterine infection, such as rubella, hepatitis, and sexually transmitted diseases; and asphyxia during birth. Low birthweight is associated with increased risk of all the prenatal and perinatal disabilities. Postnatal causes include toxins (such as lead poisoning), head trauma, severe infections (especially meningitis), severe malnutrition, and physical abuse.

Lipkin (1991) estimates that from 3% to 15% of all developmental disabilities are acquired postnatally and that many of these are preventable. A registry of all developmental disabilities in the Atlanta area (USA) for 1991 revealed that meningitis and child battering were the two leading causes of postnatally acquired disabilities in children ages 3–10 years. Injuries caused by motor vehicles ranked third. Otitis media was the primary cause of hearing impairment (CDC, 1991). The Atlanta data, of course, may not apply in rural or developing regions, but these data can raise the index of awareness and concern about these causes for health professionals everywhere.

Preventive efforts should focus on treating meningitis early, before brain damage becomes irreversible. Both bacterial infections and hemophilus influenza type B are frequent agents. Prevention of child battering, including "shaken baby syndrome," will be covered in the section on child abuse, and vehicle injuries will be covered in the section on unintentional injuries, both presented later on in this chapter.

## REDUCING SUDDEN INFANT DEATH SYNDROME (SIDS)

SIDS is of major concern in nations that have very low infant mortality rates. Where other causes for postneonatal deaths are understood and well-controlled, this residual set of sudden, unexpected and unexplained deaths baffles medical experts and shocks parents. This accounts, in part, for the large research expenditures for SIDS, despite its modest incidence by worldwide standards of infant mortality.

The definition of a SIDS case has four required findings: the death is (1) sudden, (2) unexpected, (3) occurs before the first birthday, and (4) a specific cause of death cannot be assigned despite thorough investigation, including autopsy (Smedby et al., 1993).

The fourth requirement prevents present development of an international epidemiology for SIDS. Most nations do not perform detailed autopsies on most sudden infant deaths. Nevertheless, population studies coming from a few highly developed countries with cold winter climates have identified major risk factors, as well as prevention methods that could cut SIDS deaths by more than half.

Several different pathologic processes appear able to cause SIDS, singly or in differing combinations. A breakdown in respiratory function or in temperature control, the presence of infection, and immaturity of physiologic control systems have been most often implicated (Fleming, 1994). Most SIDS deaths occur in the first 4 months of life, when the baby's self-regulating mechanisms are not adequately developed.

SIDS rates have been declining in parallel with the total of other postneonatal deaths since the 1980s in countries like the United Kingdom. There are, however, huge seasonal variations in cold climates. The United States, for example, incurs twice the SIDS death rates in winters compared to summers (American Academy of Pediatrics, 1996), and the same is true in Sweden. SIDS rates are rising in regions where increasing numbers of physicians are recognizing and reporting it. Rates have also risen when traditional cultural infant care practices are replaced with a "Western way of living" (Norvenius et al., 1993).

**Predisposing and Precipitating Risk Factors for SIDS**

1. Low birthweight;

2. Maternal smoking, either during pregnancy or after birth; smoking both times triples a baby's risk. **(See the section "Preventing Postnatal Disabilities" earlier in this chapter.)**

3. Baby sleeps on its stomach (prone); putting babies to sleep on their back is best.

4. Sleeping on soft bedding (thick quilts, pillows, waterbeds, animal skins), anything that might reduce air intake or increase rebreathing of expired carbon monoxide.

5. Covering the baby's head with bedding, or placing it such that bedding may fall over the baby's face later in the night.

6. Use of heavy blanketing or excess external heating; thermal physiology undergoes several maturational steps in the first 4 months of life, and babies can neither cool themselves enough if overheated, nor warm themselves enough if chilled for an hour or more (Fleming, 1994; Norvenius et al., 1993).

7. Allowing the baby to become chilled for an extended period. Even a warmly covered infant breathing freezing air for an extended period can experience respiratory stress and SIDS.

8. Respiratory infections, either bacterial or viral, can interact with other of the above risk factors to raise risk dramatically. A low-birthweight infant in a home with ambient smoke is more likely to die from influenza than an infant with influenza who is breathing clean air.

### Preventing SIDS

Even though the pathophysiology of SIDS is poorly understood, actions to prevent it have proven effective. Preventive steps are much like those for respiratory illnesses. For example, breastfeeding reduces risks here, too. Reversing the eight risk factors just listed is clear enough to do.

The issue of sleeping position warrants more discussion. Until infants are mature enough to roll over—from stomach to back and again to stomach—they run the risk of having fresh airflow reduced by getting the nose and mouth blocked by pillows or soft bedding and suffocating. Older babies respond to oxygen deficit by moving enough to open airflow. Second-hand tobacco smoke, carbon monoxide, or re-breathing the baby's exhaled carbon dioxide creates hypoxia. In addition, nicotine exposure is believed to impair a young baby's defense against hypoxia (Milerad and Sundall, 1993).

Programs that teach parents, nurses, and childcare workers always to place the baby on its back to sleep have been followed by declines in rates of SIDS in step with declines in the percentage of parents putting baby to sleep on its stomach. Placing the baby on either side is almost as safe. When placing the baby on its side, position the arm on the bed or cot in front of the baby to make it more likely to roll toward the back than toward the stomach when it moves. (Once the baby can roll over both ways with ease, parents need not keep repositioning the baby on its back, but should continue first laying it down on back or side.) Early concerns about the supine position possibly causing other problems have been dispelled by subsequent research, except for babies with unusual clinical problems.

Programs like the "Back to Sleep" educational campaign in England, and now being conducted in the United States and elsewhere, have a catchy title and are a constant reminder of the correct way to position the child. Such programs have had community success, resulting in 50% to 70% reductions in SIDS in several nations, including England, New Zealand, and the Netherlands. Unfortunately, most clinics and doctors offices do not give parents regular, organized education regarding how to prevent SIDS (Gibson et al., 1996), even though they may be aware that the American Academy of Pediatrics (AAP) had adopted a preventive policy. AAP has since reaffirmed that infants should sleep on their backs and has endorsed other of the recommendations included here (American

Academy of Pediatrics, 1996). Similar recommendations have come from expert consensus groups in Sweden (Smedby et al., 1993).[5]

## INCREASING IMMUNIZATION COVERAGE

PAHO/WHO's Expanded Program on Immunization (EPI) targets six diseases: diphtheria, tetanus, pertussis, measles, poliomyelitis, and tuberculosis. Some vaccines address the first two or three of these with a single injection. In 1994, the International Commission certified the eradication of poliomyelitis in the Americas (CDC, 1994).

In countries with aggressive immunization programs, diphtheria, tetanus, pertussis, and mumps have been declining steadily from year to year, but measles still has its epidemic years. In countries with lower coverage, more comprehensive immunization programs are the most powerful way to improve children's health. The international goal (such as established by UNICEF) is to achieve immunization of 80% of each community's children for all of the diseases included in EPI.

Acute respiratory infections are estimated to cause one-third of all deaths in children under age 5 years in developing countries. These 4.3 million acute respiratory deaths each year are estimated to include 480,000 due to measles, 260,000 due to pertussis, and 800,000 due to neonatal pneumonia (Tulloch and Richards, 1993). In addition to the deaths, millions of surviving children are damaged by stunted growth and diminished brain function.

The vital need to expand immunization coverage against measles and pertussis is obvious from the above data. Immunization to prevent pneumonias is not affordable in many countries, and vaccines to prevent the most commonly occurring types are not yet approved. However, hepatitis B has become epidemic worldwide in children and adults. It disables by causing liver diseases, including cirrhosis and cancer—and it spreads easily. Vaccines to prevent hepatitis B are now included in the EPI-plus program, and are also being given on a community-wide basis in many countries.

Tulloch and Richards (1993) argue that high coverage with measles vaccine is the most critical immunization to reduce both acute respiratory and diarrheal mortality in young children. The Global Burden of Disease (GBD) Study estimates that measles causes the deaths of over one million children in the developing world each year (1990 data) and that tetanus kills over 475,000, most of

---

[5] An annotated bibliography on the overall topic of SIDS was presented by Fleming (1994) and more recently by Henderson-Smart and colleagues (1998).

them under 5 years of age. Measles and tetanus vaccines are part of the immunization package used with young children. They must be promoted more aggressively in all areas where these infections are endemic.

Rubella, a major cause of congenital anomalies, can be greatly reduced by immunizing girls before they reach childbearing age. This can be achieved by using the MMR vaccine, which combines protection against measles, mumps, and rubella. Using the same vaccine with young men will provide needed coverage for measles, prevent mumps, which can have severe effects in adults, and reduce the rubella-susceptible population to levels below the percentage needed to propagate an epidemic.

The cost-benefit ratio of giving vaccines rather than allowing even a few cases of the disease to occur is well-illustrated by the cost of pertussis (whooping cough) vaccines versus the cost of caring for cases. The widespread use of pertussis vaccine in the United States has reduced incidence of this clinical disease by 99%. In a 1996 cost study conducted by the Texas Department of Public Health (U.S.A.), more than half of all pertussis cases and 67% of infant cases in 1994, required hospitalization. The median hospital charge was US$ 4,000 per case. This is 444 times the cost of a $9 dose of DPT vaccine. The cost of outpatient care for the large number of cases not hospitalized also must go into the equation (Texas Department of Health, 1996). The WHO study by Bobadilla et al. (1994) estimated that 10% of all lost Disability Adjusted Life Years in the world's children are attributable to lack of immunizations. **(Also see Chapters 2 and 13.)**

## REDUCING RESPIRATORY DISEASES

The incidence of acute respiratory infections in young children is rather similar in both developing and industrialized nations, with an average of four to eight episodes per child per year (Tulloch and Richards, 1993). There are no proven effective barriers to reduce the transmission of respiratory viruses, but there are known measures for reducing the rate at which they precipitate serious disease.

The main reason for the huge excess of child mortality due to infectious respiratory diseases in developing versus industrialized nations is the rate at which simple coughs and colds progress into pneumonia. While about 4% of children in industrialized areas develop pneumonia each year, the rate in less developed and rural areas may run between 10% and 20% (Tulloch and Richards, 1993). In the Americas the average infant mortality due to pneumonia and influenza is about 6 per 1,000, with a range from 1.5 per 1,000 in Canada to more than 20 in Haiti, Bolivia, and Peru (PAHO, 1994). Worldwide, respiratory infections account for about 20% of all deaths from birth up to age 5. In the developing world respiratory infections are the leading cause of loss of healthy life years (DALYs) among children, accounting for about 15% of the total burden experienced.

The death rates for pneumonia and influenza are much lower and continue to decline steadily for children ages 1–4 years old. Again, rates correlate closely with indicators of poverty, housing conditions, and food accessibility, from 1 per 100,000 in Canada and the United States to 224 per 100,000 in Guatemala.

The key to cutting the death rate is to prevent or promptly treat childhood pneumonias. Risk factors include low birthweight, malnutrition, indoor air pollution, and allowing infants to become chilled. There is suggestive evidence that vitamin A reduces the severity of some respiratory infections in places where diets are only marginally adequate. Pneumonias are most often viral in industrialized areas, but most often bacterial in developing areas, thus making selective use of antibiotics the treatment of choice. PAHO warns, however, that excessive use of antibiotics, as practiced in some places, actually aggravates the clinical condition of many children. WHO has developed standardized case management for childhood respiratory infections.

Universal extended breastfeeding of babies increases immunity to many respiratory diseases, as well as providing more calories and proteins than early-weaned children typically receive. Particularly important is that breast milk stimulates immunity to most of the pathogens endemic in the mother's and child's environment. A case-control study in Brazil showed that babies who had not been breast-fed had 3.6 times the risk of dying from respiratory infection than babies who had been exclusively breast-fed (Victoria et al., 1987). The mortality benefit of breastfeeding in environments where infant mortality is already low is relatively less. Adequate nutrition and protection against other diseases (e.g., diseases preventable by immunization and diarrheas) raises the host resistance of children of all ages against the worsening of acute respiratory infections.

Indoor air pollution caused either by burning smoky fuels or cigarette smoking without adequate ventilation is another correctable risk factor for respiratory disease in young children. The presence of a smoker in the household raises risk of respiratory infections in young children. In the United States alone between 150,000 to 300,000 cases of bronchitis and pneumonia in children are attributed to second-hand tobacco smoke in the home each year (United States Environmental Protection Agency, 1993).

*Universal extended breastfeeding of babies increases immunity to many respiratory diseases, as well as providing more calories and proteins than early-weaned children typically receive.*

Tobacco smoke has more lethal effects in infants, where maternal smoking doubles the rate of sudden infant death syndrome (SIDS). The combination of maternal cigarette smoking both during pregnancy and during infancy tripled the rate of SIDS in a large representative United States sample of infants (Schoendorf and Kiely, 1992).

Worldwide, it is estimated that at least 12,600 children die *each day* with diarrheal diseases (Guerrant, 1992). Of this total 4.6 to 6 million deaths per year, about 3.2 million occur in developing nations. Globally, on an average, children experience 2 to 11 diarrheal episodes per year. Children in the United States experience about two episodes per year, the same as children in affluent homes in tropical countries (Guerrant, 1992). However, among children attending day care centers the attack rate is higher. In contrast, in some impoverished areas the diarrhea attack rate averages 15–19 diarrheal episodes per child per year. In northeast Brazil, one of several examples, more infants and children die from diarrhea than all other causes combined (Guerrant and McAuliffe, 1986, pp. 287–307). In addition to high worldwide mortality, prolonged diarrheal disease can lead to serious malnutrition and stunting of growth, both of which, in turn, raise the frequency and duration of future diarrhea episodes and lower resistance to other kinds of disease. Between 1965 and 1990 mortality rates have been reduced dramatically (PAHO, 1994). This is probably the joint result of improved sanitation and increased usage of oral rehydration therapy, but there is still a long way to go in many places even in the twenty-first century.

In addition to mortality, diarrheal diseases account for about 14% of the burden of disease (a combination of early death and living with impairment) among children of the developing world (Bobadilla et al., 1994).

The WHO classification system for field use identifies three presentations of diarrheal disease: (a) acute watery diarrhea (lasting less than 14 days), (b) dysentery (with blood in the stool), and (c) persistent diarrhea (lasting more than 14 days without blood).

The key to reducing mortality or extended damage from diarrhea is to prevent acute episodes from becoming persistent, involving blood loss, or causing dehydration. Feeding oral rehydrating salt solutions continuously in repeated small doses is the main defense against dehydration. The development in 1978 of this ingenious "low tech" therapy saves about one million lives each year (Hirschhorn and Greenough, 1991). Wider usage would save even more lives.

Persistent diarrhea cases have a case fatality ratio 5.6 times that of acute cases, and dysentery cases have a fatality ratio 2.4 times the acute cases (Tulloch and Richard, 1993). The keys to reducing incidence of all forms of diarrheal disease are: (1) personal hygiene, especially with regard to fecal contamination; (2) provision of pure food and water; and (3) extended breastfeeding to build immunity. In a case-control study in Brazil, infants not receiving breast milk had 14.2 times the risk of dying from diarrhea, compared to infants fed breast milk exclusively (Victoria et al., 1987).

Preventive tasks are twofold—primary, to reduce the incidence of diarrheal episodes and secondary, to keep acute cases from becoming more serious. Both efforts depend almost entirely on changing human behavior—in the short-term, directed to parents, child-care workers, and health professionals; in the long-term, to policy makers and administrators to install pure water, food hygiene, and sewage systems. Political apathy by decision-makers, whose families are not affected by these epidemics, helps block the infrastructure investments needed to resolve these worldwide problems (Thielman and Guerrant, 1996).

The preventive interventions listed below all involve changing knowledge, priorities, and behaviors. Some may not be feasible in certain areas, depending on the climate, culture, infrastructure, and economy; other interventions may become feasible after appropriate training of health personnel. A useful guide to achieving the needed behavior changes in poverty conditions was presented by C.M. Monte and colleagues (1997).

**At least 12,600 children die each day from diarrheal diseases.**

**Primary Prevention**

1. Teach personal hygiene, especially hand washing always before handling food, always after defecation, and always after cleaning one child's defecation and before touching the next child. Use sufficient toilet paper to reduce contamination of hands. Wash children's hands often, too.

2. Provide for sanitary disposal of feces, through plumbing and sewage, through disposal of diapers in fly-proof containers, and through latrines or burying underground when in the field.

3. Encourage breastfeeding throughout infancy. Breast milk is nutritious, safe, uncontaminated and provides antibody protection. It may be necessary to modify existing employment policies in order to encourage working mothers of young infants to breast feed at work or to store breast milk in sanitary bottles so that babies can be fed while mother is away.

4. Purify drinking water, either at the community or household level. This depends upon changing the knowledge, priorities, and behaviors of political decision-makers and economic resource-providers.

5. Pasteurize or boil all dairy products.

6. Practice careful comprehensive cleanliness in food preparation at home, at day-care centers, and at commercial food preparation facilities. Keep cold foods cold and hot foods hot, if at all possible.

7. If foods must be prepared several hours (or days) before serving a large group, they should be rapidly chilled to below 4°C. Reheating foods that are a good medium for bacterial growth to 75°C or more will destroy some pathogens (e.g., *Salmonella* spp., *Clostridium perfringens*, *Staphylococcus aureus*) but not some of their toxins (Werner, 1986). Not all of these precautions can be followed in family homes, but institutions serving large numbers of people should follow them.

### Secondary Prevention

1. Maintain good nutrition to minimize the impact of diarrheal episodes.

2. Prevent dehydration and malnutrition by continuing to feed fluids and appropriate bland foods.

3. Use oral rehydration salts with plenty of fluid to maintain electrolyte balance.

4. Refer for medical care if diarrhea persists more than 14 days or stools contain blood.

### Oral Rehydration—How to Do It

The members of every social group in the world, whether they be residents of a rural island or an enclave of migrants in a major metropolis, have their own traditional definitions of each common disease and symptom complex, its possible causes, and how it should be treated. Western medicine enters the scene and overlaps its own diagnostic and treatment principles upon the folkways of local citizens. The first concern of health workers should be to transplant the new health measure—in this instance oral rehydration therapy (ORT) as the first response to diarrhea—so that it will not be rejected by the rest of the body of local beliefs and fears, so that people will "stick to it." Just as you cannot make an adhesive bandage stick to wet skin, you must prepare the "surface" before introducing a new health measure. So also with any medical innovation. (See also Coreil and Mull (eds.), 1998) for an anthropological review of diarrheal control strategies. **(Also see the discussion of strategies for behavior change in Chapter 7.)**

Teaching points to convey to mothers in the target population:

• Using local terminology, explain that ORT should be used for every form of diarrhea, whatever its cause.

• ORT may not stop the diarrhea quickly, but it will prevent dehydration—translatable as drying out, wasting away, losing strength. ORT will put life fluids, energy, resistance, and "refreshment" into the body.

- ORT involves work: feeding teaspoonfuls of ORT solution, minute by minute, for hours (feeding too rapidly may encourage vomiting). Yet it is the best thing anybody can do for the child.

- There are fewer errors in mixing ORT solution if pre-mixed packets of the dry ingredients are available for distribution. The most common error is failure to add enough water. Much of the pre-packaged ORT includes: sodium chloride, 3.5 g; trisodium citrate, 2.9 g; potassium chloride, 1.5 g; glucose, 20 g. This is to be dissolved in 1 liter of drinking water. The UNICEF package for 1 liter of ORT contains: sodium chloride, 3.5 g; sodium bicarbonate, 2.5 g; potassium chloride, 1.5 g; and anhydrous glucose, 20 g. These are robust formulas and modest deviations do not reduce efficacy, but these may be more expensive than homemade, unless packets can be given free.

- It is not necessary to boil water before making the "drink," but if the mother wishes to boil it, this should be done before the salts and sugar are added. Serve at "room temperature"—neither hot nor chilled.

PAHO (1994) reviewed data for 33 countries and found that while 70% of the people in these populations had access to ORT, only 55% of children in need received ORT properly. A comprehensive review of this topic has been prepared by Huttly, Morris, and Pisani (1997; 111 references).

## REDUCING RATES OF UNINTENTIONAL INJURIES

Unintentional injury is the term now used by public health workers to encompass what were formerly called "accidents." This is because the epidemiologic study of such events shows that injuries are not random events (as are "true accidents"), but have the same kind of predictability and identifiable personal and environmental risk factors as do diseases. They are also subject to reduction by appropriate interventions. According to the World Bank, injuries and violence accounted for 15% of years of productive life lost (before age 65) in the world. For the Americas the data are similar (PAHO, 1994, 1998, 2002). Rates are more than twice as great in males compared to females. There is a peak in mortality from this cause during the first year of life, followed by a decline until age 14. From age 15 to about age 30, a true pandemic of deaths and injuries develops.

Many volumes have been published about this area of public health, and the section that follows is merely an introduction, a source of references, and a recommendation for several high-priority interventions.

Injury is caused by the impact upon a living organism (in this section, upon young children) by a source of energy—such as blunt or sharp physical impact, moving objects (vehicles, one's own body in falls, bullets), heat, radiation, or toxins (damaging substances or chemicals inhaled, swallowed, or touched). A harmful transfer of energy is always the cause of an acute injury. The most effective preventive interventions for unintentional injuries are environmental changes, rather than trying to change human behaviors. This is especially true for children. Of course, changing the environment (whether micro or macro) for children means changing the behaviors, expectations, and vigilance of parents, health professionals, and everyone in the community.

Injuries and adverse effects (including poisoning, burns, etc.) rate as high as the seventh leading cause of infant death in the United States and similar industrialized countries. Both the death rates and burden of injury disabilities are even higher in less developed countries. In the latter countries, injuries are typically the leading cause of deaths in males from ages 5 to 44 years and in females from ages 5–24 years, after which circulatory and neoplastic diseases become the leading causes. In these countries, the leading causes of death for children ages 1 to 4 years are infectious and parasitic damage to the respiratory and intestinal systems.

In more industrialized nations, such as Argentina, Uruguay, Spain, Austria, Poland, and the United States of America, injuries are the leading cause of death all the way from ages 1 to 34 years in males and from ages 1 to 24 years in females. When indexes such as years of productive life lost (YPLL) or burden of disability are calculated, injuries become the leading cause for the entire population in most countries.

*Beyond the toll they take in death and disability, injuries exact major economic and social consequences for families and communities.*

Reducing injuries, be they intentional or nonintentional (as discussed in the following section), must become a top priority both for child health care professionals and for public health professionals. Clearly, prevention is preferable to cure, because in many cases of injury full recovery is not possible.

In addition to the toll they take in mortality and disability, injuries have major economic and social consequences for the families and communities in which they occur, including costs of outpatient and hospital treatment, absence from work (in adults), disability, lost productivity, costs of home care, and lost days from school (in children). A Swedish study of road accidents (Hartunian et al., 1980) showed that 30% of the total calculated cost for injuries was for medical care, whereas 70% was attributed to lost productivity. This ratio can probably be generalized to other types of injuries and other nations. It should be kept in mind that these costs are only short-term estimates. A severely injured child may experience a full lifetime of increased dependency and reduced work skills. Damage to the brain and nervous system can raise risks both for conduct disorders during youth and Alzheimer's disease in old age (Mrazek and Haggerty, 1994). **(Also see Chapter 11.)**

54

These are the three major determinants of whether injuries occur to children and what kind they may be: (1) the developmental age and skills of the child, (2) the dangers and protections in the child's immediate environment, and (3) the adequacy of adult supervision.

Children ages 1 to 4 years suffer more injuries than infants under 1 year old because they are more mobile—they can run and climb. Their curiosity is high; self-restraint, low; and they have inadequate experience and ability to link their actions with sometimes painful results. At ages 1 to 4, children also have more injuries than those 5 years old and older, because the latter group, although even more mobile, has learned much about household dangers, has learned to link cause and effects, and usually shows more self-restraint. The most common dangers for children aged 1–4 are burns, scalds, falls, poisons, lack of parental provision of car safety seats and restraints, and lack of smoke detectors in homes. By age 5, a higher proportion of injuries involve motor vehicles, both as passengers and while crossing streets or running from play areas into streets. Parents often expect or allow children to attempt to do unsupervised things that are beyond their developmental stage, with injuries too frequent a result.

Boys experience 150% to 250% the rate of injuries compared to girls at every age. Overactivity and aggressiveness are behavioral contributors to risk. Living in poverty is another major risk factor around the world. In Western countries, the following risk factors have also been repeatedly documented: children in families with three or more young children, single parent families, mother suffering from depression, mother is a teenager, and child has a history of injuries. Despite the validity of these predictors, intervention programs targeted at children having multiple risk factors have not, in general, been proven effective in actually reducing trauma rates (Kendrick, 1994).

Injury research across the full lifespan indicates that passive preventive measures (those not calling for continuing vigilance or repeated behaviors) are much more effective than those attempting to change repertoires of behavior. Supplying medicines or household chemicals with "child-proof" closures is an example of a passive prevention that has proven remarkably effective. Automatic seat belts for adults in automobiles, "speed-bumps" on side streets, and placing window latches that prevent a home window from opening far enough to allow a small child to crawl through are further examples of passive prevention measures.

Legislation and regulations are other effective means of prevention, providing they are enforced. Laws that mandate the use of automobile seat belts and motorcycle helmet laws and that impose heavy penalties for noncompliance—irrespective of whether an "accident" or other infraction occurs—have been often shown to save lives far beyond their cost. Laws mandating the use of approved child safety seats for all children under a specified age, coupled with systems for loaning seats to families who cannot afford them and education of parents and health professionals, have been shown to cut drastically the number and severity of injuries of young children in motor vehicles.

The third most effective approach—and one that is essential to support environmental change and legal requirements—is to pursue the sort of education that changes behavior, be it of parents, more mature children, health professionals, or community leaders (in government, school, industries, churches, and civic organizations). **(A more complete discussion of how this can be accomplished is found in Chapter 11.)**

Many careful studies have shown that health professionals working in primary care can be effective agents for change in reducing children's injury rates through counseling, facilitating small scale environmental changes in and around homes, and lobbying for "child-safe communities" with local and provincial authorities (see Bass et al., 1993; Kendrick, 1994; and Grossman and Rivara, 1992, for documentation). Several authors cited offer lists of interventions which can reduce rates of childhood injuries. The collective summary presented below is organized by the external force causing the injury.

### Preventing Impact Injuries to Children Inside Motor Vehicles

- Provide child safety seats correctly anchored by seat belts where this is economically feasible. In those states or provinces where there are laws requiring this, they should be obeyed.

- After children outgrow safety seats, keep them properly safety-belted any time the car is moving, preferably in the back seat.

- Do not allow children to ride in the back of open trucks (e.g., pickup or flatbed), unless slow speeds and great caution are used. In those states or provinces that have laws forbidding such riding, these should be obeyed and enforced. **(Also see Chapter 11 for further steps to reduce motor vehicle injuries at all ages.)**

### Preventing Impact Injuries to Children Outside of Motor Vehicles

- Children playing near streets or crossing streets should be supervised according to their age and the nature of traffic. Preschoolers might be allowed to play in unpaved streets that are free of all "through-traffic" and used only by a few responsible neighbors. Even older children will need supervision crossing highways with fast traffic, however. Parents and anyone caring for children should always use those extra ounces of caution and prevention.

- Yards where children play near home or school should be fenced if they are near streets and roads. This keeps balls and toys from rolling into the street, tempting children to run after them.

- Many young children like to play or hide around or behind cars and many have been killed by a family member backing up a vehicle over them. All drivers should always check both under and behind their vehicle (while walking outside it) before putting it in motion.

### Preventing Impact Injuries to Children on Playground Equipment or Climbing

- Many impact injuries involve falls out of trees, off porches, or from swings and slides. Adults and adolescents caring for young children should not let them experiment with doing things for which they are not ready developmentally. Often, letting a child try something new (such as a playground slide), while keeping a protective hand nearby, will allow an appropriate fear of that activity to develop until such time as the child grows further. There are also injuries associated with organized games and sports, which can be reduced by proper equipment, coaching, and a playing surface that is user-friendly.

### Preventing Injuries on Household Stairs and Windows

- Put "stops" on windows that are more than about 1.5 m (5 feet) above the ground, so that they will not open wide enough to allow a child's head or hips to fall through.

- Install folding gates or barricade the tops of stairwells with furniture to prevent young children from falling down. Even after they have learned to crawl up and down stairs, a running child can slip or misjudge the distance and tumble off the top steps. There will be many more impacts before that fall stops.

### Preventing Burn Injuries

Young children are particularly at risk to burns, scalds, and electrical shocks. Adults are so conditioned to avoiding these hazards that they forget safety has to be learned, it is not instinctive. Aside from the very old, young children are at highest risk of death due to fire, flames, and smoke.

- In climates and communities where homes catch fire, smoke detectors should be installed and regularly checked in dwellings with bedrooms without an easy exit to the outside. Even where such access is available, smoke detectors will awaken heavy sleepers so they and their families can escape in time. At least as many people die from silent smoke as from crackling flames—and smoke spreads more quickly. Properly working smoke detectors cut the rate of children dying in fires by half.

- Children should be kept well away from indoor heaters and stoves with hot surfaces. Acquire models that have protective screens or improvise barriers from materials that won't scorch or burn.

- Children's sleepwear, bathrobes, and other clothing should have snug sleeves and should be belted around the waist so they have less chance of coming in contact with heaters and igniting. Some countries require that young children's clothing be made from flame-resistant fabrics. In other nations this source of burn injury is too rare to justify a legal program, but might be included as part of parent education.

- Matches and lighters should be in places that children cannot reach. Don't allow children to play with anything that can cause a fire.

- Keep hot cooking pots and their handles out of reach of children. Many children receive second- and third-degree burns each year because they grab a pot handle atop the stove and spill boiling liquids on themselves.

- Homes with automatic hot water heaters should have the thermostat set to no more than 130° F (54° C). Most manufacturers set thermostats at 140° F to 150° F (60° to 65° C), hot enough to cause severe second-degree burns on adult skin in two seconds. Lower settings will prevent people of all ages from accidentally scalding themselves seriously. Hot tap water accounted for 24% of the scald burns requiring hospitalization in children under age 4 in a United States study. Some states have laws requiring that all new water heaters be set no higher than 130° F (54° C) (Grossman and Rivara, 1992). This paragraph would not apply to those perennially warm climates where water heaters are uncommon. The same cautions, however, must be heeded when using stove- or fire-heated water near children.

- Parents heating water for baths or washing should test the water temperatures by submerging tender skin (a wrist or cheek) in the water for five seconds before placing the baby or child in the water. Accidental scald injuries have irregular, splash-like borders, and tend to be less serious than intentionally inflicted scalds (Botash et al., 1996).

- Fireworks are another common source of burns. Children should never set off explosive firecrackers. Many children have lost fingers and eyes or have been left with permanently disfigured faces from malfunctioning fireworks. Children may also run over and touch firework fragments or wires on "sparklers" while they are still hot enough to burn. Chemical burns from hot sulphur or phosphorus cause extended pain.

- Old electrical appliances and electric cords that are frayed or have cracked insulation can cause serious shocks and burns, including house fires. In some circumstances, these may be fatal. Overloading electrical circuits by having too many appliances connected to the same outlet can also cause shocks, sparks, and fires. The visiting nurse or health assistant can look for these hazards as well as many others listed in this chapter when they make home visits.

- Children go through a stage of exploring their surroundings. Some will stick pins, keys, or other metal objects into electrical outlets, resulting in hazardous electrical shocks. Unfilled electrical outlets in children's rooms should be covered with adhesive tape or plastic covers until the child grows out of this stage.

### Preventing Poisoning

In their first year of life, children automatically and unconsciously put everything in their mouths; this, coupled with children's ability to walk and handle things in their second year, and the curiosity to open containers, adds up to a higher risk of poisoning in the ages from 1 to 5 years, than at any other time of life.

The most effective measure to reduce childhood poisonings has been legislation requiring childproof packaging of the most common, potentially dangerous substances (prescription medications, as well as over-the-counter pain killers including aspirin and vitamins, especially if pleasantly flavored). Other compounds are not protectively packaged, however, and cause thousands of poisonings. These include detergents, polishes, drain cleaners, kerosene, solvents used by painters, and farm chemicals such as pesticides, fertilizers, and chemically-treated seeds. Children should be kept away from these poisons by changing the microenvironment: poisons should be stored on high shelves or in cabinets or closets that have a complex latch that younger children cannot manipulate, and all medications should be kept in containers that children cannot open. Parents cannot watch children closely all the time, and warnings or scolding is usually forgotten by children or lost in the excitement of finding new things to do. Clearly, a passive prevention approach will work best.

> **Children from ages 2 to 5 years are at highest risk of lead poisoning.**

Children from ages 2 to 5 years are at highest risk of lead poisoning. This heavy metal, once ingested, is stored in the body, causing varying degrees of damage to the brain, nervous system, heart, kidneys, and other internal organs; depending on the dose, damage may be permanent. While there are various environmental sources of lead, the one that causes the most serious and acute damage is paint containing lead. Leaded paint was more frequently used before the 1950s. It was primarily used to paint the outside of houses and often also was used on inside wood surfaces. Any factories nearby which process lead, as well as the use of lead-glazed dishes, are other sources of this toxin. Some young children develop a habit of habitually eating non-food substances such as dry peeling paint, plaster, dirt, cloth, paper, or special kinds of clay. (This habit has been called "pica," after magpie birds who reputedly eat all kinds of junk.) Some children also dip their fingers in stove oil, leaded gasoline, or kerosene and then lick them. One can see how many kinds of poisoning might occur this way. Lead compounds apparently taste sweet to most children, so their habit is not random or due to boredom, but motivated, focused, and self-reinforced.

Therefore, parents should be taught to look for the habit of pica, to separate their children from their favorite substances, and report the situation promptly to a health professional. A child with pica will usually limit himself to two or three favorite substances. If these include lead-containing paints, painted plaster, or dirt near the house on which paint was spilled or dropped in flakes by a paint removal process, the child may, after repeated small ingestions, develop lead poisoning.

Early signs of lead poisoning in children include behavioral changes, such as becoming more irritable, crying easily, becoming more easily frightened, moving more sluggishly, having neurologic symptoms, experiencing stomach pains, and fighting with and sometimes biting playmates. In latitudes with climate change, symptoms usually worsen in hot summer.

Health professionals, when confronted with symptoms like these, should always obtain a blood lead determination. Some urban areas with old housing perform blood lead screening on all children ages 1 to 5 years, and find enough subclinical cases to initiate early treatment and to justify primary prevention for other children in those areas.

## Preventing Cuts and Lacerations

Although very frequent, these injuries are usually relatively mild; that is, unless they are intentionally inflicted. The usual causes include knives, tools, broken glass or metal pieces, and farm implements. The parent's task is to keep the child separated from such objects, until his or her developmental level (irrespective of actual age) is adequate in knowledge, self-control, and appreciation of risk to allow safe handling. Health visitors' checklists should keep them alert for such items in children's reach. Windows and glass doors should be shielded from accidental breakage and children should be prevented from cutting themselves by running into these surfaces or throwing objects that might shatter them.

## Preventing Drownings

Drowning is a surprisingly frequent cause of death among boys ages 1 to 4 years, accounting for about 20% to 30% of "external cause" fatalities in some countries, and more where the population is dense around rivers, lakes, and beaches. (Drowning again becomes a major proportional cause of death for young men 15–24 years old.)

To protect young children from drowning, they should be kept away from even shallow bodies of water unless closely supervised by a skilled swimmer. Yards should be fenced to keep children within and away from streams and ponds. Yards with swimming pools should be fenced to keep children out unless supervised. Few adults realize that small children can drown in very shallow water: infants can drown in bathtubs and toddlers, in shallow streams, if they fall down the banks and are unable to move out of a face down position. Environmental barriers and unbroken parental alertness are key factors in preventing drowning.

When children become developmentally ready, teaching them to swim and to float—to manage in deeper water without fear, but with healthy respect—is another well-proven preventive from drowning.

## Dealing with Insect and Animal Bites

In tropical climates insect bites can transmit such damaging diseases as malaria, yellow fever, river blindness, and Chagas' disease. In addition, many people, including children, have allergies to insect bites, which can precipitate shock or even death if not treated. Ideally, doors, windows, and other openings should be screened. If this is not affordable, it is essential to use insect netting on beds and hammocks. Careful use of insecticide sprays in homes also is effective, but this can only be done safely by a trained person. For especially susceptible children, insect repellents may be used during waking hours when mosquitoes and other vectors are most evident.

Animal bites are less frequent but more serious in areas where cats and dogs are not immunized against rabies. Children should be cautioned repeatedly never to chase or touch strange animals and not to threaten or hurt household pets. Again, a fence around play areas will keep pets and children in and other animals out.

Everyone should avoid animals that are acting strangely, that appear in a rage, or those that have lost muscle coordination—they may have caught rabies from another animal. Natural reservoirs for rabies include wild foxes, wolves, coyotes, raccoons, bats, and skunks. In developing countries, dogs are the principal reservoir. Although rabies is mainly a disease of animals, it can be spread to humans by bites or animal saliva. When rabies is not treated promptly with the correct injections, it is usually fatal to humans.

Other less severe diseases can also be caused by animal bites or saliva. Preventive measures are the same as described above, primarily separating children from unfamiliar animals. First aid involves washing the wounds immediately with soap and water, enclosing the animal (or killing it, if wild) for laboratory examination, and taking the bitten person to a health professional for examination and treatment (Chin (ed.), 2000).

### Preventing Strangulation/Choking

Choking in young children usually occurs in one of three ways:

* by children putting small hard objects, such as balls and toy parts, in their mouths and letting them fall back into their throats;

* by ingesting pieces of food that are too large to swallow unless the food is thoroughly chewed—remember that young children tend to gulp;

* by putting very young children into cribs, playpens, or other enclosures or porches where the bars or posts that form the sides are far enough apart for the child to wedge his head through. The child may then turn or twist enough to be unable to retract the head through the openings, and in the ensuing panic cut off air flow through the neck.

The extent of choking/strangulation as a cause of death is great; in recent years it accounted for 16% of all injury mortality under age 5 years in a large U.S. state.

Such injuries can be largely prevented by educating parents to modify the child's microenvironment in selection of cribs, playpens, and toys, and to cut solid foods very small before feeding. Some states or countries require labeling of toys, telling of any danger to any age groups.

### Preventing Suffocation

Like strangulation and choking, suffocation causes death by anoxia, but it does not involve compression of the neck or blockage of the trachea. Suffocation occurs when properly oxygenated air is no longer available to a person. This can occur when a closed room or automobile accumulates an excess of carbon dioxide or monoxide from heaters or engines which burn up the oxygen. It also often occurs when young children play with plastic bags, plastic sheeting, or rubber balloons in such a way as to block their nose or mouth. In infants, reduction of air intake, such as may be caused by resting face down on thick blankets or comforters, may precipitate sudden infant death syndrome.

Large airtight containers, such as discarded refrigerators, freezers, or storage trunks, are attractive playthings for children. Every year some get caught inside and suffocate before they can escape. Many communities have laws requiring that the doors (or lids) of all such containers be removed before they are discarded or left unattended. This should become a universal safety practice.

### Preventing Firearm Injuries

The epidemic of gun-related injuries and deaths really begins at about age 15 in males; there is no such epidemic in females. Review of cause-specific mortality rates across 10 countries (8 in the Americas) shows male-to-female homicide rate ratios for ages 15 to 54 ranging from 3 to 1 to 15 to 1. In the United States it is estimated that there are at least five nonfatal shootings for each fatal one. Hospital and police costs also are tremendous. A report to the United States Congress in 1989 estimated that the average total cost for each firearm fatality (homicides, suicides, and unintentional injuries) was $373,000. Nonfatal injuries cost much less, as does the financial impact per case in other nations.

You may wonder why we have included this in a section on pediatrics. Unfortunately, guns are increasingly reaching down to younger ages to reap their victims. In 1990, in a large United States state, 16% of total injury mortality in children under age 5 years was attributed to homicide and an additional number to unintentional firearms injuries. For children ages 5 to 9 years, the total trauma mortality included 5% due to "accidental" firearm injuries and 7% of deaths due to homicides, most of which were caused by firearms.

Still, in the pediatric age range—ages 10–14—this large state with a good mix of urban, suburban, small town, rural agriculture, and industrial areas, attributed 9% of injury mortality to unintentional firearm discharge, 13% to suicide, and 16% to homicide due to guns. That totals 38% of all traumatic fatalities, equal to the total caused by motor vehicles in this age group and location.

The rates of violent death vary greatly from country to country, and the proportion due to firearms differs by the number of handguns available to the general public. Nations with more restrictive policies and laws concerning handguns have fewer gunshot injuries and deaths due to suicides, homicides, and unintentional "accidents."

Preventive measures include keeping guns out of the home and teaching children not to play with others who have personal access to guns. If guns are kept in the household, they should be kept in locked cabinets—cabinets that even 14-year-olds cannot open—and they should be kept unloaded with ammunition stored in a separate locked place. It should be noted that long-barreled guns (rifles or shotguns) are involved in proportionally fewer unintentional injuries, suicides, and homicides than are smaller handguns. Teaching the dangers of guns, how to handle them safely, and why never to get near them when emotionally upset, may be valuable, if the lessons are internalized. Here again, environmental change is more powerful than teaching safe behaviors, because strong impulses can melt away past learning at least for short intervals. The extra few minutes it takes to unlock both guns and ammunition may allow enough cooling off to prevent disaster.

## CHILD ABUSE AND NEGLECT

Child abuse and neglect are part of the larger problem of violence in modern society. At least 150,000 children aged 0–4 years are intentionally killed each year worldwide (Murray and Lopez, 1996, p. 468). (Because persons of any age can be the victims of violence, this topic will be addressed at each stage of the life cycle. At all stages the victims suffer physical and/or psychological and/or social trauma and require the services of health agencies and possibly other sectors of community services as well.) Abuse and neglect can create physical and emotional damage that will express itself again in future years. Preventing abuse and neglect not only saves lives and prevents disabilities, it also is a vital part of promoting future mental health and social adaptation.

Child abuse and neglect are either becoming more severe and more prevalent in most nations or they are becoming more often recognized and classified as "non-accidental." Creighton (1988) estimates that the incidence of physical abuse of children increased by 70% in the United Kingdom between 1970 and 1986. Whatever the reason, the rates of intentional injury and related mortality in children have risen to the point where national and international health authorities have ranked abuse and neglect as major public health problems. This is because psychosocial pathology causes abuse, violence is transmitted like an epidemic, and the resulting damage endures for years and places great demands on health professionals, emergency care facilities, rehabilitation services, and mental health treatment.

Abuse—whether of children, adolescents, partners, or the elderly—can take place in a wide variety of forms: physical trauma, psychosocial damage (such as threats of injury or death, a constant barrage of insulting or belittling accusations, loss of trust in everyone, exposure to unpredictable uncontrolled rage, being isolated or abandoned), and sexual abuse (both actions and threats).

Neglect also can take several forms: failure to provide the necessities for life and normal development, such as food, clothing, shelter, communication, self-acceptance, and encouragement of learning, and failure to protect from environmental and household hazards, excessive cold or heat, and social or sexual exploitation. Child abuse and/or neglect includes any act of omission or commission that endangers or impairs a child's physical or emotional health and development (Kerfoot, 1992).

## Prevalence and Severity of the Problem

Relatively few nations systematically collect child abuse data, and for those that do, reports often underestimate the true incidence of this problem. The American Association for Protecting Children reported an abuse rate of 34 per 1,000 children in the United States for 1987 (cited in MacMillan et al., 1993). Another national household survey reported about 10% of parents admitted at least one "severe violent act" against a child in the previous year (Straus and Gelles, 1986).

The severity and long-term impact of child abuse is also generally underestimated. Homicide is the leading cause of injury-related deaths in infants in some nations. According to the American Academy of Pediatrics (AAP) physical abuse is the leading single cause of head injury in infants (under age 1 year) (American Academy of Pediatrics, 1993). Many intracranial injuries in infants and young children show no fractures or surface bruises, but rather subdural, subarachnoid, or retinal hemorrhages and a cluster of clinical neurological signs and symptoms. This clinical presentation includes "shaken baby syndrome." The cited report reviews the radiology, pathological findings, and long-term disability from such injuries. In a United States case series, 80% of deaths from head trauma in children under 2 years of age were intentionally inflicted. Often the only visible signs of less severe shaking of the baby are intraocular hemorrhages and clinical indicators of possible cerebral edema, neurologic signs, or light coma.

> *Abuse and neglect can create physical and emotional damage that will express itself again in future years. Preventing abuse and neglect not only saves lives and prevents disabilities, it also is a vital part of promoting future mental health and social adaptation.*

In a series of infants who were comatose when initially examined, 60% either died or suffered continuing profound disabilities. Most cases present with less severe findings, mimicking more common disorders; as a result, they are not correctly diagnosed at first (American Academy of Pediatrics, 1993).

As seen in the section "Preventing Postnatal Disabilities," earlier in this chapter, in a major metropolitan area, the second leading cause of child disabilities originating after birth is beating of children.

## Cross-cultural Considerations

Rates of child abuse in less industrialized nations than the United Kingdom, Canada, and the United States are mostly unknown. In many traditional agrarian cultures, children are perceived somewhat more as their family's property, and raising and disciplining them is considered a private family matter. Actions considered abusive in some nations are considered acceptable in others. This is changing in many places, as Western industrialized cultural norms and values spread.

An important consideration to be weighed into each community's position on injuries from abuse, is the extent to which the entire community recognizes both the short- and long-term costs of current child abuse and neglect. Costs for the community include the death of some children and the permanent disability of many others that may emerge as crippling brain damage, psychiatric disorders, the spread of violence around the neighborhood when the abused or neglected children reach adolescence, and the transmission of violence to the next generation when the children become parents.

Being a victim of repeated childhood maltreatment or experiencing physical or sexual assault, confers a heavy risk for psychiatric disorders later in life, including depression (Mrazek and Haggerty, 1994, p. 165). A review of prevention of mental disorders commissioned by the United States government, also reports a doubled rate of juvenile delinquency in youth who in their younger years were abused or neglected, compared to a control group in the same communities (25% vs. 13%) (Widom, 1989; Mrazek and Haggerty, 1994).

Some cultures, particularly in Africa, believe that it takes a whole village to raise a child. This communal involvement takes pressure off parents and allows a sharing of concern and responsibility. It also serves a preventive function by allowing parents a chance for respite and help on those days when stress brings their emotions near the boiling point.

## Clinical Signs of Child Abuse

It is very difficult to predict the onset of abuse to a given child, because the risk factors, while known, are too non-specific. In fact, they label far more parents "at risk" of abusing than ever go on to traumatize their children, and this mislabeling can be hurtful to families. Once child abuse is discovered in a family, however, both that child and its siblings can be considered at high enough risk of further abuse to warrant secondary preventive efforts. Hence, identification of existing cases is of critical importance.

The following general clinical signs in an injured child raise the suspicion that intentional injury may have occurred, once other more probable causes have been shown to have been unlikely (taken from Kerfoot, 1992).

**Damage to surface tissue.** Suspect abuse when the child has multiple bruises and the bruises are in places unlikely to be inflicted by an accidental event. Children too young to walk are unlikely to incur multiple bruising. Moreover, abuse often damages the head, face, and middle of the back on both sides of the spine. Look for sets of small bruises which might result from a tight grip with thumb and fingers, enough pressure to cause a small internal bleed.

**Black eyes in a young child are rarely accidental.** If two black eyes are present and there is no injury of corresponding severity to the middle of the forehead or bridge of the nose, the black eyes may have been inflicted separately and intentionally. Look for patterns in the bruises, such as the outline of a hand, small pairs of bruises from pinching, or linear welts or C or U shapes from a belt or its buckle.

**Lacerations and abrasions.** These also warrant the health professional's examination and careful thought. Lacerations of the lip or inside the mouth are suspicious, but could be the unintentional result of a child falling with an object in his or her mouth. Lacerations on the back of the hands are more likely to be intentional than those on the front of the hands, but once again, the explanation given by the adult must make sense.

**Burns and scalds.** These are common injuries, and only about 2% of heat injuries in young children are intentional. Kerfoot points out that the typical instance of a child pulling a pot of hot liquid off the stove results in the child sustaining burns under the chin and around the armpits and torso. When an adult uses this scenario to explain scalds in a different part of the body, more inquiry is needed.

**Children who instinctively and quickly pull away from pain.** This gives truly accidental burns irregular edges. Burns without evidence of withdrawal are suspect. The shape of a burn gives a clue as to the object involved. Cigarette burns,

---

**THE EXPLANATION**

An adult who brings in a child for care will always have an explanation for the child's condition. The health professional should determine whether the story makes sense in light of the nature, number, and distribution of the observed injuries. A medical examination provides an opportunity to observe the child's entire body for scars, old bruises, and other signs of past damage. This might best be done with parents or other accompanying persons out of the room. If the child can talk, this provides an opportunity to obtain the child's version about the incident and other findings. It is advisable to check also the child's buttocks and genitalia, without drawing attention to them, in the course of the examination. Those are common sites for inflicted injuries. If more than one adult accompanies the child, have them interviewed separately about circumstances of the injury. A hastily concocted false explanation may not be told consistently unless it was planned and rehearsed between the adults.

especially if multiple, generally signal abuse. Carelessness or abuse involving hot water, such as in the bath, often presents as scalds having a glove or stocking configuration with straight edges on hands, feet, or buttocks. More criteria for the diagnosis of intentional intracranial injuries and fractures are found in recent textbooks.

### Child Neglect

In impoverished communities, many children may appear to be neglected to an outside observer, as the family may be unable to provide desirable levels of material needs. In these situations, responsibility for upgrading the support of children lies with the community, state, and nation. There is no better investment in a nation's future than removing barriers to the physical and mental development of its children.

Each family should be able to supply its children with the most fundamental of needs: love, concern, nurture, self-acceptance, social support, and protection from the adverse aspects of the physical, biological, and social environment.

The absence of psychosocial caring often manifests itself in deficiencies in shelter, food, and clothing for a given child that are worse than those of the adults or other children in the home, and worse than demanded by the level of resources available to that family as compared to others nearby. Sometimes a family unconsciously selects one child as a scapegoat for its troubles, and only that child shows signs of abuse and neglect.

Educating parents about how better to manage available resources and of the specific needs of very young children may improve circumstances. Sometimes it is useful to review the family's priorities and move the child's basic needs to a higher level. The forces of consumerism encourage families to buy a television set rather than repair a leaky roof or provide children with shoes and sweaters for cold weather. Health professionals may need to counter such messages and bring health priorities to the forefront in meetings with schools, local groups, churches, and individual families. Providing the media with news stories of positive things parents can do will extend outreach even further.

---

**CHECKLIST OF SIGNS OF POSSIBLE NEGLECT FOR HEALTH PROFESSIONALS**

The following conditions, if severe or noted repeatedly over time, should initiate further inquiry or possibly a home visit, not for the purpose of inspection but rather a friendly visit to become acquainted with how things are going at home.

**Dwelling Place**
- Does the home have adequate sanitation, including proper disposal of excrement, refuse, spoiled food, and trash?
- Is the home protected against rodents, insects, and other animals, as well as cold or rainy weather?
- Are sleeping areas clean, comfortable, and not too crowded?
- Is the home free of fire hazards and risks for falls, poisoning, scalding, etc.?

**Nutrition**
- Is food quality adequate and the diet balanced?
- Are food and eating utensils kept clean and free of spoilage and vermin?
- Are meals prepared for children and served at reasonably consistent times?
- Do the children always seem hungry or sleepy?

**Personal Hygiene and Care**
- Are the children usually dirty and lacking in hygiene?
- Are their clothes usually dirty and not cared for (e.g., mended)?
- Are their clothes appropriate for the weather conditions?
- Do the children lack needed medical and dental care? (If these are not accessible, affordable, or acceptable, perhaps changes are needed at the community level.)
- Are underage children left unsupervised for long periods of time or supervised only by other underage children?

---

**Tertiary Prevention**

If further investigation shows that young children are being chronically abused or neglected, health or welfare agencies may need to intervene on their behalf, such as by removing either the abuser or the victim from the dwelling. The systems for dealing with such problems differ across communities and cultures. The primary concern must be for the child's safety, health, and well being. If the child's own family can be helped to do better, that might be the best choice.

However, case reports and newspapers all too frequently tell the story of a child dying of further abuse after being sent back to his or her own family after one or two previous visits for emergency medical care.

### Secondary Prevention of Abuse and Neglect

**Demographic risk factors:**

- children born to single parents or to teenagers;

- children who were unwanted pregnancies that continue to be resented;

- children born to parents who are chronically in conflict;

- adults living in the home who use alcohol and drugs to the point of losing control;

- children living in homes of lowest socioeconomic status or whose parents have attained only low education levels;

- the family's daily life is seriously disorganized and unpredictable (often a result of earlier items mentioned);

- the child is between 3 months and 3 years (time of greatest vulnerability);

- children who appear different from the average, children who cry a lot, and those with handicaps are most likely to be targeted for harsh treatment.

**Psychosocial risk factors:**

- parents who were raised in abusive or neglectful homes and reenact these behaviors with their children;

- male partner's jealousy and fear of losing "first place" in the woman's attention and love for the child

- inadequate knowledge of child development, both for normal children and developmentally handicapped children. Failure to recognize the wide variability in reaching developmental milestones and the inability of the very young "to control themselves" may lead to unreasonable parental demands, outrage that they are "not being obeyed," and, finally, child abuse.

### Primary Prevention of Child Abuse and Neglect

The fundamental strategies for primary prevention of this worldwide epidemic are all psychosocial in nature.

- Adults and teenagers (the next generation of parents) should be educated in infant and child development and its wide variability from child to child. This will replace ignorance or wrong ideas and expectations about child development and children's mental and emotional capacities at early ages. What a parent or prospective parent expects of children will influence how they react. Much child abuse originates from adults placing demands on children that they control behaviors (e.g., crying, toilet training, grabbing and dropping fragile items) that they are too immature to manage well all the time. This is why children who are developing more slowly than the average child strain their caretakers' patience and endure an undue share of punishment.

- Parents should be educated about how children may best be rewarded and punished at each age, thus making behavior change more efficient and less frustrating both for parents and children.

Some parents or political or religious groups argue that programs to prevent child abuse take away parental rights to punish their children, leaving them with unruly children. This is a false argument. Discipline is intended to teach the child, not as a way for the adult to discharge his or her anger. Modern behavioral science has found many ways to correct those behaviors that the child is developmentally able to control, based on timely scolding, non-damaging physical contact, brief periods (minutes) of isolation, and the rewarding of "good" behaviors so the child can substitute them for "wrong" behaviors. Reinforcement—positive or negative—is most effective in very young children when done within seconds of the event calling for it. Only when children have grown to have an adequate cognitive recognition of past time and the behaviors they performed can they respond properly to punishment or rewards for acts done at other times and places.

*There is no better investment in a nation's future than removing barriers to the physical and mental development of its children.*

Babies and young children are biologically programmed to fret and cry when in pain or sick in some way. They often cannot turn off crying, any more than they can turn off vomiting or bleeding. The first task of the parent confronted with crying is to find out what is causing it. Often guidance can be obtained from an older, more experienced parent. If excessive crying persists, diagnosis and care by a health professional may be required. After reaching the age of 1 or 2 years some children use crying, not only to signal illness, discomfort, or grief, but also to change parental behavior in the absence of a real problem. Such crying is better stopped by ignoring the child until the crying stops, rather than by physical punishment. If such crying spells become unduly extended or repetitive, assistance from a health professional is warranted.

Most first-time parents do not realize how much average infants cry every day. Botash and colleagues (1996) cite four studies of infants' crying. St. James-Roberts (1991) reported that 29% of infants cried more than three hours daily during their first three months. Brazelton found that 50% of normal, full-term infants cried or fussed more than 2.75 hours daily. Baildam et al. (1995) found that crying reached its peak at around six weeks of age. Removing fussing and crying spells lasting less than 5 minutes resulted in a range of 0 to 26 crying episodes 15 minutes or longer, with an average of 4.4 spells per child per day.

Parents and prospective parents need to expect those ranges of crying durations, and should not punish the baby for its normal organic responses. Crying time decreases in most infants as they get beyond 2 or 3 months of age. This is both because the infants' physiological controls and back-up systems gain greater capacity, and because parents learn what various cries mean at different times (e.g., when hungry or after defecating), and thus can correct the cause of the crying more promptly.

A clinical study showed that when experienced mothers, given brief training in behavioral management, were assigned to give telephone guidance to new mothers with babies younger than 6 months of age, the behavioral management counseling over a term of three to four months reduced daily crying and fussing by about 51%—from a baseline average of 346 minutes to a post-counseling average of 169 minutes (cited in Botash et al., 1996).

Such counseling programs could be incorporated into community health activities directed against all manner of childhood illnesses and injuries. Because these efforts are carried out by volunteers, they are inexpensive to conduct. The only costs are for a professional to train the volunteers, to encourage participants, and to receive referrals of difficult cases.

- It is critical to educate the community, including women's groups, men's groups, health professionals, school teachers, and schoolchildren, about the differences between legitimate discipline and physical, psychosocial, and sexual abuse. This will help define and raise consciousness about community norms for child-rearing. Children should learn about these matters in an age-appropriate way, because people outside their nuclear family, such as baby-sitters or more distant relatives, may abuse them. Sexual abuse is often inflicted on children ages 5–12 years and often has long-term negative effects. Hence, it is important that young schoolchildren learn what kinds of "games" and intimate touching are unacceptable. Children who are aware may also be able to protect younger siblings from physical abuse and neglect. As stated by many, it takes a whole village to raise a child safely.

- Parents and other adults who are in contact with children should receive assistance in impulse control. The previous three interventions deal with the cognitive aspects of prevention; this step addresses the emotional-behavioral components. Many parents and child-care workers may have all the essential knowledge regarding child development and teaching behaviors, but their environmental frustrations and unruly tempers allow them to strike out at children in dangerous ways. Both men and women are at risk. One approach reported to be successful (but documentation is not available at this time) in strengthening impulse control is organizing anger management groups of parents who feel themselves at risk of hurting children, plus those with a record of being abusive, along with a group counselor trained in impulse management and group therapy. Members of the group share their problems/situations (including triggers to rage) and also their coping methods under the guidance of the counselor. More evaluative studies need to be done to test alternative approaches.

- Parents must learn to take "time-off." Social service programs that reduce the load—or overload—of parenting also are useful, at least during crisis periods. Such programs may provide volunteer baby-sitters (including "volunteer grandparents," day care, or after school activities on one or more half-days per week) to allow an overloaded parent to get rest, respite, recreation, or recuperation. This strengthens the parent to cope more effectively the rest of the week.

Prevention or early treatment of child abuse and neglect has lifetime benefits for the mental health and social adjustment of the children being helped. Child abuse and neglect can be reduced dramatically and the future of each community and nation uplifted.

## SCREENING SUMMARY FROM BIRTH TO AGE 4 YEARS

The last several sections have covered issues common both to infancy and ages 1–4 years. We previously have given screening suggestions for pregnant women and newborns. Now we present suggestions for screening children ages 1–4 years, as a summary of the sections dealing with specific disease groups, injuries, abuse, and neglect.

Items 10–13 are important foundations for a child's future mental health. If these issues are amiss in a group of children, they may become less able to contribute to the community's future productivity, even if they have good "physical health." Their bodies can be viewed as well maintained vehicles in the hands of impaired, reckless, or purposeless drivers.

**SCREENING CHECKLIST FROM BIRTH TO AGE 4 YEARS**

1. Ask how often the child has respiratory infections (using local terms), and find out how severe they get and how are they treated.
2. Ask about diarrhea. How often has the child experienced episodes and how long did they last; was there any blood in the stool; was the child treated with ORT?
3. Check height, weight, and head circumference to measure development and identify stunting or obesity.
4. Check for iron deficiency anemia.
5. Make sure immunizations are up to date for diphtheria, tetanus, pertussis, polio (if outside of eradicated areas), measles, mumps, rubella, hepatitis B, and other diseases of local importance.
6. Do tuberculosis test if family is at high risk.
7. Ask about the habit of "pica" (the chewing and swallowing of non-food substances). It is a major risk factor for childhood poisoning, including often fatal toxicity from lead, which damages the heart, liver, kidneys, and especially the brain, resulting in lowered mental function and behavior disturbances among survivors.
8. Ask about smoky air in the home, either from tobacco or cooking or home heating.
9. Review injury risk to toddlers: hot water temperatures; access to stove (and hot utensils), heating sources, matches, firecrackers, soaps and cleansers, kerosene, heating oil, chemicals, pesticides, un-gated stairways, unscreened high windows. All medicines should be kept in childproof containers. Firearms, if any, should be kept unloaded, stored, and locked where children cannot reach them.
10. Ask about how children are punished when naughty. Is it age-appropriate? Is it too severe for the wrong that was done?
11. Be alert for signs of child neglect and abuse, including poor hygiene, continual hunger, chronic unusual fatigue, inadequate clothing in cold weather, bruises, cuts or burns on face, neck, back of hands, back, buttocks, or genital area.
12. Is there continuity of care by the same few adults, all of whom uphold consistent standards of care and provide the child a predictable and loving environment?
13. Is the child's human and physical environment stimulating to sensory and cognitive development?
14. If the child rides in motor vehicles, are child safety seats used during the child's first few years of life and are seat belts used later? Children should ride in the back seat.
15. Provide fluoride supplements to children in areas where water has less than 0.7 ppm of fluoride.
16. As soon as the child can respond appropriately (preferably before age 3 or 4 years) check hearing and eyesight, if sensory limitations have not previously been reported. This may be done simply and clinically if testing equipment is not available.
17. In climates where injury by fire or smoke is a concern, encourage or assist in obtaining smoke detectors if dwelling is at risk of fire, or if escape may be delayed.
18. Check blood pressure (using child cuff and norm data).

As babies and children mature through youth and adulthood, they carry the patterns of interactions and expectations learned first in the family into later interactions with playmates, school peers, teachers, and adults in the community. Hence, to be most effective, efforts to promote mental and social health, as well as physical health, must be started early in childhood.

# FROM AGES 5 THROUGH 14 YEARS

## MAJOR HEALTH PROBLEMS

The world over, death rates for children aged 5 to 14 years are 50% to 80% lower than for children 1 to 4 years old in the same country. Larger declines occur in those countries that have the highest mortality in the early years. These mid-to-late childhood years are the healthiest of the entire life-span, both in terms of mortality and permanent disability.

Those children who survive past age 4 years have built up biological immunity, physiological reserves, improved homeostatic controls, and the mental skills (including experience and communication) to avoid most danger. This benign health situation changes for the worse with the coming of puberty, however.

In the Region of the Americas, mortality rates for this age level range from about 23 per 100,000 in Canada to somewhere around 150 per 100,000 in some areas in Central America—more than a six-fold difference. Six nations in the Americas had rates higher than 100 per 100,000 in 1985–1989 (PAHO, 1994), as do many other countries elsewhere in the world. In nations with low overall death rates, "external causes" (injuries, both intentional and unintentional) are the leading single cause of death. In nations with less developed health infrastructure (lack of pure water, sanitation, vector control, immunization, primary health care coverage) infections and parasitic diseases are the prime causes of death, with external causes second. Tropical diseases still are major disablers and killers (PAHO, 1994, 1998, 2002; Murray and Lopez, 1996).

Gender differences become more pronounced in these ages, with boys having 30% to 90% greater death rates than girls. The excess in death rates among males comes primarily from injuries. This is the age at which interventions should begin at the social and cultural levels—particularly with boys—to deglamorize risk-taking, assaultive, and destructive behaviors. This is important to address now because over the next 20 years of the life cycle the male-to-female death ratio becomes even more skewed, with many countries experiencing a 3 to 1 male excess at ages 15 to 24 and/or ages 25 to 34 years. The difference is largely due to trauma and violence. Health professionals must become more active in helping educators, parents, and the media to instill the important distinction between constructive manliness and ignorant, destructive machismo.

In most areas where motor vehicles are widely available, they are the major contributors to traumatic death in middle and late childhood. This includes children walking or playing near roadways, as well as those riding in cars or trucks or on motorbikes. **(Also see sections on preventing impact injuries inside and outside motor vehicles earlier in this chapter.)** For many nations, drowning is the second most common traumatic form of death, especially in boys. **(Find more detail in section "Preventing Drownings," earlier in this chapter and in Chapter 11.)**

## HEALTH PROMOTION OPPORTUNITIES

Children and youth between the ages of 5 and 14 years are at an ideal stage to be taught the values and practices that will promote good health throughout the rest of their lives and to have those tenets reinforced. Children in this age range are learning rapidly and developing firm beliefs and standards. Schools, recreational and social groups, and families can fill this fertile time of development with positive and healthy role models, knowledge, and lifestyles. Too often, unfortunately, the news media in the 21st century reinforce the opposite.

Earlier in this book we emphasized the importance of providing very young children with human relationships that are loving, supportive, trustworthy, and consistent. These teach the child self-acceptance, a sense of self-worth, and expectations that other people are nurturing and helpful. This learning takes place at the level of feelings and expectations. After age 5, a child is better able to process cognitive learning about specific health-promoting and damaging factors influencing physical and mental health and social relationships.

Ages 5 to 14 years are the ideal ages to reinforce one of life's most important skills: how to get along—to interact constructively—with other people. This begins in infancy with immersion in dependable, loving care—learning that people bring good things, including comfort and pleasure; that dependence shifts with development to independence and interdependence. Controlling anger and respecting others also must be learned for future social, psychological, and physical health. In their important work, *Anger Kills*, Williams and Williams have comprehensively dealt with this issue (1993). The ideal social setting provides social interactions that are fair and that benefit all concerned; in other words, "win-win situations."

*Studies have repeatedly shown that groups that consume many whole grains, vegetables, and fruits develop fewer cancers and heart diseases.*

Healthy social learning in childhood will prevent many problems at each later stage of life. **(See also the sections "Conduct Disorders/Delinquency" and "Positive Mental Health" in Chapter 7 for a comprehensive discussion.)** A program for anger control among schoolchildren has been developed and tested by Olweus (1991). A major review was prepared by Feindler (1990).

These are the ages in which to teach—and personally demonstrate—healthy eating habits; personal hygiene; avoidance of unsafe food, water, and sources of parasites; how to reduce risks for injuries; the value of learning; how to deal with troubling feelings and troublesome people; social amenities; and problem-solving in an equitable manner. The child should be praised and taught how to reward himself or herself for these positive attitudes and behaviors. In these years children learn most deeply the values esteemed by the family, their religious faith, and the benevolent, responsible segments of society.

This is also the time to teach avoidance behaviors and to attach negative judgments to the objects of avoidance—including rejecting health-damaging substances such as tobacco, alcohol and other drugs, and inhalants; high-risk behaviors; peers who urge aggressive or self-destructive problem-solving; premature or unsafe sexual activity; feelings of helplessness, hopelessness, or violence; self-debasement to the point of impairing one's achievement; and distrust of others to the extent of isolation, paranoia, or alienation. These strong internalized personal foundations will promote physical, mental, and social health for a long and valuable lifetime.

These childhood years are the prime time for children to develop tastes in food. When older adults talk about vegetable stew or chocolate cookies "the way Mother used to make them," they are remembering the experiences of these childhood years. The message to us is that this is the time to create a taste for many kinds of vegetables, fruits, and whole grains. If meal times are happy times, all the foods of childhood will be enjoyed more and will continue to be experienced throughout adulthood with pleasant memories. Similarly, this is the age in which to discourage the eating of fatty foods, candies, and junk food, which appears attractive but contains too much fat, sugars, or salts, and lacks fiber and essential nutrients. Parents can better reinforce such eating habits in their children—as well improve their own health—by eating the same healthy foods.

Clinical and community studies have repeatedly shown that groups consuming many whole grains, vegetables, and fruits develop fewer cancers and heart diseases than groups eating more empty calories: refined grains, fatty meats and cheeses, and other saturated fats. Excess alcohol consumption appears to raise the risk of cancer at six different physical sites, an added reason to teach alcohol avoidance at these ages (Trichopoulos and Willett (eds.), 1996). **(Also see Chapters 9 and 13.)**

The period between ages 8 and 12 years has been recognized by schools as the most effective time to teach about the dangers of smoking cigarettes and chewing tobacco. Many, perhaps most, adult smokers begin this habit before age 15 years. Teaching the facts alone has proved ineffective in delaying or eliminating tobacco use. Facts must be supplemented by "inoculating" attitudes: presenting pro-tobacco arguments of peers and immediately countering these with arguments favoring abstinence. These counterarguments and refusal skills appear to be best taught by role-playing among classmates, guided by teachers or older peers who themselves are non-users. With regard to motivations, having a stained smile, bad breath, and immediate negative effects on sports performance provide much stronger avoidance motives than the risk of cancer or heart disease 40 years hence. Preventive teaching curricula are available in major languages. **(See also section "Tobacco Use" in Chapter 13.)**

Health professionals should take the initiative to work with local educators and parent groups to reach the public with the many small but important steps they can take to save children from trauma and disability. This unit on child health and safety might well be included in health and home economics courses in secondary schools and in parenting classes.

# 4. Adolescents and Young Adults 15–24 Years Old

## NURTURING THE SEEDS FOR A HEALTHY FUTURE

Planting the seeds for a healthy future was first discussed in the preceding chapter. Those early seeds include teaching children (by adult example) the high value of good health and how to build it through continuing health promotion and self-care. We included cleanliness to avoid infection, healthy eating, adequate exercise and sleep, keeping dangers out of household and play areas, avoiding careless and risky behaviors, and respecting and esteeming others as well as oneself.

Adolescence is the time to revisit these principles. Health concerns in this age group have changed, and young persons are beginning to take over the responsibilities formerly borne by their parents, including that of promoting their own health and self-care for minor health problems. This, then, is the time to consider the following:

- Have healthy principles taken root? If so, they need encouragement so they can flourish and meet the needs of the coming decades.

- On the other hand, if harmful behaviors and attitudes threaten to encroach, then pruning or clearing out may be called for at this time.

Youth have entered a new season in their lives, and the tasks of those advocating for health within the family and in schools, the workplace, and the community must change with them. The overall purpose is to establish inner controls and outer goals that maintain a lifestyle which prevents disability and postpones the chronic diseases that are so common and damaging in adults of middle and older age. It has become the fashion for youth's mentors to face this stage of life with apprehension, and for good reason.

*If birth is the "launching pad" of life, adolescence, with its accelerating power and rapid changes, represents the "booster-rocket stage" that will determine how high the future orbit will be. Adolescence holds the potential for great lives.*

The physical, psychological, and social transitions that youth go through revolutionize both their ways of living and their health problems. In agricultural areas and in areas where industrialization is first beginning, childhood ends when boys and girls become large enough physically to be put into full-time work. A shift in health problems occurs quickly, as the number of work injuries and exposures to illnesses increase markedly. Heavy demands are placed upon incompletely grown bodies; farm or factory machinery is placed in inexperienced hands and operated by workers whose prudence, judgment, and continuous self-control have not yet matured. The result is injuries on the job and while traveling on the roads by bicycle or motor vehicles to and from the worksite. In addition, psychologically immature youth may be abused by others.

To the extent that youth working long hours are drained of energy and physiologic renewal beyond what their available nutrition and sleep can restore, youth's growth, maturation, and sexual development may be impaired. This was endemic during the Industrial Revolution in the 19th century, and still may often be seen today, if looked for in communities where child labor rather than schooling is the norm.

According to data from UNICEF (1992) close to 20% of all the world's children aged 10–14 years are working full-time and not attending school regularly. These figures run higher in developing and economically troubled areas. Furthermore, most of youth 15–18 years old are not going to school or receiving training in most regions. Worldwide data reveal strong links between low education and poor health in adulthood. Therefore, this loss of schooling is breeding a new generation in which a high proportion of adults will experience health vulnerabilities both in themselves and in their families. Education is the "admission ticket" to the changing new world and to the best chance for good health. Nations cannot leave their next generations facing the world with only the last generation's skills.

*Education is the "admission ticket" to a changing world and to the best chance for good health.*

Epidemiologic studies show that youth (up to age 18) incur more physical damage to their bodies than do adults when exposed to the same levels of environmental toxins, especially silica, benzene, pesticides, and solvents. Youth also sustain more neurological damage from exposure to heavy metals than do adults. Some studies have found that workers under age 18 absorb more pesticides than do the adults working beside them in agricultural jobs. Why this is so has not been explained, but the message is that better training, better tools, and/or better protection are urgently needed (PAHO, 1994, p. 124).

Many urban children ages 10–14 years work, and sometimes live, on the streets. They eke out a living by selling small items, washing cars, watching cars, and running errands. In rural areas, more of these children work on farms. In both urban and rural areas many young children work in the construction trades— and construction and mining are the industries responsible for the highest rates of injury, disability, and mortality. The International Labor Organization is promoting many legislative and regulatory efforts, but many nations resist enacting and enforcing these protective steps, largely influenced by economic pressures.

All over the world, young people strive for independence from their families from puberty onward. They look to their peers for how to appear and behave, handle their sexual drive, try out their increasing physical and mental potency, and engage in risk-taking to impress others and challenge their own limits. Each of these developmental thrusts helps prepare youth for their roles as adults and also determines the forms of morbidity, disability, and mortality they experience. More and more, the exposure of children and youth to television, cinema, and now to the Internet, from distant parts of the world, teaches personal behaviors, values (or *anti* values), and lifestyles that may conflict with the local family culture, sometimes with destructive consequences. This chapter will review the major forms of mortality and morbidity for ages 15–24 years, as well as the psychosocial causes of the most common diagnoses and essential rational-emotional learnings, as a way to lay the foundation for good health both currently and later in life.

> *Nations cannot leave their next generations facing the world with only the last generation's skills.*

## MAJOR HEALTH PROBLEMS AT AGES 15–24

### MORTALITY

By age 15 mortality rates are starting their sharp rise that will continue for the remainder of the life cycle. From lifetime's age of lowest mortality—5 to 14 years—death rates rise by 50% to 100% for ages 15–24 years. Nevertheless, mortality remains below 100 deaths per 100,000 young women and between 100 to 200 per 100,000 young men in most parts of the world.

The leading cause of death both for males and females in these ages is trauma and injury. Motor vehicles are the leading cause for non-intentional deaths, especially in those countries where vehicles are widely used. For young men homicide and suicide are major killers. Homicide is a severe epidemic in the Region of the Americas. In a 1994 survey of 34 nations around the world (nine in the Americas) that reported such data in the *World Health Statistics Annual*, only eight nations had male homicide rates greater than 10 per 100,000 for ages of 15–24. The top seven of these were in the Americas, and their rates ranged from 17 to 75. In contrast, Spain's rate was only 1.5. Middle Eastern Crescent nations also have elevated homicide rates among males.

Rates of fatal biological disease creep up slightly from ages 15–24 years, with cancers and heart and blood vessel pathology being the two most common. However, a review of 16 nations in the Americas that report cause-specific mortality shows that for ages 15–24, the median percentage of all male deaths due to external causes is 72% (range 57% to 81%). For women ages 15–24, external causes account for a median of 34% of all deaths (range 22%–68%).

Suicide first appears as a major cause of death starting at age 15. In most countries, more males kill themselves than do females. The predisposing cause of most suicides is depression. Experiences of loss, defeat, frustration, humiliation, or hopelessness often trigger this destructive act. And, for each completed suicide there are many unsuccessful suicide attempts, with ratios varying widely by gender and nation. Hispanic countries have particularly low rates both for attempted and completed suicides. China has especially high suicide rates among young women, as well as very high rates for very old adults of both genders. **(Also see Chapter 11 for further discussion of suicide, homicide, and violence.)**

Since a suicide attempt is the strongest predictor of a future completed death, all attempts should be treated seriously. The young person who attempts suicide should receive counseling, and the circumstances of the attempt should be studied and the environment should be changed, if possible, to reduce risk of recurrence. A major determinant of whether a suicide attempt is fatal is the weapon used. Guns have the highest fatality ratio. In addition, having a gun in the home raises the risk of suicide for all family members. It also raises risk of homicide for all. In homes with guns—usually intended to protect the family—family members or friends have a 30 times greater chance of being shot by those guns than does an intruder or robber.

With disease mortality rates so low during age 15 to 24 years, the focus of health-promoting efforts shifts to reducing current morbidity and disability, as well as working to reduce the risks of the major chronic diseases, which strike people mostly after age 40 years.

## MORBIDITY AND DISABILITY

For every youth killed in vehicle accidents and for every homicide there are many young persons temporarily or permanently injured. Thus, because of their larger contribution to both morbidity and disability, external causes deserve intensive prevention and control efforts. Injured survivors cost the community more resources in terms of medical care, and those killed cost the community all they would have produced during the years of productive life they lost. In most WHO regions, death rates for the total of accidents and violence are two to seven times higher in males than in females. Chronic diseases are infrequent, but some, such as AIDS and other STIs, tuberculosis, asthma, and diabetes, can cause serious disability in young adults they affect.

Most of the other underlying causes of illness and disability in youth also are of social-behavioral origins—use of tobacco, misuse of alcohol and narcotics, sexually transmitted diseases, and unwanted pregnancies, many of which are aborted. Habits developed during youth set the direction toward either a longer healthier life or strong risks for chronic disease, disability, or earlier death from cardiovascular, respiratory, or cancerous diseases.

## Risk Behaviors

**Tobacco Use.** The greatest single life-long health gift families and communities can present to their youth is freedom from tobacco addiction. Tobacco is nature's vehicle to deliver nicotine, a sly drug that briefly calms the nervous, reactivates the tired, and has become a symbol (in some places) for social sophistication. Nicotine then leaves the body with a craving for more. The chemical craving for nicotine among heavy smokers creates a rapid relapse rate for those who quit smoking that is quite similar in its speed to the relapse rate of addicts who have just quit heroin.

Most tobacco by far is consumed through cigarette smoking. Pipe and cigar smoking are less common, and apparently less lethal. Tobacco also can be consumed as "snuff" or by chewing it, sometimes mixed with other substances and in other ways, depending on the local culture. Consuming smokeless tobacco gives rise to cancers of the oral cavity, head, neck, esophagus, pharynx, and larynx, and it raises the risk for stomach cancer. **(Also see section "Cancers of the Oral Cavity, Esophagus, Larynx, and Pharynx" in Chapter 9 and text on primary and secondary prevention in section "Tobacco Use" in Chapter 13.)**

Smoking turns tobacco's carcinogens into aerosol form. The smoke—which contains carbon monoxide, hydrocarbons, hot gases, and tiny ash particles—moves through the breathing apparatus and deposits itself in the lungs. From there, the soluble portions, including nicotine and its metabolites, and carbon monoxide, pass into the bloodstream, which then carries them to the entire body.

Scientists studying tobacco smoke have found in it 43 different carcinogens among an estimated 4,000 compounds. Most of these compounds have not been adequately tested for their possible cancer effects.

The distant bodily effects of tobacco smoke are demonstrated by increased rates of cancer of the bladder and uterine cervix, plus all the respiratory organs and some digestive organs. The recovery of a nicotine metabolite (cotinine) from vaginal secretions, the damage to peripheral arteries in hands and feet, and the numerous effects on the fetuses of pregnant women who smoke tobacco add to the evidence of the far reach of tobacco pathology.

The effects of environmental tobacco smoke (ETS), or exhaled smoke, have been proven repeatedly. Exhaled smoke in the home harms everyone living there. Similar dangers, ranging from respiratory infections to asthma, cancers, and heart attack, are present in smoky workplaces.

The litany of tobacco-related diseases is long, but this information seldom persuades teenagers, because the truly serious health maladies do not occur immediately, or even in five to ten years. The incubation, or latent period, is long, 20 to 40 years, and most teens live for today and next month rather than for the far future.

The best leverage for primary prevention of tobacco is to base the argument on signs that occur immediately: bad breath, stained teeth, stained fingers, diminished ability to taste pleasant foods, loss of endurance in sports and other activities, shortness of breath, and the feeling of being under the control of a relentless habit.

In many cultural groups young people have decided that smoking or chewing tobacco is "not smart," "not cool," not a habit that the more successful youth share. Building such a social norm, or reminding youth that such negative evaluations are around them, are ways to advance primary prevention.

Chapter 3 stated that the ideal time to start teaching anti-tobacco information and values is between ages 8–12 years. The teen years are when most smoking addicts begin their habits. The earlier the age of starting, the earlier the likelihood of debilitating disease. The United States Surgeon General has estimated that one-third of youth that start smoking tobacco in their early teens will eventually die of a tobacco-related disease.

*The greatest single life-long health gift families and communities can present to their youth is freedom from tobacco addiction.*

The cigarette smoking epidemic began in the industrialized nations. The prevalence of smokers increased rapidly between 1914 and 1918 and again between 1939 and 1946. These were the years of the two world wars, during which tobacco companies provided free cigarettes to military personnel from European nations and the United States. The growing surge of women's independence, coupled with clever and targeted advertising, recruited many women into the ranks of smokers. Meanwhile, the rates of pipe and cigar smoking and use of smokeless tobacco increased modestly. As cash income increased in developing nations, their younger people sought to mimic Western lifestyles and rapidly experimented with tobacco—and then got hooked. Without question, tobacco is an addictive drug.

A smoking pandemic has swept areas that are in the early stages of industrialization. At the turn of the twenty-first century, nearly 70% of Chinese men smoke, and the rates are similarly high elsewhere in Southeast Asia. Rates in Europe and Latin America range around 50% for men. In the United States, the United Kingdom, Switzerland, and other similar countries, smoking rates have decreased. In most places women have a lower prevalence of smoking, especially in traditional cultures. The rates for teenage girls are higher than for boys in some urban areas, especially where advertising glamorizes the habit. This warrants special programming.

The tobacco epidemic's decline is tracking the same course as the epidemic's emergence: smoking is declining in highly industrialized nations, with the greatest quitting rate among the more educated professional workers and the lowest quitting rates among less-educated laborers and women.

As new knowledge and attitudes about smoking damage spread through areas and nations, the prevalence of tobacco use declines. Using this information in tobacco prevention programs gives teachers added leverage in promoting healthy future-oriented lifestyles in youth. Information and knowledge, however, are not enough to change most behaviors. **(The additional required forces are presented in Chapter 12.)**

**Misuse of Alcohol.** This chemical abuse or dependency is a diagnosable disorder by itself, but far more often it serves as a gateway to other serious problems. Chapter 7 presents further information about the health consequences and the prevention and treatment of alcoholism. Studies searching the histories of narcotics addicts typically report that tobacco was the substance first used for its chemical effect, then beer, followed by drinks with higher concentrations of alcohol. Most youth stop at that point, but some go on to marijuana (cannabis) and fewer of these move to opiates, cocaine derivatives, or other designer drugs, depending on the addicts' local environment and available money.

Low self-esteem; fearfulness; feelings of sadness, boredom, and social conflict or rejection; and the desire to feel and even to be different than one is—especially in the presence of peer pressure—provide the fertile ground from which each year's crop of new substance abusers springs up. This is a one-sentence oversimplification of a complex set of problems that have been studiously researched and voluminously reported from many parts of the world.

Alcohol lowers self-control, dissolves good judgment, distorts perception, and impairs physical skills. Drinking alcohol, even at amounts below clinical intoxication, raises the risk of all of the following:

- *Unsafe sexual behavior.* This can lead to unwanted pregnancy, uncared for pregnancy, the risks of abortion, and sexually transmitted diseases, including HIV infection. None of these outcomes can be known—or ruled out—in the days or first weeks after the exposure. This may provoke fears, remorse, self-condemnation, or related psychological problems for months to come, even if the worse fears do not come true.

- *Motor vehicle and pedestrian injuries.* Even partial intoxication impairs perceptual and motor skills enough for fatal results. Autopsy and blood and breath analyses for alcohol show it to be involved in about 50% of fatal roadway crashes, as well as 50% of fatal small boat crashes in many countries.

- *Drownings.* Many drownings among persons over age 15 (mostly males) are due to alcohol-induced poor judgment or show-off behavior. Keep in mind that warm weather raises the frequency of drinking and swimming.

- *Occupational "accidents."* These occur mostly (by count) in the absence of psychoactive chemicals, but the chances of their occurring are very high among the few people who either have alcohol or drugs in their bodies or are hung over or trying to recover from a recent exposure to alcohol. Power-driven tools are most dangerous to chemically influenced persons both in factories and on farms.

- *Assaults and homicides.* Both occur at highest rates when the attacker or the victim, or both, are under the influence of alcohol. This is more prevalent where the assaults and homicides are not primarily due to gang wars, narcotics dealing, or paramilitary violence.

- *Suicides.* These account for a higher percentage of mortality between ages 15–24 than at any other time in the life cycle—and alcohol is involved in many of these deaths. Persons suffering from depression and having suicidal ideas often do not take the fatal step until after alcohol has made them feel even more mental anguish, washed out their psychological defenses and better judgment, and reduced their fear about performing the killing act.

- *Development of life-long chemical dependencies.* Use of alcohol as self-medication or escape from problems first creates a psychological dependency, usually followed by a chemical dependency. Most persons in all cultures can use alcohol occasionally and moderately in social settings, either to celebrate or relax. However, an important minority (estimated at about 10%) start from the periodic "social drink" and move to alcohol craving, frequent drinking, binge-drinking, the acute traumatic crises described above, anti-social behavior, trouble with the police, loss of job, separation from family, and loss of mental and physical health. The important issue is that many chronic adult abusers of alcohol and drugs began their habits while adolescents.

**Use of Illegal Drugs.** Narcotics and illegal drugs are used to change emotional states, fears, thoughts, urges, self-perceptions, and social interaction or to reduce pain. Unfortunately, not all of the changes that occur are pleasant or anesthetizing, even though that is what the user seeks and expects. Especially after repeated or high-dose usage, drugs start to lose their effect, what is known as habituation. Then emotions may become more painful, thinking more fragmented, and withdrawal symptoms severe. Urges and goals focus only on getting more drugs, and fears center on not getting drugs. Social relations become strained or break, as the user, now an addict, has love only for his chemical and love-hate for the persons that supply it.

Drugs used differ by culture and geography, but they infiltrate all socioeconomic levels. Some drugs are smoked, some are taken as pills, some are injected into veins, and some are inhaled (glue, acetone, solvents that vaporize). All recreational drugs are used because they change brain function; unfortunately, they can often leave permanent brain damage after the thrill is gone. Some drugs, such as cocaine, can create addiction after only one or two uses. Since addiction treatment often fails, prevention is clearly the path of choice.

Although marijuana (cannabis) is a milder drug, it can serve as a gateway for more damaging drugs. Public health and education professionals should be concerned about cocaine in its several forms; heroin; amphetamines and other uppers; inhalants such as glue fumes, acetone, and aerosols; drugs injected by needles; and steroids used without a doctor's prescription. Each of these damaging chemicals has many slang names; use those common in your area when inquiring about drug use in the street.

Most drug use leads to drug tolerance: in other words, the usual dose does not give the usual effect, and increasing amounts are needed at ever increasing costs. Among men, this primarily leads to such crimes as assault and theft to get more money; secondarily, men may turn to prostitution, usually servicing men. Women often turn to prostitution for money, although they also may turn to theft.

Because drug use confuses mental function, it also raises the risk of such trauma as from motor vehicles, falls, and burns. It can cause permanent damage to the brain, heart, and other systems; overdoses may cause death. Drug users financially support illegal drug suppliers, their crimes, and corruption. They damage families and communities. Health officials must realize that these chemicals travel a long distance, not only to damage individual bodies and minds, but also families, communities, public safety, and the body politic itself.

**Unsafe Sexual Behavior.** In adolescence, sexual interests and impulses first become prominent drivers of behavior, and sexual drives remain strong throughout young adulthood. To quote a biologist-poet, adolescence is "the efflorescence of gonadal dominance." At every age risky sexual activities can cause any one or more of over 20 sexually transmitted diseases (STIs), but the most vulnerable period for acquiring STIs is between ages 15 and 44 years. Some STIs can be treated successfully if discovered and treated early. Others can never be cured: they either leave permanent damage, as do herpes, papilloma, and hepatitis virus, or they lead to premature death, as does HIV.

Chlamydia causes almost nine times as much disability in women as in men, and the prevalences of gonorrhea and trichomoniasis also are somewhat higher among women. HIV, however, remains more common in men. Most of the disability from HIV and other STIs is sustained in the 25–44 year age range, but ages 15 to 24 years are when promiscuous habits are formed and most of the infections are first contracted.

Strength of sexual urges, their control, and their circumstances of expression are determined by a multiplicity of biological, psychological, and social forces, past learning, social values, and peer behaviors. All of these factors can be modified to help channel behavior towards safer and healthier ways. Development of socially desirable beliefs, attitudes, and behavioral standards is most successful when begun in childhood, well before puberty. This is not a call for early sex education in terms of anatomic and fertility information, which should be initiated when locally appropriate. Rather, it affirms that beliefs and attitudes toward sexuality, respect for self and others, and restriction of sexual behavior to a permanent monogamous relationship can begin well before the biological urges and social pressures complicate this learning process. The section on "Unsafe Sex" in Chapter 13 discusses the worldwide epidemic of sexually transmitted diseases and presents approaches to primary and secondary prevention and treatment for all age levels.

*Improving the fitness of a population by increased exercise is the second most powerful way to reduce future disease.*

**Lack of Regular Exercise.** Children naturally enjoy active play, whether it be running, jumping, lifting, carrying, pushing, and digging. It's enough to wear out adults watching them. This energy level usually continues through adolescence, then tapers off, as young adults become more mature and sedate. If, however, regular aerobic exercise—serious enough to raise the heart rate and require heavier breathing—can become a life-long habit, much weakness, tiredness, overweight, and vulnerability to illness can be prevented.

Regular aerobic exercise (at least 30 minutes, four or more times per week) burns fat, converts dangerous cholesterol to a safer form, helps control blood pressure, strengthens muscle and bone, and improves respiratory function and intestinal activity. It also helps remedy mild depression. Improving the fitness of a population by increased exercise is the second most powerful way to reduce future disease. Moderate exercise, such as walking, has almost the same beneficial effect as running or strenuous exercise. Walking also has less risk of strains or injuries to muscles and joints. Thirty to forty minutes of walking four or more times a week—if done at a speed to raise heart rate and increase the pace of breathing—will have great benefits, including reducing the future risk of adult-onset (Type II) diabetes.

Youth is the time to develop skills and interests in activities that can last a lifetime—hiking, bicycling, tennis, swimming, and weight training. Doing work that exercises muscles, lungs, heart, and maintains strength and flexibility adds to fitness. The sports of children and youth (e.g., games that involve running, such as soccer and basketball) are a great way to start. A favorite "active" activity should be maintained throughout the life span. Later, in adulthood, sports may be less competitive and less strenuous, but with age-grouped sports, there are "senior competitions" such as swimming meets and tennis tournaments for people in their seventies and eighties. Too many people become sedentary too soon. In the US in the 1980s and 1990s the one risk factor producing the most excess cases of coronary heart disease was lack of physical exercise. **(See the section on "Major Health Problems" in Chapter 6 and the section on "Physical Inactivity/Sedentary Lifestyle" in Chapter 13.)**

**Unhealthy Eating Habits.** Some areas experience seasonal or year-round food shortages. In these areas, the goal for adults in times of plenty is to consume enough calories to prevent major weight loss and enough protein to maintain organ and muscle functioning, even through seasonal shortages. In more areas of the post-industrial world, however, seasonal shortages are a thing of the past. It is "overnutrition" that has become the problem. In these areas, restriction of caloric intake is the goal, while maintaining adequate protein, mineral, vitamin, and fiber consumption. In many cultures, recreational foods—sometimes aptly dubbed junk food—have become popular with both young and middle-aged adults. They are full of calories but relatively empty of essential nutrients, such as amino acids, vitamins, minerals, and anti-oxidants. Candy, carbonated sodas, beer, fried chips, pastries, and cakes are examples of junk food. Health is promoted by restricting—or altogether avoiding—foods heavy in fat (especially saturated fat), sodium, or "empty calories." Regular consumption of whole grains, vegetables, salads, fruits, and protein sources low in saturated fats (lean meats, fish, poultry, milk products, and many kinds of beans) represents a health-giving dietary pattern appropriate from early childhood to old age, unless a medical problem leads a physician to recommend a temporary change.

**Psychologically-driven Eating Disorders.** Particularly in economically well-developed nations where food is plentiful, several psychologically-driven eating disorders have developed, especially among girls and young women. Women aged 15–34 years old have the highest prevalence of eating disorders, manifested either as abnormally high or abnormally low caloric intake. Anorexia nervosa, bulimia nervosa, binge-eating, and chronic excessive eating leading to obesity are the most commonly seen eating disorders.

*Weight-losing Disorders.* Women have a tenfold higher frequency of weight-losing disorders compared to men. In earlier generations, eating disorders were limited to a few post-industrialized countries, but with the spread of modern urban culture by movies and television, anorexia nervosa, in particular, may occur almost anywhere. Anorexia nervosa at onset is a mental health problem of several origins.

The primary risk factor both for anorexia and bulimia is "dieting," the intentional major restriction of caloric intake in order to lose or maintain weight (Hsu, 1996). The prevalence of dieting is about 50% in American women and 40% in Swedish women (Hsu, 1996); the prevalence of dieting is low in developing countries, but increases with Westernization.

Whatever the psychodynamics and tactics for "self starvation," most patients with anorexia compulsively pursue physical activity, thus burning up more calories. Their dieting approaches a food phobia. At some point in the weight loss process, metabolic changes progress, leading to amenorrhea and other more serious biological changes. These can even result in death, if the patient is not hospitalized to receive metabolic as well as psychiatric care.

A related disorder is bulimia nervosa, characterized by binges of overeating, often followed by self-induced vomiting (purging). This behavior also has a complex psychogenic origin, and is now suspected to have some neurobiological roots. Bulimia has profound biopsychosocial effects on patients, overlapping with those of anorexia. Affective disorders, such as anxiety and depression, are common co-morbidities both for bulimia and anorexia. Both these weight-losing disorders cause malnourishment symptoms similar to those found in groups suffering from famine. L.K.G. Hsu's review (1996) estimates the prevalence of eating disorder cases in local populations sampled from the United States, the British Commonwealth, and Scandinavia to range from 0.1% to 0.8% for anorexia, and from about 1% to 3% for classic bulimia, ranging up to 7% for full and partial bulimia combined (this last figure from Virginia, USA).

The frequency of dieting nearly doubles between ages 14 and 18 years in Westernized girls. Although dieting and weight loss are benign for more than 95% of girls and young women, communities or health clinics seeing enough cases of full or partial anorexia or bulimia can screen for these problems inexpensively by identifying persons who are following severe caloric restriction. Only about half of those on diets are overweight by weight-height tables, and those who are markedly underweight for their height are at highest risk for an eating disorder. Female gymnasts or dancers also tend to be at higher risk. Girls on diets see themselves as "too fat," whereas boys on diets are usually trying to increase muscle mass.

One can help prevent eating disorders by targeting group-based educational programs to young women, to try and get them to adopt more healthful and natural "ideal body images," adopt nutritionally sound eating patterns, and learn the present and future nutritional dangers inherent in most of the constant and rapid fire parade of "crash diet" fads streaking through the culture.

*Weight-Gaining Disorders—Obesity.* Chronic overeating rests somewhere between an eating disorder and a noxious lifestyle; when coupled with a lack of adequate physical activity, the result is obesity. The prevalence of obesity continues to rise mostly in industrialized nations, and transitional nations are now starting this pattern. (In much of the developing world, undernutrition and starvation remain the overriding problems). In industrialized areas, obesity is increasing more rapidly among families with low education, less income, and among people of color. This appears to be tied to the fact that starchy and fatty foods are cheaper than vegetables, fruits, and protein-rich foods; long-standing cultural food preferences; and—in a potentially healthy twist—devaluing the "ultra-slim" body image favored by rich, urbane Caucasians.

Overeating may sometimes be encouraged by parents who have experienced food shortages. They continually urge their children to eat more at meals and to eat snacks, perhaps driven by a fear that food shortages may occur again, or perhaps in the belief that fat children are healthier. Often when families immigrate from areas of food shortages to areas where food is plentiful, there are substantial weight gains for everyone in the family. These gains are healthful until the normal range of weight (for height and age) is reached. Beyond that, adding more weight does not increase health nor enhance the appearance of success.

Williamson (1995) estimates that about 34% of adults in the United States are overweight. Prevalence is slightly higher in women than in men and increases with age. Prevalence of overweight also is high in Western Europe. Overweight, as measured by Body Mass Index (BMI=weight in kg divided by height in $m^2$), is not as specific a health threat as obesity. Some persons with higher BMIs, usually men, carry much of their weight in muscle mass—witness physical laborers and athletes. Obesity can be inferred from weight and height, but the determination is more validly based on estimation of percentage of weight that is fat. This can be most simply calculated from measures of skin fold thickness (surface fat).

> *Adolescence may be the best time to mount primary and secondary prevention programs against obesity, because this is the age at which individuals become more independent in their food choices and also when many cases of chronic overeating begin.*

Childhood obesity has been increasing in the United States at least since 1960. Population surveys taking skin fold measures estimate that about 20% of the country's children are obese. The health implications are worrisome: for example, obesity appears to be the leading cause of childhood hypertension (Dietz, 1995), and obesity is associated with unhealthy serum lipid profiles both in children and adults. Although survey data is quite scanty, obesity appears to be less common in developing countries. The greater amount of physical exertion and reduced access to high calorie, low nutrient "junk food" in developing countries may help account for this.

The most common medical complications caused by obesity in adults are hypertension, adult-onset diabetes mellitus, dyslipidemia, ischemic heart disease, gallstones, cholecystitis, respiratory impairment, arthritis, gout, and perhaps some cancers. Fat distribution affects the complications of obesity, with heavy fat deposits in the central abdominal area being most harmful physiologically. It also promotes a negative self-image and psychological discomfort in many younger adults.

Adolescence may be the best time to mount primary and secondary prevention programs against obesity, because this is the age at which individuals become more independent in their food choices and also when many cases of chronic overeating begin. Further, many youth "develop a taste" in childhood for foods that are rich in fats, sugars, and calories. Their new independence should be accompanied by social experiences in sharing more healthful food choices.

**Psychologic/Psychiatric Concerns.** While the foundations for psychological and behavioral health are established in childhood, enduring psychological disorders are usually not recognized clinically until adolescence. Mental deficiency and some rarer disorders, such as autism, are usually discovered in early childhood, but the more common emotional and behavior problems of childhood are generally "outgrown" far before the teen years.

Most schizophrenic syndromes first manifest themselves between the ages of 15 and 34 years. Their incidence varies widely across nations and social classes, with the most disadvantaged generating the most cases. Severe psychoses remain relatively infrequent in most places, with prevalence under 2%.

The most common emotional-behavioral problems in youth, as well as in adults, are depression and anxiety. Eating disorders, which particularly beset young women in some populations, are usually accompanied by conflicts involving anxiety and depression. Anxiety, specific fears, depression, and feelings

92

of low self-worth all make interpersonal relationships uncomfortable. This often impairs the social skills required for successful adjustment to work, school, and family. Anxiety, depression, and hostility, when long-lasting, also interact with neurophysiologic, endocrine, and immune system functioning in ways that may cause or worsen "physical" illnesses, such as gastrointestinal, cardiovascular, endocrine, and dermatologic disorders.

Young people are more likely to act out their frustrations and unhappiness than to repress or discuss them. This "acting out" often leads older adults to complain about the younger generation—a dynamic that has been occurring at least since early Egyptian times.

Many risk factors have their source in impulsive behaviors. Unfiltered by knowledge or experience and unmediated by "common sense," these rash actions are sparked by feelings, attitudes, impulses, or peer pressure, without forethought about potential harm. Examples of these impulsive and risky behaviors include taking chances in roadways as a walker, cyclist, or driver; taking one too many alcoholic drinks; experimenting with drugs; being chronically angry; provoking fights; spending leisure time among persons who carry weapons; engaging in rash sexual behavior; neglecting to fasten seat belts in an automobile; failing to use safety and protective work gear; "playing with fire" in any of its forms. All these risks involve misjudging oneself to be more invulnerable and the laws of nature more forgiving than is the case in either. **(Public health approaches aimed at generating mental and social resources for impulse control and positive mental health are discussed in the sections "Conduct Disorders/Delinquency" and "Positive Behavioral and Mental Health" in the section "Malnutrition" in Chapter 13.)**

## PSYCHOSOCIAL FOUNDATIONS OF MOST HEALTH PROBLEMS AT THESE AGES

Changes in "the whole person" that is trying to emerge out of each youth during adolescence include exposure to a different road map for life from the one learned at home during childhood. Helpers in this "map making" venture include other youth, teachers, the mass media, media-made "heroes," and other groups at school, at work, in religious groups, and on the streets. In an effort to shed the restraining values and habits imparted by their families, youth may turn to any of these sources of influence—for better or for worse. Other strivings also mold youth—to be accepted, liked, popular; to prove one's independence, maturity, and talents.

For young males, the surge of endocrines and the pressure from male peer group competitiveness derail rationality and give rise to "machismo"—a brash display of dominance, toughness, competitiveness, reckless showing off, and possessive sexuality. Machismo finds expression in every culture, and every culture has a name for it. It leads to aggressiveness and intentional violence, which is an increasing threat worldwide and locally. Intentional violence causes more than 1.4 million years of life with disability (YLD) worldwide each year, and men sustain more than five times as much of this damage as do women (Murray and Lopez, 1996, p. 540). **(See further discussion in Chapter 11.)**

Young females rebel, too, and fall prey to the urge to be their "own persons," usually accompanied by a yearning to be accepted, popular, and to receive recognition—or seize it, if necessary—but now from sources outside the family. This usually involves exchanging the family's standards and goals for those of the peer group and the media's heroines. Often young women also take increased risks, often sexually, and may become "oppositional" to authority.

Young men and women also share these other complicating traits:

- **A sense of invulnerability**. Young people feel they can "beat the odds" and not be hurt by being reckless on the road or taking risks with alcohol, drugs, boasting, fighting, and careless sex. Some may also assume they can learn without studying or achieve without adequate commitment.

- **Living only in the present.** Youth focus on immediate possibilities and gratifications, paying far less attention to the years ahead. It is important to note that young adults with more education have a greater future perspective than less educated ones, who live more in the now.

- **Impulsiveness in making choices.** Adolescents and young adults tend to make quick decisions and act upon them promptly. Both their sense of invulnerability and their living in the present contribute to this, as well as the tendency of many to think primarily about themselves. In addition, many of youth's choices that affect their health are not made with health in mind. In fact, the reasons may be far different—to display independence, to express rebellion, to win attention, to impress peers, to get a thrill, to test their limits. This is important to understand, because it means that giving more health information will not change behavior until health motives become a part of the decision-making equation.

> *Having a fully developed time perspective enables persons to better plan for the development of their family, career, middle age, and older years. It also equips them to respond to public health programs that have future payoffs for individuals, families, and communities.*

All these are limitations in young people's approach to living that youth themselves—and those who care about their healthy development—must seek to overcome. But the behavioral vulnerabilities and health crises in millions of young people cannot be solved by every adult becoming a good role model or teacher to an adolescent at a time—or even to whole class-

BUILDING BETTER HEALTH

rooms at a time. Actually, young people not attending school experience far higher rates of health and social problems. To succeed, prevention must have a wider reach. It must also work through the social and cultural environments. In almost every populated place in the world, persons ages 15–24 years are sufficiently protected from the physical environment and have developed resistance to harmful aspects of the biological environment. Cause-specific morbidity and mortality data support this conclusion.

The environmental levels most responsible for the maladies of this age group are the *interpersonal,* the *social/economic,* and the *cultural/ideological.* Youth culture, fueled now as never before by the mass media, contains new ideas; new kinds of "heroes"; and novel ways of dressing, talking, and rebelling, around which subgroups can rally and identify themselves with. Much of the "cargo list" in the cultural environment is beneficial, much is harmless passing fad, and the remainder—to borrow infectious disease terminology—acts as an agent-infecting behavior, so as to raise risks to the health problems of this age group.

To continue the infectious disease analogy, these ideologically toxic agents of unhealthy behavior are transmitted in the *interpersonal environment* by person-to-person contact. For example, youth learn to use illegal drugs mostly by personal contact with other users. The mass media may serve as a vector to disperse the agents far and wide. Often, however, the media simply lower host resistance to the behaviors until an "infected" carrier makes personal contact. Finally, the *social/economic* level of the environment may unwittingly reinforce and institutionalize destructive values and damaging behavior. For example, schools may allow some children to bully or attack others. In factories, managers may make sexual advances on subordinates, unless the organization or the community enforces policies with punishments to forbid this. Or, a community police force may enforce alcohol, illegal drug, or reckless driving laws only some of the time, or only against poorer youth. Further, consumerism and materialism lure people of all ages into believing that well-being and happiness are just one more purchase away. People who go that route to boost their low self-esteem may well bankrupt their families' economic future, or even steal to get the money, to buy unrealistic and momentary "satisfaction."

Even as the environment's *psychosocial* and *cultural/ideological* strata can spread and encourage problem behaviors, so must the work be done within, to change these environments and promote good health for the total person, family, and community. The following section deals with that work.

## CONVEYING LEARNING AND VALUES TO OVERCOME HEALTH VULNERABILITIES

How, then, can rational, emotional, valuing, and conduct skills, which are so necessary to healthy adults, be absorbed by youth? This has been a key question that has preoccupied parents in early tribes and prehistoric civilizations, as well as parents of today and parents of tomorrow. Perhaps ancient cultures came closer than we have to the answer; at least they were more sure of the answers they taught. Today, in our pluralistic, multicultural world there are so many sets of values, ways of doing things, and standards of behavior that no matter which is chosen, the parental generation is less certain which one is correct, and the younger generation is less sure the other is wrong. Furthermore, cultures and their ways of living and thinking now change much faster than ever before.

The epidemiological triangle explored in the section "Strategies for Identifying Causes" in Chapter 2 gives clues about approaches that might be used to encourage young people to build healthier, less troubled, more productive lives for themselves. Young people, then, would be regarded as the "host"; the environment, as before, would be multi-layered; and the "agents" could be of two types, either damaging or protective forces.

### HOW TO DEVELOP SYSTEMATIC HEALTH PROGRAMS FOR YOUTH

**Protective agents and behaviors.** Their advantages and rewards should be emphasized, as should the idea that these *healthy behaviors* are coming into style, that everyone will soon be thinking and acting in these ways. These are the *adult* things to do.

**Damaging agents and behaviors.** Emphasize that although they may be momentarily exciting, in the long term they are, in a word, dumb. The best way for a young person to show independence and personal power is by not going along with dumb, self-defeating actions. The program should teach and publicize true information about the harmful outcomes of damaging agents. It is essential to not exaggerate, or the critical public—the youth—will dismiss your whole message as biased.

**The "hosts."** The target audiences for attitude and behavior change are, in fact, many different subgroups. Prepare separate messages for each subgroup, considering varying psychosocial characteristics such as culture; education; place of residence; and attitude differences such as group-oriented, solitary, rebellious, apathetic, or cooperative tendencies.

**The environment.** Send energizing, constructive messages through institutions and groups in the social environment that reach to and are accepted by the target groups. (Look at the list of twelve channels of communication in Chapter 12. Consider which ones can become "vectors" or transmitters of positive messages.)

At the family and neighborhood level use the media to show and disseminate health-promoting, non-violent—*nontoxic*—resources and activities. Promote those social events, spare-time recreation, and small informal groups of friends that share a family's positive ways of thinking and behaving. Parent groups also can work together toward such goals. Youth groups with a civic-betterment or religious orientation usually provide an uplifting, health-enhancing environment. Parents must keep in touch with what their children are doing, and with whom, whether the children are at home or away, where oversight may be lax. (Also see Chapter 12.)

At a more individual level, schoolteachers, group leaders, and parents not only should talk about healthful living, but their lives should demonstrate it. They can be role models, encourage youth to join in, and praise and reward successful behavior patterns. Notice that teaching by telling people what to do, or what not to do, without living it oneself, often fails. It may even spark rebellious urges to behave in the opposite way.

> *Cultural and subcultural differences are critical in leading people toward healthy, productive, and loving personal lives.*

Many excellent books have been published recently on adolescent development, health marketing, and self-directed behavior change. Interested persons are urged to consult these sources during program planning.

## PROTECTIVE FACTOR: PROMOTE THE UNIVERSAL VACCINE

Is education the universal vaccine? The amount of schooling youth receive has a powerful effect on their present and future health and life expectancy. We can only guess at how and why this happens, but there is no guessing about the worldwide power of this effect on nearly all kinds of health outcomes. Without a doubt, increased lifetime income and increased social participation in mainstream community activities play a part. Therefore, encourage young people to continue their full-time school for as long as is customary for the middle-class in their community. For economic reasons, this may entail fewer years in developing countries or poor areas than in economically better off areas. There is something about formal schooling, even in job-skill curricula, that improves health throughout the life cycle.

Compared to adults who had had more years of schooling, adults in the United States who had completed 12 or fewer years of schooling:[1]

- had higher total age-adjusted death rates;

- had twice the age-adjusted chronic disease death rate;

- had two to three times the death rates due to injuries;

- had higher death rates due to infectious diseases;

- were twice as likely to die of HIV-AIDS;

- had 1.8 to 3.7 times the rate of suicide;

- were more likely to report "heavy alcohol use";

- were more likely to smoke cigarettes;

- were more likely to be overweight by a ratio of about 2 to 1, although these ratios are changing in light of the current unhealthy weight-gain epidemic in the country;

- were more likely to have sedentary lifestyles; and

- experienced more avoidable hospitalizations.

In a Middle East nation, babies of women with some primary education sustain more than double the infant mortality rates as women who completed secondary school or more. This mortality gradient by mother's education remains equally strong for children through age 5 years. Many nations in the Americas show equivalent trends.

---

[1] Data derived from United States Public Health Service reports on social inequalities in adult health. Similar data have been reported for many of these indicators from the United Kingdom.

Why does added schooling confer such strong and widely different health benefits? It does not appear to be the result of the few hours of health education included in some curricula for teenagers. The adage, "Every year of learning adds to later years more earning" can, in part, be traced to the following:

- More experience in thinking through problems completely;

- Exposure to a wider range of possible solutions to problems and more helpful resources—in other words, more choices;

- The ability to include a future dimension when considering outcomes of today's actions;

- Development of a sense of responsibility and "self-efficacy"—a sense that "I can change things, or save things in my life, that I am not a passive pawn of fate";

- Supervised practice in interpersonal skills such as cooperative work, anger control, negotiating skills, winning and losing;

- All day interaction with a peer group in an adult-led environment where there is reasonably adequate (or better than that) control of the transmission of values, content, objectives, and reinforcement of these.

Higher incomes also are associated with better health, but the income effect on health seems to follow the education effect. Education occurs first. Of course, education and economic levels are two sides of the same coin. Economically advantaged families see that their children get more formal education. And, young people with more education obtain the kind of work that pays more money. Another partial explanation is that more education raises self-esteem, a sense of personal worth, the feeling that one can overcome fate or chance, that one has the knowledge about how to stay healthy and the skills and judgment to avoid injuries and violence, as well as the cognitive tools to keep learning more. Longer schooling also increases the strength of friendships and the range of one's social network—contacts that can be helpful during adult life. Emphasizing the schooling of girls and young women brings these fruits of education not only to them, but also to the infants and children they will bear and care for.

> The health sector and the education sector need to work together more of the time and with more enthusiasm. What is exciting is that better health makes better learning possible, and more education brings with it better health. Both together spell economic development for the community!

*(Text continues on page 105)*

## SCREENING CHECKLIST FOR AGES 15 TO 24 YEARS: BY INTERVIEW AND OBSERVATION

Most of the items in this checklist apply to many subpopulations. In certain cultural settings some problems may not be relevant, or it may not be economically possible to correct them.

### Dietary Practice

Are meals eaten regularly according to local custom and are meals shared with other people (for biological as well as psychological and social benefits.)

### Daily Food Intake

Does daily food intake include adequate amounts of whole grains, fruits, vegetables, and protein sources?

### Daily Unhealthful Food Intake

Does daily intake restrict the amount of saturated fats, salt, refined sugars, and "junk food" (i.e., recreational foods lacking in essential nutrients)?

### "Dieting" Behavior

Does the person or group engage in exaggerated dieting so as to cause unhealthy weight loss or malnourishment? Are there any signs of eating disorders? Does the person ever fast for more than 24 hours? Does the person vomit to help lose weight?

### Caloric Intake and Exercise

Is there an imbalance between caloric intake and exercise utilization of calories such that obesity is developing? Obesity in children and young people is now an epidemic in industrialized nations.

### Exercise

Does the person or group engage in sufficient daily physical exertion at work, school, or elsewhere so as to increase aerobic fitness for cardiovascular, respiratory, and musculoskeletal systems? Adequate aerobic exercise involves sufficient activity to make one breathe harder and increase heart rate for 25–35 minutes, repeated regularly 3 or 4 times per week. Is this maintained even during seasons of inclement weather?

### Tobacco Use

Family and peer group usage is the strongest predictor for individual use. Is the person exposed to groups where smoking or use of smokeless tobacco is the norm? If so, can the family habits be changed, or can the person spend more time with nonsmoking peers? Does the individual use tobacco? What forms? How frequently? How much per day? Ask both for smoking and smokeless tobaccos (a major cause of oral cancer).

### Alcohol Use

Ask about alcohol use, including binge drinking, in the peer group. In some groups, weekends are the time to drink until passing out or losing control. Involvement with such groups is one major individual risk factor. Persons are more likely to answer accurately about their groups than about themselves. For the latter use a tested set of questions like the CAGE questionnaire listed below (Ewing, 1984, plus recent reviews).

- Have you ever felt the need to Cut down on your alcohol drinking?
- Have you ever felt Annoyed by criticism of your drinking?
- Do you ever feel Guilty about drinking?
- Did you ever take a drink first thing in the morning—an "Eye opener"?

These questions are usually asked orally, later in an interview. Straight "Yes" answers are less frequent than "partial positives," such as "partly, occasionally, a little." The format "have you ever" will also elicit positive responses from past drinkers and recovering alcoholics who no longer have the problem.

Additional useful screening questions include: About how many days in the past 30 days did you have an alcoholic drink? How often do you have five or more drinks within a few hours? **(See also the pertinent item in the "Screening Checklist" in Chapter 5.)**

### Use of Other Mood-altering Substances
This, too, is a sensitive matter. Usually, good rapport or a sense of trust with the subject is necessary to obtain a "straight answer." One approach is to ask: Do any of the people you spend time with ever take pills, or drinks, or smoke or inject things to make them feel better, more excited, more calmed, or just to get away from boredom? Positive responses or requests for clarification or examples can be pursued. Sharing hypodermic needles is a mark of advanced drug abuse as well as risk of HIV. Then the questions can be shifted to the respondent. For example, "And which of these do you do too?" "How often?" Again, peer group usage is the main risk factor, and perhaps even a subclinical indicator, of personal use or of high chances of starting use.

### Sexual History
An individual may engage in sexual relations with persons of either sex or with both sexes. Taboos on sex and its discussion lead young people especially to use local slang for particular anatomy and actions. Be sure the interviewer fully knows and understands the local glossary. It may differ by age groups. "Having sex" means different things to different folks. Again, rapport and trust are critical to obtaining better information. A nonjudgmental approach using open-ended questions, such as at first asking "what else?" may work best initially. This can then be followed by specific, direct questions to "pick up loose ends." Always, consider both denials and acknowledgements only as approximations to the truth. Find out whether the person has ever had a "sexual experience." What did that involve? What activities did the person engage in during the last six months? About how many partners has the person had so far?—many partners could be a strong clue to risk of sexually transmitted infections (STIs). Was STI protection used? All the time? **(Also see section "Unsafe Sex" in Chapter 13.)**

### Pregnancy Prevention
Unwanted pregnancies are all too common in youth, especially as cultural and family restrictions on sexual behavior become looser or are ignored. This process has been speeded by young persons migrating away from their families for jobs. Unwanted pregnancies occur throughout the fertile years, including among married couples who already have as many children as they desire or can support economically. Family planning (control over pregnancy) is valuable for all these people, including its use to space pregnancies at least two years apart for the health of all concerned.

Extended breastfeeding delays the return of fertility and menstrual periods, but it is not a reliable way to prevent pregnancy. Contraceptives prevent the start of a pregnancy with greater certainty, but only avoiding sexual intercourse entirely is 100% effective.

Oral contraceptives (either containing progestin alone or combined with estrogen) can be injected, implanted under the skin, or taken orally (one every day). The injected and subdermal implants are about 99% effective. The effectiveness of the oral pill also reaches 99% when used correctly and consistently. The failure rate rises when usage is less than optimal. Each of the hormonal contraceptive methods brings a small risk of side-effects which need to be monitored, with consideration for changing the prescription (United States Preventive Services Task Force, 1996).

*(Box continues on next page)*

Condoms have a failure rate of 3% when used correctly every time, but in fact, they have about a 15% failure rate among average users. Other barrier protection methods, such as diaphragms, have a failure rate of 6% under the best circumstances, but about 20% in average population circumstances. Cervical caps have similar protective effectiveness. Keep in mind that many contraceptive methods provide no protection against sexually transmitted diseases, and that some barrier methods which prevent infection have too high a failure rate for dependable pregnancy prevention.

The United States Preventive Services Task Force's *Guide to Clinical Preventive Services* (1996) recommends periodic counseling both about contraceptive methods and prevention of sexually transmitted infections for all sexually active women and men. Nations with family planning priorities have programs and materials in place to move toward such goals. Matters of contraception are influenced by culture, belief, family circumstances, and personal factors. Consequently, they need to be worked out individually between a woman or a couple and the clinician.

### Sexual Risk Behaviors
Seven major risk factors for sexual infections are:

- Activities allowing exchange of genital or anal fluids or contact with blood without barrier protection (e.g., a condom). Fluids such as tears and perspiration are safe.
- Activities exposing skin or oral, anal, or genital mucosa (especially if abraded or broken) to body fluids, sores, rashes, warts, or possible parasites.
- Anal penetration is very dangerous both to the passive and the active partner. The rectal area is an incubator for many pathogens.
- Having multiple partners over time multiplies risk of infection.
- Having partners who themselves have multiple partners (including sex workers).
- Having unprotected sex with a stranger (or even a friend!) exposes one to the diseases that person's partners have.
- Using alcohol or drugs to the extent of impaired judgment in settings where the person might become vulnerable to the sexual risks above.

Persons engaging in unsafe sexual practices or those with a history of sexually transmitted diseases may benefit from testing for gonorrhea, syphilis, chlamydia, and HIV, as well as behavioral modification to reduce future risks. **(See also the section on "Unsafe Sex" in Chapter 13.)**

### Risks of Motor Vehicle Trauma or Injury
The following questions will help determine the level of risk of motor vehicle trauma or injury. **(For a more comprehensive review, see Chapter 11.)**

- Does the person ever ride with drivers who have just drunk alcohol? Does the person ever drive after consuming alcohol?
- Has the person or any friends recently been charged with traffic violations (a predictor of a future injurious crash)?
- Has the person or a friend had a vehicle "accident" (depending on circumstances it might predict future mishaps)?
- Does the person ride motorcycles or motor scooters without a helmet? Falls are inevitable, and risks of permanent disability, especially neurological, are great.
- Does the person ride in autos or trucks without using seat belts?

### Risks of Occupational Injury

Ask the following questions:

- Does the person work with machinery similar to that on which other workers have been injured from time to time? Can the problem be reduced by protective changes in machinery? Can protective gear or garments be distributed to workers? Can workers be retrained or trained differently? (The work group's recent experience is a good predictor for future individual risk.)
- Is the worker exposed to dust, chemicals, or biological agents that can accumulate acutely or chronically to impair health?
- Does the worker do heavy lifting or engage in labor that involves twisting or maintaining a poor posture for hours? These are all common causes of musculoskeletal injury and disability, which may be largely prevented by worker training or re-engineering of work tasks.

### Risks of Home and Leisure Trauma

Find out about the following issues.

- Ask about hobby and recreation activities. Home workshops or farm plots may involve the risky use of power machinery, paint, solvents, or pesticides. Check for safety habits, including eye, hand, and inhalation protection.
- Does the person like to "take risks" in daily activities or competitions? Does the person race motorcycles or cars? Try to get as specific an answer as possible.

### Risks of Injury from Violence

Get answers for the following questions.

- Does the person (especially if male) spend time with groups or in places where arguments, fights, or violence occur? Where street drugs are sold or used?
- Does the person belong to a gang or a group to help protect himself/herself from other people or gangs?
- Does the person or friends carry knives, clubs, guns, or other weapons to protect themselves?
- How often in the past year has the person been involved in a physical fight?
- How often has the person been threatened or attacked while at school or at work, or while traveling to or from such places?
- Has the person been hit or hurt by a boyfriend or girlfriend? (Young women are at particularly high risk from men they date, as well as from family members.)
- Has the person been forced into any kind of sexual behavior against his or her will, including sexual assault, rape, and related trauma? Was this an isolated incident or a repeated occurrence? **(See also the section on "Special Issues for Women" in Chapter 5 and see Chapter 11).**

### Social Supports

Find out if the person lives in a stable household. Are household members, or other family or friends, able and willing to help the person if injury, illness, loss of job, or other life crisis occurs? Are both practical assistance and emotional acceptance readily available?

### Sleep Habits

Does the person usually get an adequate amount of quality sleep? Young adults typically short-change themselves on sleep, and this can lead to reduced immune function, mental judgment, and motor coordination, as well as long-term effects on the cardiovascular system.

*(Box continues on next page)*

## Immunizations

Is the individual and group up to date on immunizations? Young women must be immunized against rubella before entering childbearing years. Both genders should receive booster shots for diphtheria and tetanus every ten years.

## Signs of Physical Abuse

Young women are at particular risk of physical or sexual abuse. Ask about it sensitively but directly. Look for signs of new or old injury to the face, hands, and arms. If a physical examination is done, look for bruises, cuts, or burns on the back, buttocks, breast, abdomen, and genitalia. (For specific guidance on how to do this, see Aciero, Resnick, and Kilpatrick, 1997.)

## Sunburn

Urge fair-skinned persons to avoid skin exposure to mid-day sun and to use creams that block ultraviolet light. Three instances of severe sunburn, especially if blistering results, constitute a risk factor for malignant melanoma—a usually fatal skin cancer. For persons with much exposure to sunlight, look for malignant skin lesions. **(See also pertinent section in Chapter 9.)**

## Mood Disorders

Adolescents and young adults are at higher risk for depression, suicide, and anxiety disorders. Groups can be screened by standardized questionnaires. With individuals, such problems can also be estimated by direct observation and interview. These mood reactions may either be generated by fluctuations in brain chemistry or by life crises, particularly the loss of a loved one, defeats, or perceived damage to one's self-worth. **(See also Chapters 7 and 11.)**

Reassure the interviewee that many people have "ups" and "downs" (using local idioms for pleasures and troubles), then proceed with questions such as "How has it been for you?" "Have you had big changes to deal with?" "Have you felt sad at times? Discouraged? Upset? Angry?" "How often?" "How strongly?" "How recently?" "Have you ever (or recently) felt so sad or troubled that you stopped doing some of the things you ordinarily like to do?" "How long did this last?" "As you look ahead a year or so from now, do you think things will be better? Worse? The same?" ("Worse" may be a clue to hopelessness.)

There are also standard brief questionnaires that can be used as screening instruments to assess general mental health, anxiety, or depression in groups. A "general well-being scale" also can be used, and then followed up with interviews with low scorers.[2] None of these scales is diagnostic of any condition and they can be answered falsely. They are useful as a quick screen, however.

## Family Issues

Find out if the person is responsible for the health or well-being of children or other dependents. If so, review with them the screening checklists for those age groups that are included in this handbook's pertinent chapters.

---

[2] See Ware, Johnston, and Davies-Avery, 1979, and in Bradburn, 1969, for several examples of scales, one of which is still widely used.

Is education the "universal vaccine" for the 21st century? Not totally, of course, but its widespread health advances have been sufficiently documented around the world. Indeed, we can achieve sizeable health benefits in the intermediate to long-term by believing—at least part of the time—that education is the universal vaccine.

## A SCREENING QUESTIONNAIRE

The "Youth Risk Behavior Survey," which is available from the U.S. Centers for Disease Control and Prevention,[3] is a well established system for asking about behaviors that greatly influence health in adolescents and young people. The self-administered survey form includes questions targeted mainly to middle-class children and youth in the United States, most of whom attend school and are familiar with such questionnaires. The questions will need to be adapted for use in other cultures or languages.

The section below summarizes the survey according to major topics of inquiry. A few widely applicable types of questions will be listed under each topic where appropriate.

In clinical situations, an interview with a health professional or a trusted neutral person who develops rapport with a youth will generate more reliable data than a self-administered questionnaire. Another approach is to lead a small group of ten or fewer persons in answering the questions, perhaps reading some of the more difficult items. When questionnaires such as this—which ask for personal and sensitive information—are administered to large groups, young people often react by inciting one another to give false or frivolous answers.

### INQUIRY TOPICS FROM THE "YOUTH RISK BEHAVIOR SURVEY"

1. **Individual Personal Information.** This includes age, gender, year in school, height, weight information.

2. **Vehicle Safety.** Use of helmets on motorbikes and bicycles, seat belts in autos and trucks. Use of alcohol by drivers. **(See the section on risks of motor vehicle trauma or injury in Chapters 4 and 5; the section on alcohol abuse and dependence in Chapter 7; and the section on motor vehicle injuries in Chapter 11.)**

3. **Risk of Violence.** Missing school or work from fear of assault. Carrying weapons such as knives, clubs, or guns. How often does the person feel

---

[3] http://www.cdc.gov/needphp/dash/survey99.html

threatened? How often is the person involved in a physical fight? Has the person been slapped, hit, or attacked by a boyfriend or girlfriend? Has the person been forced into sexual activity against his or her will? **(See relevant items in the "Screening Checklist" in Chapter 4; the sections on "Special Issues for Women" and "Special Issues for Men" in Chapter 5; and the section on "Suicide and Violence" in Chapter 11.)**

4. **Depression and Suicide.** During the past year, has the person felt sad or hopeless for two weeks or more? Has the person recently felt that life is not worth living? If the answer is "yes," then ask, Has the person considered suicide or planned to kill him- or herself? **(See the section on "Major Health Problems" and relevant items in the "Screening Checklist" in Chapter 4; the sections on "Recognizing and Dealing with Depression" and "Suicide and Violence" in Chapter 7.)**

5. **Tobacco Use.** (This topic covers both smoking and chewing tobacco or snuff.) How many days has the person smoked in the past 30 days? On average, how many cigarettes has the person smoked or how many times has the person used other forms of tobacco per day? **(See the subsection on tobacco use in the section on "Risk Behaviors" and pertinent item in the "Screening Checklist" in Chapter 4; pertinent portions in section on "Head and Neck Cancers" in Chapter 9; and section on "Tobacco Use" in Chapter 13.)**

6. **Alcohol Abuse.** How many days in the last 30 days has the person had a drink containing alcohol? Use local names for such drinks, and cover beer, wine, and distilled liquor. How often has the person had more than five alcoholic drinks within a few hours? **(See the section on "Pregnancy" in Chapter 3; pertinent text in section on "Risk Behaviors" and pertinent items in "Screening Checklist" in Chapter 4; pertinent items in "Screening Checklist" in Chapter 5; section on "Alcohol Abuse and Dependence" in Chapter 7; and section on "Alcohol Use" in Chapter 13.)**

7. **Use of Marijuana.** After developing trust with the person being interviewed, ask how frequently the person has used marijuana in the last 30 days and how much. When did the person last use marijuana? **(See pertinent text in the section on "Risk Behaviors" and pertinent items in the "Screening Checklist" in Chapter 4; and pertinent item in the "Screening Checklist" in Chapter 5.)**

8. **Use of Other Mind-altering Drugs.** Drugs in this entry include heroin, amphetamines and other "uppers," cocaine and its derivatives, inhalants, steroids without prescription, strong pain medication such as morphine and other "downers," hallucinogens, and new designer drugs such as Ecstasy. Ask such questions as "Have you ever used _____ (identify the drug by its

local name)? How recently? How often? How did it affect your mind? Your body? How often have you injected something into your body by a needle? (never, one to five times, more than 5 times)." **(See pertinent text in section on "Risk Behaviors" in Chapter 4; pertinent item in the "Screening Checklist" in Chapter 5; pertinent text in the section on "Eleven Crossroads where Risk and Protective Factors Meet" in Chapter 7; and Table 13.1 in Chapter 13.)**

9. **Sexual Risks.** Because sexual issues are considered shameful or secret in most cultures, each group develops its own slang or group language to talk about sexual organs and actions. Be sure to use local wording when asking for information. Ask especially about possible exchange of body fluids (especially genital secretions or blood); skin contact with sores, pimples, or warts; and penetrations involving mouth, vulva, or anus. Ask about the approximate number of partners the person has had in the last year. Ask for history of sexually transmitted infections (STIs) and pregnancies. Ask about methods used to prevent STIs and pregnancies. How consistently were these used? **(See pertinent text in section on "Risk Behaviors" and pertinent items in "Screening Checklist" in Chapter 4; pertinent item in "Screening Checklist" in Chapter 5; and section on "Unsafe Sex" in Chapter 13.)**

> *The World Bank lists illicit drug use as the eighth leading cause of death in industrial countries and the tenth in developing regions. It also ranks as the eighth leading cause of disability in industrial countries and ninth in developing regions.*

10. **Body Weight.** This topic deals with preventing obesity, the risk of excessive weight loss by dieting and purging, and the risk of anorexia nervosa and bulimia. **(See pertinent text in section on "Risk Behaviors" in Chapter 4.)**

11. **Nutrition.** Promote the consumption of vegetables, salads, fruits and fruit juices, whole grains, and milk products, so that they comprise much of the person's regular diet. Find out how frequently junk foods and junk drinks—whose calories come mostly from fats, sugars, or alcohol—are consumed. Discourage their consumption. **(See pertinent text in section on "Children 5 through 14 Years" in Chapter 3; pertinent items in "Screening Checklist" in Chapter 4; pertinent item in the "Screening Checklist" in Chapter 5; and section on "Malnutrition and Hunger" in Chapter 13.)**

12. **Physical Activity.** This topic gathers information about frequency of vigorous exercise (causing sweat and hard breathing), milder exercise (such as walking or housework), strength building exercise, participation in sports teams, and hours spent sitting during an average weekday (a summary in-

dicator of sedentary lifestyle). **(See relevant text in section on "Risk Be-haviors" and relevant items in the "Screening Checklist" in Chapter 4 and in the "Screening Checklist" in Chapter 5.)**

13. **AIDS.** The survey asks only one question on this topic: "Have you ever been taught about AIDS or HIV infection in school?" There are many other ways to learn about AIDS. The key issue, however, is consistent use of safer sexual practices.

Young people 15–24 years old are poised at the early middle of their life cycle. They carry with them health assets and deficiencies acquired during gestation and childhood. And in their teens and twenties they will also accumulate further risks and benefits, strengths and damages that will persist into the rest of their lives. Their risk behaviors either accumulate and are remodeled or stopped over years of experience. A human life, much as the life of a tree, shows growth rings that reveal sequences of good and bad years. There can be damaging years of drought and there can be boon years of nurtured growth. Each season of life is important and presents the opportunity to build better health. Make the best of each one.

# 5. The Prime of Life: Ages 25–64 Years

In this wide window in a human's lifespan, some have argued that there really are two stages involved—a younger and an older stage. The two stages share such vital common features, however, that this book will deal with them in a single chapter.

People between ages 25 and 64 years are the community's "machinery." They propel and steer the economy and provide direction for the community's lifestyle and future. They are the community's decision-makers and key movers in developing and attaining social and health improvements in their localities. Many persons in their prime of life are parenting children, doing the family's work, earning the money and acquiring the goods needed to care for dependents, participating in organizations, and being neighbors. By age 50, many also begin to care for aging parents, becoming responsible for their shelter, personal care, or economic help.

Indeed, these prime years are the most productive ones for most people, and so, this generation needs vital good health to carry out its social and economic tasks in the community, especially where the median age is very young. In those circumstances this relatively small fraction of the population must support a larger aggregate of young dependents and, increasingly, of older dependents as well.

Preventive medicine goals for this age span include preventing injury and disability and postponing or preventing chronic degenerative diseases. Successful promotion of health at these ages is the foundation for the economic development of communities and nations.

## THE GROWING IMPORTANCE OF ADULT HEALTH

Throughout the last century, public health efforts have been remarkably successful in reducing disease, disability, and death among infants and children. This success has meant that in developing countries, 85% of children live to their fifth birthday, and in fully industrialized countries, nearly 99% of them do (Feachem et al. (eds.), 1992). As a consequence of these gains in infant and child mortality, the population of adults older than 15 years old is growing rapidly, especially in developing regions—developing nations were home to 2.05 billion adults in 1985, with increases each subsequent year.

**TABLE 5.1.** Median percentages of 15 year old youths projected to die before their 65th birthday, by gender, region, and economic development.[a]

| National groupings | Men | Women |
|---|---|---|
| Asia Pacific 36 nations and areas | 23.1[b] (12.2–47.8)[c] | 16.7 (5.7–43.8) |
| Latin America and the Caribbean 40 nations and areas | 20.2 (13.6–32.3) | 13.4 (7.0–26.4) |
| Middle East and North Africa 25 nations and areas | 22.8 (11.0–39.9) | 18.8 (7.3–40.5) |
| Sub-Saharan Africa 31 nations and areas | 37.5 (20.5–53.5) | 32.7 (14.4–51.5) |
| Industrialized socialist[d] Eastern Europe 9 nations | 22.4 (14.2–27.7) | 10.0 (7.8–12.7) |
| Industrialized free-market 28 nations and areas | 14.2 (11.3–18.7) | 7.3 (5.7–13.2) |

*Source:* Adapted from Feachem, Kjellstrom, Murray, et al., 1992:297–301.
[a] Mortality projections are based on World Bank model estimates calculated from data from 1985 or later (157 nations and areas) or from 1980–1984 (12 nations and areas).
[b] Median of group.
[c] Range of group.
[d] Economic system at the time of data collection.

*Improving adult health is more essential now than ever before because:*

- *there are now more adults in the world than ever before;*
- *adults are responsible for raising children and teaching them to become healthy and responsible citizens; and*
- *adults are society's "economic engine," producing the resources to lift communities out of sickness and poverty into health and greater overall life-satisfaction.*

The World Bank has compiled data on survival rates for nearly 200 nations and geographic units (Feachem et al. (eds.), 1992), and that institution's statisticians have developed and cross-validated models to estimate the probabilities of live-born babies to die before age 5 and of youth 15 years old to die before age 65 years. Table 5.1 shows the probability of death between the ages of 15 and 64 years, by gender, for six aggregations of nations and reporting areas at all stages of economic development.[1] (Only data from the 169 national units with mortality data from 1980 and later were used in the table.)

The differences in probability of survival at each of these life stages are surprisingly large between sexes and across aggregations of nations. Differences appear to be due largely to environment, which would suggest that a large portion of the inequalities—and of the inequities—could potentially be remedied.

---

[1] For data on individual nations the reader is referred to the World Bank's 1992 report: *The Health of Adults in the Developing World,* or to subsequent updates of that publication.

A striking observation about the large differences in the median chance of dying (between one's 15th and 65th birthdays) across the world's regions is that the rank order of these differences closely mirrors the degree of economic development within each region.

The second remarkable feature is the great range of values seen within each region. For example, in the Asian-Pacific region there is a fourfold difference in the percentages of men dying and a near eightfold range in chance of death for women, depending upon the area of residence: Hong Kong, for example, has by far the lowest rate in all the Asia-Pacific region. The industrialized—read "richer"—countries have the lowest mortality, followed by Latin America and Eastern Europe.

If we take a closer look at the Region of the Americas countries and reporting areas (Pan American Health Organization, 1994, pp. 8–19), the rank ordering of death rates at most age strata has a nearly perfectly linear negative correlation with gross national product (GNP). In other words, each step of increase in economic production is accompanied by a step of decrease in age-specific mortality rates throughout the life cycle. In the Americas, the major exception to this rule is Cuba—despite its relatively low GNP in terms of external currencies, the country has low mortality rates comparable to much richer nations. This may well be the result of the high priority Cuba has given to universal health care and education.

The gender differences in death rates across regions and reporting areas show a nearly universal excess of male deaths, and this is true not only for ages 15–64, but for other ages as well. Males have higher death rates than females at every age from the prenatal period to the end of life. After infancy, the excess in male mortality is largely attributable to behavioral causes: risk-taking; fighting; violence; greater alcohol, cigarette, and illegal drug use; occupational injuries and diseases; less use of health care when needed; and inadequate self care. In theory, the male flight toward death could be subdued substantially by psychosocial, subcultural, and behavioral change. Could this ever happen?

## MAJOR CAUSES OF DEATH

As younger adults enter the 25 to 64 year age range, they bring along the full array of risk factors and health problems they were exposed to while younger. For men, the rates of unintentional and intentional trauma, injury and disability, continue to hold sway until after age 35. Actually, external causes—trauma inflicted from outside the body—remain the leading causes of both mortality and disability for men until at least age 35 in most of the world's nations. Between ages 35 and 65 years, cardiovascular disorders, cancers, and respiratory diseases become the major causes of death and disability for men. For women ages 25–34 years, external causes, malignant neoplasms, and cardiovascular disorders are the leading causes of death, all with quite low and very similar rates. As one reviews statistics in the *World Health Statistics Annual* in the 1990s, these three causes almost always rank as the top three causes of death for women in industrialized nations, although in no consistent order.

In industrialized nations chronic diseases are responsible for about three-quarters of all deaths in both sexes. Cardiovascular diseases and cancers are the major killers of both men and women in the prime of life. Among those who smoke cigarettes, tobacco-related diseases rise to prominence, and the cardiorespiratory disability they cause also makes prognosis poorer for all other major diseases. Clinicians treating smokers should urge their patients to stop smoking. **(Also see Chapters 12 and 13)**. They should also screen for risk factors and early signs of ischemic heart disease; peripheral vascular disease; emphysema; bronchitis; reduced expiratory volume; and signs of cancer of the head, neck, bronchus, and lung **(see Chapter 13 for a full list of tobacco-related diseases)**.

Other common risk factors—and each one of them contributes to various disorders—are worth checking and correcting in adults. These include sedentary lifestyle, obesity, alcohol misuse or overuse, high blood lipid levels, and high blood pressure. In this age group, digestive cancers become more frequent clinically. In developed countries the most common cancer sites are lung for men and breast for women.

## CARDIOVASCULAR DISEASES

In developing countries, cardiovascular diseases also is the leading cause of death for both men and women in the prime of life. Cancers and infectious and parasitic diseases rank second and third for women, and third and second for men. In 1990, tuberculosis accounted for the majority of infectious deaths, estimated at 586,000 in men and 320,000 in women 30 to 59 years old annually in developing countries. Among cancer deaths, cancers of the cervix and breast were most common in women, and cancers of the liver and lung in men. Unintentional and intentional injuries were major killers in men, together accounting for about 775,000 deaths in 1990 in the defined groups (Murray and Lopez, 1996).

Cardiovascular diseases in the prime of life differ in industrialized and in developing countries. In the former—in post-industrialized and sedentary countries—they tend to be mostly ischemia caused by atherosclerosis; but in most developing nations, diseases of pulmonary circulation, cardiomyopathy, sequellae of rheumatic heart disease (including heart valve damage), inflammations, and "other cardiovascular" disorders predominate. As people in developing countries increase their cigarette smoking and add more saturated fats to their diet, atherosclerotic diseases will increase. By the same token, as developing countries reduce the incidence of those infectious and parasitic diseases that affect the heart and reduce the contributors to pulmonary hypertension, the burden of non-atherosclerotic cardiac diseases will decrease. **(Also see Chapter 8.)**

## TUBERCULOSIS

Tuberculosis (TB) is becoming epidemic again, especially in developing countries. The highest TB death rates occur between the ages of 30 and 59 years, accounting for nearly half (46%) of the nearly two million TB deaths each year (Murray and Lopez, 1996). The tubercle bacillus, while required for diagnosing this disease, is by no means a sufficient cause. In some economically advantaged areas only 1% or 2% of infected people (diagnosed by PPD skin test) become clinically ill in the next decade. Yet, in some disadvantaged areas more than 50% of infected persons may become clinically ill. Clearly, tuberculosis as a cause of disability and death unleashes its full force in those localities that have inadequate sanitation and public health programs—places where people live in crowded, substandard housing, work under unhealthy conditions, and have poor nutrition. Professor George Comstock (in Last, 1986) calls tuberculosis "to some degree a barometer of social welfare." In industrial nations, TB also is on the rise again, especially among the poor, homeless, and poorly nourished, as well as among those with impaired immune function. For example, about one-third of HIV cases in the world are expected to have tuberculosis listed as their final cause of death.

The main reasons for the worldwide resurgence in TB appear to be: reduced levels of public health attack on the disease by screening (by skin test, chest X-rays, or sputum culture, depending on circumstances); failure to treat active cases promptly with antibiotics (thus permitting the infection to spread); and failure to deal with the great increases in susceptibility caused by poverty and malnutrition.

> *The main reasons for the worldwide resurgence in TB appear to be: reduced levels of public health attack on the disease by screening; failure to treat active cases promptly with antibiotics; and failure to deal with the great increases in susceptibility caused by poverty and malnutrition.*

TB takes a greater toll on men. Moreover, because it strikes early in life, with elevated death rates from age 15 onward, TB can inflict greater damage on developing communities than can chronic diseases whose impact becomes serious only after about age 50. TB is ranked as the sixth leading cause of loss of healthy life-years (DALYs) in the developing world for 1990—18.5 million per year for ages 15–59 years only and nearly 40 million for the entire age span. No improvement is projected through the year 2010.

Treatment with antibiotics stops the advancement of TB in the patient and also greatly reduces the chance of the disease spreading to others. It is one of the most cost-effective public health interventions, costing only $3 to $7 per year of disability or lost life prevented. Given the cost of TB, starting with two million lives per year plus uncounted disability, lost production, broken families, etc., a much higher priority should be given to its prevention.

## MAJOR CAUSES OF DISABILITY

Women and men experience quite similar durations of disability as a proportion of their average life spans. Worldwide, however, differences are substantial, and they are linked to economic development. People in established market economies live about 8% of their lives disabled; in Latin America and the Caribbean, the figure rises to about 12%; and in Sub Saharan Africa, it is about 15%, even though they die much earlier on average (Murray and Lopez, 1997).

The causes of disability differ substantially from the causes of death in the "middle years." Table 5.2 lists the rate of DALYs per 1,000 population for ages 15 to 59 years, for men and women, in two geo-economic regions: highly industrialized market economies and Latin America and the Caribbean, with its mix of developing and market economies and tropical and temperate climates. The

**TABLE 5.2. Major causes of loss of health for men and women 15–59 years old, in Disability Adjusted Life Years (DALYs) per 1,000 population in that age group, by gender, in established market economies and in Latin America and the Caribbean, 1990.[a]**

| Causes of health loss | Established market economies | | Latin America and the Caribbean | |
|---|---|---|---|---|
| | Men | Women | Men | Women |
| Cardiovascular diseases | 17.7 | 7.7 | 17.7 | 15.6 |
| Malignant neoplasms | 14.7 | 12.9 | 7.8 | 12.2 |
| Digestive diseases | 6.4 | 3.9 | 11.2 | 7.9 |
| Musculoskeletal (mostly arthritides) | 4.5 | 8.1 | 7.8 | 12.6 |
| Maternal problems (pregnancy and delivery) | — | 1.3 | — | 13.4 |
| Neuropsychiatric disorders | 44.4 | 37.7 | 60.8 | 46.0 |
| Unintentional trauma | 19.2 | 6.5 | 40.4 | 12.1 |
| Violence and self-hurt | 8.6 | 2.9 | 25.2 | 5.6 |

*Source:* Table entries are abstracted from data in Annex Table 9a,g in Murray and Lopez, 1996.
[a] The four columns of rates are based on data from about 750 million persons.
— Not applicable.
**Note:** Two regions defined by the GBD Study were selected to represent industrially developed and developing areas. Established market economies includes nations in Northern and Western Europe and Canada, the United States of America, Australia, and New Zealand; former socialist republics are not included. Latin America and the Caribbean includes all of the Region of the Americas south of Canada and the United States of America. Some of the Latin American and Caribbean nations are advanced in development, but included here.

Latin American and Caribbean region was not chosen as an "opposite" to the established market economies. Rather, it was chosen because it is a region in transition, shifting economically, socially, and epidemiologically toward what is now considered full development. The table presents data for ages 15–59 rather than for the age group 25–64 years old, as is done everywhere else in this chapter, because data for the latter age group was not readily available.

The top reasons for loss of healthy life years for men and women in established market economies and in Latin America and the Caribbean are neuropsychiatric conditions. This broad category includes unipolar major depression, bipolar disorder (formerly manic depressive psychosis), schizophrenia, alcohol abuse or addiction, drug abuse, post-traumatic stress disorder, panic disorder, obsessive-compulsive disorders, as well as the more neurological disorders of dementia (at all ages), Parkinson's disease, multiple sclerosis, and epilepsy.

Neuropsychiatric conditions account for more health loss among both men and women 15–59 years old than any other diagnostic category. According to the GBD Study, this holds both for worldwide data and for six of the eight separate regions covered (established market economies, India, China, Southeast Asia and Pacific Islands, Latin America and the Caribbean, and Middle Eastern Crescent). In the former socialist economies, neuropsychiatric causes account for most DALYs in women, but rank second to unintentional injuries in men in these ages. In Sub-Saharan Africa, the leading causes of lost health in adults are infectious and parasitic diseases, intentional and unintentional injuries (in that order in men); and infections, parasites, and problems of pregnancy and delivery in women.

The most common and damaging specific psychiatric condition worldwide is unipolar major depression. Women are particularly hard hit. In some places alcohol abuse ranks first for men, but unipolar depression is always a major problem. Overall, combining genders and all ages, the ranking of neuropsychiatric conditions by years of health lost is as follows: unipolar depression, alcohol abuse, bipolar disorder, schizophrenia, and dementia. Each of these (in sequence) subtracts between 50.8 million to 8.5 million healthy life years (estimated DALYs) from the total world experience each year. The magnitude of these figures gives added priority for research and prevention of depression. **(Also see Chapter 7.)**

The second and subsequent causes of lost health differ in men and women aged 15–59. For women in developed nations, malignant neoplasms rank second. The reasons for this are twofold—on the one hand, other major health risks have been brought under better control; on the other, clinic facilities that can diagnose malignancies are widely available. In transitioning and developing nations, as exemplified by Latin American and Caribbean nations, cardiovascular and maternal problems, malignancies, and unintended injuries all account for at least 10 DALYs per year per 1,000 population aged 15–59 years old. Clearly, the major causes of death and disability overlap in some categories, but differ in others. Both outcomes must be taken into account when planning preventive health programs.

## SPECIAL ISSUES FOR WOMEN

Family violence is a major preventable cause of nonfatal injury in women in these decades of life. This burden of disease is greater in developing countries where male dominance holds sway. Physical and sexual abuse do damage well beyond what emergency clinics can treat. In addition to the bruises, internal bleeding, and musculoskeletal harm the victim sustains immediately, international research has now demonstrated that episodes of abuse give birth to long-lasting physical illness complexes, often in the gastrointestinal or genitourinary systems (Acierno, et al., 1997 and Resnick, et al., 1997). Experiencing violence, even the threat of violence, can plant the seeds for post-traumatic stress syndrome, chronic fears, and depression. Men who are violent with their wives or partners often also bully and attack their children. **(Also see the section on "Child Abuse and Neglect" in Chapter 3.)** Sadly, women appear to be at an especially high-risk for assault injuries when they are pregnant.

The *American Psychologist* devoted its 1999 January issue to a review of the prevalences of domestic violence and the shelter and treatment programs worldwide. The issue, which includes information from Argentina, Chile, Greece, Israel, Japan, Nicaragua, Mexico (a demonstration project), Russia, and the United States of America, is a rich resource for agencies planning to establish preventive programs.

Reproductive health is a major issue for women throughout their childbearing years. Bearing too many children (some experts see four as the healthy maximum), or bearing them with fewer than two years between pregnancies, has been proven to create serious health risks for the mother and her babies in many countries. **(See pertinent text in section on "Risk Behaviors" in Chapter 4.)** This means that a variety of effective family planning techniques should be made available and accessible as part of primary health care. The same program that teaches the woman about contraceptive use also should work with her partner, appealing to him to opt for a few strong and healthy children rather than many unplanned children, at least some of which are likely to be sick or impaired. **(Also see the section on "In Pregnancy" in Chapter 3.)**

*Health promotion and care for women can have a multiplier effect when women are taught in a practical, experiential way how to preserve their health and that of their children, spouses, and older adults.*

Women's disability caused by complications of pregnancy and delivery is pandemic in more slowly developing regions (as shown in Table 5.2). In Sub-Saharan Africa, India, and the Middle East Crescent, these maternal problems account for 24%, 19% and 28%, respectively, of all years of lost life or impaired health in women 15–44 years old. As more and more women enter the workforce each decade, occupational injuries and toxic exposures are becoming more significant the world over.

Health promotion and care for women can have a multiplier effect when women are taught in a practical, experiential way about how to preserve their health and that of their children, spouses, and older adults. This should be an ongoing process, which, if done in an interactive group setting, keeps teaching relevant, allows immediate clarification of uncertainties, and multiplies community diffusion of knowledge.

## SPECIAL ISSUES FOR MEN

The onslaught of intentional and unintentional trauma expands to an ever larger proportion of total deaths as traditional infections get reduced. In developed nations, injuries account for 22% of all deaths in men between 30 and 59 years old and for 12% in women in those ages. In developing regions total injuries in 1990 accounted for 19% of men's deaths (775,000) and 9% of women's. The largest proportion of all deaths attributable to injury (all ages, both sexes) occurs in China (11.5% of total deaths there).

The cost to men in DALYs also is astounding. Worldwide, the GBD Study estimates that about 28% of all healthy years lost by men aged 15–59 are caused by injuries. The injury burden suffered by men ages 15–44 is much higher proportionally than that suffered by older men. The greatest proportions of disabilities due to intentional and unintentional injuries occur in Sub-Saharan Africa (41%), the former socialist republics (32%), and the Middle Eastern Crescent (30%). In Sub-Saharan Africa and the Middle Eastern Crescent, more than half of injury disability is intentionally inflicted. War is the largest single component in the Middle Eastern Crescent, and organized violence outranks war for the male burden in Sub-Saharan Africa. Even in fully industrialized countries intentional injuries make up 30% of total injury disability. Without a doubt, this is a golden opportunity for socially meaningful prevention.

Is the carnage from external causes a public health problem? Or, are the high percentages of disabilities inflicted intentionally? Certainly, the lost years of life and health are major public health problems. But economic disasters are not far behind, when young adults, in whom 15 to 20 years of child rearing and educating have been invested, lose part or all of their economically productive years to trauma.

What about the etiology? Who is working to identify the agents, the vectors, the environmental contributors to this pandemic? Table 5.2 shows that all injuries (combining unintentional trauma and violence/self-hurt) rank first and second—right alongside neuropsychiatric disorders—as a contributor to lost health in the men who are the economic backbone of most communities in the world. In addition, the disabled who survive require professional and family care and resources, at considerable expense.

*Hostility and aggression are the cultural diseases that lead to violence. Failure to value the lives and rights of others is a moral deficiency disease that multiplies the destructive effect.*

Obviously, no conceivable vaccine can treat this public health pandemic of violence that only threatens to worsen. The GBD Study predicts that by 2010, the total damage caused both by unintentional and by intentional injuries will increase among men and women. Only serious, intense, resource-utilizing cooperation among major governmental sectors might begin to reverse this tide. Raising the level of education already has a proven track record in reducing many kinds of health and social problems; it may do the same for injuries. Improved motor vehicle safety, too, can save lives and disability through enforcing traffic safety laws and mandatory use of seat belts, preventing persons who have drunk alcohol from driving, and removing structural hazards on roadways and at intersections (Evans, 1991, Chapter 13). Better worker training and the mandatory installation and use of protective and safety gear is another approach for the workplace. Finally, studies can be undertaken about local trauma risks, to be followed by actions to reduce them. **(Also see Chapter 11.)**

Steps can also be taken to curb intentional injuries, including self-inflicted wounds and suicide, violence against others. Heightened awareness of depression and hopelessness by lay persons and professionals alike could help relieve the disability of depression. Referring a depressed person for medical help and accompanying him or her to and from the treatment site can also help prevent suicide attempts. **(Also see Chapters 7 and 11.)**

Hostility and aggression are the cultural diseases that lead to violence. Failure to value the lives and rights of others is a moral deficiency disease that multiplies the destructive effect. Families, schools, religious and ethical organizations, businesses, civic organizations, the media, and the government need to work together and motivate each other to uproot and disown the culture of violence. Teaching non-aggressive problem-solving using mediation and negotiation, searching for solutions where both parties win, and teaching the sanctity of human life can all reduce violence. Reducing despair may reduce emotional pressure and give cognitive approaches a better chance. Violence often follows frustration and desperation, but violent behavior is learned through interpersonal and social experiences. Under the right circumstances, problem-solving can be learned instead. But for all these approaches to work, they must be taught in early childhood and modeled throughout the lifespan. The National Academy of Sciences in the United States prepared an integration of violence prevention literature and recommendations (Reiss and Roth, 1993, Chapter 3).

And, if we can learn to do this as individuals, as families, and as communities, perhaps—just perhaps—national and regional leaders can learn these skills too. That would cut down the third great cause of intentional injuries: war. Wars caused an estimated 502,000 deaths and countless suffering and permanent disability in 1990, with similar losses seen in each subsequent year (Murray and Lopez, 1996).

## AVENUES FOR REACHING ADULTS WITH PREVENTIVE PROGRAMS

Traditionally, public health programs have focused on children and their mothers. The statistics in this handbook demonstrate that these programs have been successful to the point that in most nations the major disablers and killers are now found in the adult population. The causes and risk factors for these health problems are known, programs of prevention have demonstrated success, and the same general approaches so successful with children are waiting to be put in motion for people of all ages.

But children might be seen as a captive population. The vast majority can be reached through parents, child-clinics, health professionals, child day care centers, and schools. Places in which to reach and treat adults in the prime of life are not that well defined.

Many working people think that making a special trip to a clinic or physician for a health reason, when they feel just fine, is just too much trouble, so it might be best to "catch" people where they go on a regular basis. In that light, the workplace is a prime site for screening and prevention activities. This requires the support of an employer, who might be persuaded by arguments that better health means better productivity and less absenteeism. For day laborers, the place may be where they congregate prior to being hired. And many women and men go to a market each week to barter, sell, or buy. A community market is a convenient place to reach people of all ages with health services.

In the Americas, the Middle East, the Far East, and much of Europe, religious observance is common. Most faiths set aside a day of worship and this day, or other times when people gather at places of worship, may be well suited to reach people for whom the workplace is not convenient. In urban areas, other regular gathering places such as sports stadiums, theaters, and other public buildings or open areas, may be considered for promotion and health prevention activities.

Networks of social connectedness can be employed to "fish for" those adults not caught by the above networks. Convincing leaders of extended families and kinship groups of the importance of a new health action and of how it can strengthen the whole family in the future, is a first step. Getting those leaders to accept responsibility for teaching and bringing in their entire group to participate in the health programs is the second.

> *Involving friendships and occupational and interest groups helps health program participation greatly, especially in more urban settings where kinship ties are weakened.*

Involving friendships and occupational and interest groups helps health program participation greatly, especially in more urban settings where kinship ties are weakened. Worker groups, women's organizations, sports clubs (both for active participants and their older family and friends), church groups, civic clubs, political organizations, neighborhood improvement groups, farmers' cooperatives—all these are already existing social networks that can be "borrowed" to serve a health purpose. **(Also review the twelve channels of communication presented in the section "Presenting Programs Successfully" in Chapter 12. These can help put health improvement on the agenda of even more people.)**

## SCREENING BY INTERVIEW

### TOBACCO USE

Cigarette smoking damages nearly every body system. The problem with smoking *only* a few cigarettes is the extremely powerful chemical urge to smoke more and more; abstinence is actually easier to maintain. There is less evidence for health damage from minimal occasional cigar or pipe usage.

Chewing tobacco or betel nut and the like, leaves carcinogens in contact with the mouth's mucosa for many hours, damaging the mouth and nearby tissues. Cessation of tobacco use is the biggest single contribution one can make to the health of the individual, the family, and the community. **(Also see Chapter 13.)**

### EATING HABITS

Ascertain what the person and his or her family usually eat at home and away, such as in school and at work. Optimally, people should be eating several servings of vegetables, salad foods, and fruits each day (for cancer prevention), as well as whole grains and protein sources having minimal saturated fat. Eating habits should minimize consumption of fatty meats, butter, salt, and lard for cardiovascular health. Dairy products are healthful, especially if their fat content is reduced below "natural" levels. People should keep calorie intake balanced by physical exertion so that a healthy weight is maintained.

## REGULAR EXERCISE

What is the person's usual amount of physical exertion—on the job; at home; in other activities? From ages 10 to 75 more strenuous exercise is better, exercise that involves large muscle groups, such as bicycling, swimming, working on the farm or in a garden, or engaging in active sports. In the older years, exercise should continue: daily 30-to-40 minute walks yield benefits for the whole body, including the brain (Paluska and Schwenk, 2000).

## ALCOHOL CONSUMPTION

Evaluate both the usual amount consumed in a week and the maximum amount taken at any one occasion. The CAGE questionnaire will screen for drinking problems in cooperative persons (Schofield, 1988). Drinking five or more alcoholic drinks on any one occasion, or drinking to the point of losing control or coordination, are signs of binge drinking and loss of control. Regular consumption of more than two alcoholic drinks per day (equivalent to 2 oz of ethanol) can raise resting blood pressure over time. Continuing this modest level of daily drinking for 10 years or more raises the risk of alcoholic liver damage. **(Also see the "Screening Checklist" in Chapter 4.)**

Continued alcohol use for many years also raises the risk of peptic ulcers; congestive heart failure; cancers of the head, neck, liver, and pancreas; and damage to the nervous system resulting in psychiatric and neurologic disorders. Alcohol also releases impulsive aggressive behaviors; causes family breakups; and raises risk of injuries, legal problems, assault, and suicide.

Ask especially about driving vehicles after drinking. In most industrialized nations, if a person's blood alcohol concentration (by weight) is 0.10% or higher, he or she is considered legally intoxicated. Tests in driving simulators show individual differences in the blood alcohol concentration at which people start losing coordination and skill, ranging from 0.05% to higher than 0.20%. In many places, legal codes are based on blood chemistry, not behavioral condition. Death and disability due to trauma are not fully curable, but are largely preventable. Alcohol abuse exacts a heavy price from the family and community in physical and mental health, social welfare, and economics. **(Also see the section on "Alcohol Use" in Chapter 13.)**

## USE OF OTHER MOOD ALTERING SUBSTANCES

Prevalence of drug abuse declines after age 35, but more people begin misusing over-the-counter and prescription drugs after that age, especially for pain relief. It is worth asking: "What kinds of drugs, medications, or other remedies do you take to help you feel better?" Then evaluate the substance, and its frequency and quantity of use. Be aware that respondents often underestimate or deny usage. **(Also see pertinent item in the "Screening Checklist" in Chapter 4.)**

## SOCIAL AND EMOTIONAL WELL-BEING

The dark side of this coin is the wide prevalence of neuropsychiatric disorders, and the even wider spread of life crises, losses, sorrows, and nervousness that are the common colds and mild fevers of the psyche.

Some useful exploratory questions might include: "How are things at home?" "How do you like your job?" "When was the last time you felt so sad that you cried?" "Can you tell me more about that?" "Does nervousness run in your family?" "How often do you feel nervous?" For women especially, probe further on the issue of depression with questions such as: "Are there times when you cannot get going?" "Times when you just don't care anymore; when everything is going badly?" For men, probe alcohol, depression, and aggressiveness: "Do you spend time in places or with groups where people get drunk, or start arguing or fighting, or perhaps carry weapons?"

Ask the interviewees where they expect to be and what they would want to be doing five years from now. If respondents don't know, ask them to guess. This probe also can be done with groups of adults responding in writing on a printed form. Answers may reveal any of the following: depression, hopelessness, unrealistic goals, fatalism, a sense of dead end in the person's life, an inability to go beyond living only for the moment, a desire to flee the present situation, or destructive wishes. On the other hand, answers may show persons to be satisfied with their present lot and having positive expectations and plans for the future.

*Sexually transmitted infections inflict a heavier toll of disability on women.*

These suggestions are not intended to replace the need for mental health workers in screening in the health services. In fact, when such interviewing, or questionnaire screening, is done routinely, the need for trained counselors and preventive programs may become much more apparent.

## SEXUAL PRACTICES

This issue, as is alcohol consumption, is where the people in greatest danger are more likely to understate their behaviors. Sometimes, more truthful answers may be obtained by prefacing the questions with a permissive statement such as: "These days people are engaging in many kinds of sexual activities. Can you tell me about the people you know or associate with? What kinds of sex do they have?" (Record replies.) Follow up with questions such as: "Which ones of these have you engaged in?"[2] **(Also review the suggestions made for this topic in the "Screening Checklist" in Chapter 4.)**

Be aware that sexually transmitted infections inflict a heavier toll of disability on women. Pelvic inflammatory disease, sterility, and other tissue damage are common sequellae. Men often bring sexually transmitted infections home—to leave them with their wives or partners.

This line of questioning is intended to identify those risks that put future health in jeopardy, such as having multiple partners; having sex without protective barriers (such as latex condoms) to prevent infection by exchanging body fluids or tissue friction; having sex with persons whose sexual history is not well known; having anal contact; and having oral or genital contact with sores, pimples, or warts that may contain herpes and viral or bacterial agents. The goal is to make all sexual behaviors safe. Just one unguarded occasion could deliver a lethal sexually transmitted infection. **(For an in-depth discussion, see the section on "Unsafe Sex" in Chapter 4.)**

Women and couples should be questioned regarding family planning and contraceptive use and counseled about the several options available. This is particularly important for women who already experience health problems relating to the reproductive system or whose families already exceed their emotional and physical resources. **(Further information about family planning can be found in the item on pregnancy prevention in the "Screening Checklist" in Chapter 13.)**

## RISKS OF MOTOR VEHICLE TRAUMA OR INJURY

- Does the person ever ride with drivers who have been drinking alcohol?

- Does the person himself ever drive after alcohol use?

- Has the person or any friends recently been charged with traffic violations? (A predictor of a future injurious crash)

---

[2] There is controversy about how best to ask questions about alcohol, illicit drugs, sexual activity, and other possibly illegal or embarrassing behaviors. For ideas on this issue, see Sudman and Bradburn (1982 and later editions). Chapter 3 in this source deals with asking potentially threatening questions about behavior.

- Has the person or any friends had vehicle accidents? (Depending on circumstances, it might predict future mishaps.)

- Does the person ride in autos or trucks without using seat belts? Seat belts do not prevent collisions, but do protect the human body from fatal concussion impact and ejection out of the vehicle.

- Does the person ride motorcycles or motor scooters without a protective helmet? Bicycles and motorbikes contribute to many injuries. These may result from being struck by a car or truck, hitting a stationary object (post, curb, wall), striking a hole in the road, or sliding and falling on sandy or wet surfaces. Helmets prevent facial and brain injuries—the latter, of course, being incurable.

## RISKS OF OCCUPATIONAL INJURY

- Does the person work with tools or machines similar to that on which other workers are injured from time to time? Can this problem be reduced by protective changes in the machinery? Should workers be given protective gear or garments? Should workers be trained differently? (The recent experience of the work group is the best predictor of near-future individual risk.)

- Is the worker exposed to dust, chemicals, or biological agents that can accumulate either acutely or chronically in the body and impair health?

- Does the worker lift or carry heavy loads, or perform work that involves twisting or holding poor posture for long periods? These are all common causes of musculoskeletal injury and disability, which may be prevented by worker training or minor re-engineering of work tasks. Back injuries are increasingly common and can be disabling. In fact, many industries sponsor brief "back schools" to train workers how to prevent such injuries.

## SOCIAL SUPPORT NETWORK

Persons should be asked how many adults and children live in their household. How many people are able to offer help if problems occur in the family (problems such as no one to care for children if the mother gets sick, the roof leaks, the family temporarily runs out of enough money to cover its needs, needing help to send a message or do an errand)?

Ask also if there are one or more persons with whom the interviewee can discuss worries or share feelings. From how many individuals does the person feel comfortable enough to seek information or advice? If the answer in any category is "none or one," discuss with the person how to increase the social support network. To assess the quality of the social context, the interviewer might ask: "How are things at home?" or, "Overall, are the people you are with every day a source of encouragement and help or a source of trouble and worry?" (Often the honest answer is both, in which case the relative balance should be assessed.)

## HEALTH PROBLEMS IN OTHER FAMILY MEMBERS

Make appropriate referrals to health clinics or social agencies. Studies have shown that untreated health problems in any one family member are associated with increased vulnerability for the rest of the family to other kinds of illnesses and life difficulties.

## HOME SAFETY

Do stairs or porch railings need repair? Are smoke detectors and alarms installed if appropriate; have they been recently tested? (If there are young children in the home, see the "Screening Checklist" in Chapters 3 and 4.)

## SCREENING BY OBSERVATION

### APPEARANCE AND BEHAVIOR

During the time spent with the individual or group, the clinician should remain alert for:

- signs of emotional depression (also see the section on "Recognizing and Dealing with Depression" in Chapter 7);

- signs of fearfulness, anxiety, or hyperactivity;

- signs of schizoid thinking or bizarre appearance;

- signs of physical abuse or neglect (also see the section on "Suicide and Violence" in Chapter 11);

- signs of respiratory difficulty (also see Chapter 10); and

- other physical signs or behaviors of health relevance.

Information for the items listed above may be gathered from groups by using questionnaires, or by a group-administered interview, wherein the questions are read to the group. The answers are given on individual answer sheets with numbered questions and boxes for checking the multiple possible replies. Questions also may be read to the respondents, asking them to mark in box 1, 2, 3, 4, etc., to indicate their answer. These latter options allow rapid collection of information from large groups having limited literacy.

## CLINICAL AND LABORATORY SCREENS AND PROPHYLAXES

This is an ideal list. What is routine in any given place will depend on the major health problems of local men and women, clinic facilities, cost-effectiveness, and available resources.

### HEIGHT AND WEIGHT MEASUREMENT

This is a preliminary indicator for either obesity or undernutrition. Either condition could aggravate other diseases.

### BLOOD PRESSURE MEASUREMENT

Measure blood pressure three times during the visit. If the average falls in the hypertensive range for adults (systolic blood pressure ≥140 mmHg or diastolic blood pressure ≥90 for borderline hypertension; systolic blood pressure ≥160 or diastolic blood pressure ≥95 for definite hypertension), have the client come back in a week or so for another set of measurements. A single measure (or a single occasion) is too unreliable for clinical decision-making. **(Also see the section "Hypertension and Hypertensive Heart Disease" in Chapter 8.)**

### MAMMOGRAM

In the United States this diagnostic test is recommended every year in women ages 50–59 (United States Preventive Services Task Force, 1996, Chapter 7). This will not be possible in some communities and nations, and may not be cost-effective in areas where breast cancer rates are very low. Where mammography is not available, clinical breast examinations should be done for women aged 50–70. In many cultures this is most acceptable if performed by a female clinician. **(Also see the section "Breast Cancer" in Chapter 9.)**

### PAP SMEARS

In sexually active women perform a Papanicolaou smear every one to three years, if economically feasible. Every adult woman should be tested until two consecutive tests are fully negative (United States Preventive Services Task Force, 1996). If there is an increase in the number of her sexual partners, Pap smears would be resumed.

### SKIN LESIONS

Look unobtrusively at arms for needle marks from use of injected drugs. Look also for the beginnings of skin cancers in persons heavily exposed to sunshine. **(Also see the section on "Skin Cancers" in Chapter 9.)**

### TUBERCULOSIS

Do an appropriate test for tuberculosis if the person is in a social group where rates are elevated or for whom a family member, close friend, or coworker has been recently diagnosed with TB. Be alert for reactivation of old TB lesions in people experiencing malnutrition, extended hardship, social upheaval, or chronic infections.

### ORAL HEALTH

Check the mouth for tooth decay, gum disease, oral hygiene, and mucosal lesions suggestive of oral cancers or immunosuppression. **(Also see section on "Head and Neck Cancers" in Chapter 9.)**

### SEXUALLY TRANSMITTED INFECTIONS

Persons whose behaviors put them at higher risk for sexually transmitted infections should be examined, given laboratory tests as appropriate, and counseled regarding dangers of HIV and other sexually transmitted infections. **(Also see the section on "Unsafe Sex" in Chapter 13.)**

### ISCHEMIC HEART DISEASE

Where there is high prevalence of ischemic heart disease, do a non-fasting test for total serum cholesterol, starting at age 35 in men and at age 45 in women, and continuing until age 65. Repeat the test about every five years, more often if cholesterol is high, less often if low. Persons with total serum cholesterol higher than 200 mg/dl should be counseled to reduce dietary intake of fats, especially saturated fats. Persons with total serum cholesterol higher than 240 mg/dl should be referred for medical review in addition to dietary guidance (United

States Preventive Services Task Force, 1996). (Also see the section on "Ischemic Heart Disease" in Chapter 8.)

## TETANUS-DIPHTHERIA

A tetanus-diphtheria booster shot should be given early in adulthood and every 10 years thereafter. Puncture wounds or deep cuts may require an immediate injection of tetanus antitoxin, followed later by a tetanus booster.

*These screening checklists are not intended to advise physicians on how to care for their patients. Rather, they are intended to alert public health and preventive medicine professionals and planners to a broad list of health issues at each stage of life, toward which locally appropriate programs may be directed.*

## HEPATITIS B

Hepatitis B vaccine is strongly recommended for high risk persons, such as those with frequent exposure to blood or blood products or recipients of blood transfusions. In areas where hepatitis B is epidemic and a major cause of cirrhosis and cancers of the liver, health officials are promoting mass immunizations at younger ages.

## DIGESTIVE CANCERS

Be alert for signs or symptoms of digestive cancers. Ask about tarry stools. After age 50 do tests of fecal occult blood, both for colon and stomach cancers (United States Preventive Services Task Force, 1996). (Also see the section on "Stomach Cancers" in Chapter 9.)

These screening checklists are not intended to advise physicians on how to care for their patients. Rather, they are intended to alert public health and preventive medicine professionals and planners to a broad list of health issues at each stage of life, toward which locally appropriate programs may be directed.

# 6. The Older Years: 65 to 100

## HEALTH GOALS FOR THE LATER YEARS

The most rapidly growing segment of the world's population is the oldest. Centenarians are the fastest growing group proportionally, followed by persons aged 80–99 years old. Throughout human history, people living to these ages have been few, indeed. Over time, with the conquest of the major infectious epidemics, the number of older persons edged upward. And now, given medical science's breakneck advances, especially in pharmacology, "senior citizens" are coming into their own. It has been forecast that in the 21st century, the growing population of persons older than age 85—the "old-old"—with their tremendous consumption of medical services, will spark major economic, medical resource, and ethical crises for developed and developing nations alike.

The field of gerontology has been running fast to keep pace with this demographic transition. In field studies gerontologists and geriatricians have shown that many of our long-held "common sense" beliefs about the old and aging are simply wrong. The older a group of people gets, the more variety they show. In fact, the elderly show much greater variation in physical, mental, and social functioning than any other age group.

Functional declines with age can be postponed by maintaining an active physical, mental, and social life. And so, the goal of health promotion programs for older people is not to prolong life indefinitely, but rather to put as much life as possible into the years that remain for each person.

One way to help reduce the heavy consumption of health care resources by the older population is to compress the period of terminal morbidity. The objective here is to keep people active and caring for themselves independently until as close as possible to their death. This would minimize the duration, although not necessarily the intensity, of the medical care they require. But it clearly reduces suffering and limits the feelings of decline for the elders and their caretakers and family.

The economics of intensive medical care for the elderly are increasingly under debate. When medical resources are inadequate for the entire population, who should get the priority? The elderly? Young adults? Developmentally damaged babies? Pregnant women? Or, should the best care be given only to those who have enough money to pay for it, regardless of age or prognosis?

Medical economists report that in post-industrialized nations, about 18% of an average person's lifetime medical expenses are spent in the last year of life. How much of these resources, spent when life expectancy is only perhaps one year, should be instead spent upstream in the river of life, to provide preventive services to younger productive people earlier in their voyage?

The economic arguments about the degree of emphasis on geriatric care involve a debate as to whose benefit is most important, the individual or the community as a whole. Does the money spent keeping a 70-year-old alive deliver as much benefit as the same amount spent to provide intensive care in a coronary unit for a 50-year-old with myocardial infarction? Or, say, to provide hospice care for a 30-year-old with AIDS? Or, orthopedic surgery and rehabilitation for an 18-year-old with multiple fractures from an automobile crash? Quickly, moral as well as economic judgments enter the discussion.

*The goal of health promotion programs for older people is not to prolong life indefinitely, but rather to put as much life as possible into the years that remain for each person.*

On the benefit side of the equation, extending the life span into later decades has been accompanied by well-maintained mental capacity, physical strength, and community productivity in most older people. In nations where retirement benefits are available at age 65, many people stop working when they reach that age. Yet, a surprising number draw their pensions but go out and get jobs, often pursuing occupations that demand less physical strength or carry less stress. In more agrarian settings, men and women continue to work at farming as long as their strength holds out.

The bottom line of this discussion is that there are many opportunities—often overlooked by society as well as by individual—for older folks to contribute economically, socially, or interpersonally to their families and their communities. For example, in communities where young mothers commonly enter the workforce, adequate parenting may be in short supply. Enter the grandparents: the experience and patience of the "grandparent generation" suits them well for providing supplementary parenting. Given the many problems of today's children and youth, grandparenting—even as unpaid work—may well be one of the greatest economic and social gifts anyone can give his or her community. And I'm sure we all can come up with additional examples. The important psychological, social, and cultural benefits provided by older community residents are just beginning to be discovered.

What can health workers do to help older persons realize their full potential—and to reduce their need for high-tech medical care?

# MAJOR HEALTH PROBLEMS AT THESE AGES

## MORTALITY

Life expectancy is the age to which the middle person (in terms of age) in a population cohort survives. Since most economically developed countries have life expectancies at birth of more than 65 years, more than half of all deaths will occur in the 65-years-and-older age stratum. Thus, the causes of death in this age stratum will dominate the total for the nation as a whole. This means that it is essential to study the causes of death and disability separately for each stage of life—as earlier chapters in this Handbook have done—to guide focused preventive efforts earlier in the life cycle.

It is not surprising, then, that crude death rates for nations, based heavily on deaths of old people, show that cardiovascular disorders, cerebrovascular diseases, malignancies, obstructive lung diseases, and pneumonias are the leading causes of death in most regions of the world. This holds true for nations both early and late in their economic evolution.

The acceleration of mortality speeds up as the decades of life pass. From ages 25 to 34 years, the rates of mortality from all causes double for each successive decade, for both men and women in most nations. In every decade, men's death rates (per 100,000) are clearly higher than those for women.

For some causes, the multiplier is even greater per decade. For total cardiovascular diseases in most countries, mortality is two to three times as high at age 65 years as it is at age 55, and again multiplies four to five times from age 75 and older. Cerebrovascular accidents (strokes) show a similar acceleration of rates after age 55. Total cancers double between ages 55 to 65, and again after age 65. All this means that death rates are speeded up 10 to 15 times over the last three or four decades of the life cycle.

This information on the acceleration of death rates at older ages reveals three important facts:

- the rapid acceleration of vulnerability among older people.

- the potential societal gains from effective earlier prevention programs. These programs could delay this surge of disease and death until later in the life cycle.

- the huge increase in costs for medical care and nursing-home care in the large number of older people who remain disabled and dependent, often for years before dying from their disease conditions.

Many older people suffer through years of disability—feeling and functioning poorly—before they die. Now we know that much can be done to reduce risks and severity of disabling conditions, maybe not for all but certainly for many. The major causes for suffering and frailty include the leading reasons for death, and also other kinds of health problems.

Up to 1990, the world's population over age 60 years was still smaller than that of other age groups. Women outnumbered men by a ratio of 123 to 100, and gender differences in the relative weight of different causes of disability were much less than among middle-aged people. For all of the world's regions, 80% to 95% of disabled years are attributed to noncommunicable diseases. Overall, the impact on disability from communicable, maternal, perinatal, and nutritional conditions falls from 46% for ages 0–4 years to 6% in persons 60 years old and older. Similarly, the impact of all injuries on disability falls from 18% for ages 0–4 to 2.5% in ages 60 years old and older (worldwide YLD data taken from Murray and Lopez, 1996, Annex Table 8).

## LEADING NONCOMMUNICABLE DISEASE CAUSES OF DISABILITY WORLDWIDE

**In Older Men**
* respiratory disorders (mostly chronic obstructive lung disease),
* cardiovascular diseases (mostly ischemic heart disease and stroke), and
* neuropsychiatric conditions (mostly dementia).

**In Older Women**
* neuropsychiatric conditions (mostly dementia, with major depression also),
* respiratory disorders (mostly chronic obstructive lung disease),
* cardiovascular diseases (stroke and ischemic heart disease), and
* visual loss from cataracts and glaucoma.

Malignancies are a prominent cause of death in both older men and women, but contribute smaller numbers of disabled life years than the above conditions.
**(The factors which lead to and protect from neuropsychiatric, respiratory, and cardiovascular diseases will be examined in depth in Chapters 7, 8, and 10.)**

## RISK FACTORS FOR MAJOR CAUSES OF DEATH AND DISABILITY

* Cigarette smoking is a strong contributor to the development of ischemic heart disease (heart attack), cerebrovascular disease (stroke), chronic obstructive lung disease, bronchitis and/or pneumonias, and many cancers. Smoking ups the ante for the potential amount of sickness and suffering and determines the type of death. There is only one solution—stop smoking.

- High fat diets raise the risk of colon and prostate cancers, and possibly other cancers. They also powerfully increase atherosclerosis, which expresses itself in heart attack and stroke.

- High blood pressure is the strongest contributor to stroke (both hemorrhagic and thrombotic), helps cause heart attack, and when severe will also damage the kidneys. The solution is to lower blood pressure, by using medications or improving one's lifestyle. **(Also see the section on "Hypertension and Hypertensive Disease" in Chapter 8.)**

- Obesity burdens the heart and lungs. It raises blood pressure and is associated with increased low-density lipoproteins (bad cholesterol); it promotes adult onset diabetes mellitus. Obesity also raises the risk of colon, kidney, and endometrial cancers. And, by putting excessive weight on the lower limbs, it aggravates arthritis in the joints. The solution—lose weight and maintain a low healthy weight; exercise and reduced caloric intake will help.

## PROTECTIVE FACTORS FOR MAJOR CAUSES OF DEATH AND DISABILITY

Yes, even the oldest age groups can enhance protective factors. Recent research repeatedly has shown that regular physical exercise continues to provide much greater benefits at a much later age than common sense would have predicted. For example, a research study randomized 70 to 79 year old persons into a walking group and a control group. After 26 weeks, the walking group had increased their maximum oxygen uptake by 22%. This is a striking rejuvenation in view of the fact that from about age 30 onward maximum oxygen uptake for most people declines by an average of 1% per year. In fact, walking may be one of the best forms of exercise for older people.

*The longer in a lifespan that risk factors for these diseases can be kept low and protective factors can be kept high, the fewer adults that will die prematurely; the better health adults will carry with them into this period, thus postponing terminal decline; and the less medical services they will consume.*

Older persons can derive important improvements from exercise programs, especially endurance training and resistance training. Just keeping physically active alone helps control diabetes and reduces the risk of stroke. In a large cohort of older women, those who spent fewer than four hours a day on their feet had double the rate of hip fractures, compared to those who were up and about four or more hours. These benefits not only postpone death, but they also reduce risk of falls, prevent disability, and increase stamina. And the good news is that moderate exercise is almost as beneficial as hard exercise, and carries much less risk of injury (Carlson et al., 1999).

There are many different published exercise prescriptions, but most share the following points:

- exercise regularly, preferably four or more times per week,

- do it with enough zest to make you breathe faster and your heart beat faster,

- continue to exercise for 20 to 30 minutes,

- slow down if you are breathing too fast to carry on a conversation, if you gasp for breath, or if you feel any pressure, heaviness, or pain in your chest, shoulder, neck, or left arm.

Another important protective factor is to consume a healthy diet. Eating a variety of foods will give a person the full range of nutrients. Vegetables, fruits, clean salad foods, whole grains, and low-fat dairy products should be eaten every day, if possible. Lean meats should be eaten in moderation and fats that are solid at room temperature should be avoided. Weight should be kept at a healthy normal level. During food shortages, an elderly person should try to consume enough calories to maintain a normal body weight. If possible, vegetable sources of protein should be included in the diet, as well as the foods listed above.

## MUSCULOSKELETAL CONDITIONS

Musculoskeletal conditions—arthritis and osteoporosis—are associated with hip and spinal fractures. Taken together, they are major causes of disability and limitations of mobility, especially in elderly women living in highly developed nations. Arthritis, an inflammation in joints and adjacent tissues, will, over time, destroy cartilage and change the shape of the bone. It can affect hands and arms, feet and the legs, and the back or neck. Both ostheoarthritis and rheumatoid arthritis become more prevalent and more severe with advancing age. These conditions are two to three times more common in women than men. The arthritides are reported to be the major cause of limitations of mobility in the elderly in some industrialized nations.

### Arthritis

True rheumatoid arthritis appears to result from a wayward immunologic process in which antibodies, whose job is to fight off outside infection, falsely identify some of a person's own cells as outside invaders. The fight that follows causes inflammation and, after months or years, ends up as a chronic disease.

The full etiology of rheumatoid arthritis is not known, nor have primary preventive measures been established. The disease has a genetic component, and oral contraceptives seem to reduce symptoms in some women. One step to reduce the progression of rheumatoid arthritis (secondary prevention) is for the patient to take nonsteroidal, anti-inflammatory drugs to reduce inflammation, pain, and fever, because they are thought to increase damage to tissues in the joints. Care must be taken to avoid overdosing these medications because they can damage other organs.

Osteoarthritis is the more prevalent type, and its frequency increases rapidly with age. Redness of adjacent skin, joint swelling, morning stiffness, and pain at night are its core symptoms. Trauma to joints or repetitive stress and strain on joints are thought to set off many cases. Obesity makes matters worse, by overloading joints. Secondary prevention involves reversing these two risk factors. Proper exercise can be a protective factor that can reduce the amount of disability and pain. Exercise should be gentle and daily to improve flexibility of joints without overloading them. An "Arthritis Self-Management Course" has been developed which has been shown to significantly reduce pain, doctor visits, and hospitalizations (Lorig et al., 1999).

The economic and personal costs of arthritis and other musculoskeletal impairments are rapidly rising worldwide. Occupational health specialists can help to prevent or delay many of these cases (especially disabling back injuries) by ergonomically readjusting work activities, thus reducing the frequency and intensity of work movements that repetitively strain joints, especially in the spine.

### Osteoporosis

This condition mostly affects people over age 65, and it is more prevalent in women than men—almost all women over age 75 have X-ray evidence of osteoporosis in their lower spine. Pathologically, it consists of a loss of calcium from bones, which weakens them to the point of easy fracture. Osteoporosis spells the difference between a fall that is uneventful and a fall that ends in fracture and permanent disability. Most such fractures occur in the arms, legs, hips, and spinal column.

**Risk Factors for Osteoporosis.** (1) A sedentary lifestyle, (2) a diet low in calcium, (3) smoking tobacco, and (4) decreased estrogen in postmenopausal women.

**Protective Factors for Osteoporosis.** All of these are especially effective when practiced continually from an early age. (1) Exercise regularly—weight bearing exercise, such as walking or running, is particularly beneficial. Putting the body's weight on the bones presses calcium into the bone matrix, and strengthening the leg muscles helps prevent falls; even standing is more beneficial than sitting. Swimming greatly benefits the heart and lungs, but does little for osteoporosis). (2) Have an adequate dietary calcium intake. (3) Consider estrogen replacement, if a physician advises it.

**Environmental Protections.** Since falls and other injuries become more common again in later years, elders—and others—should be protected by providing the following (Haber, 1994):

- provide plenty of light where there are steps or slopes,

- install handrails on stairs if there are none,

- apply adhesive strips or a rough surface in bathtubs and showers,

- install strong bars to hold onto in the bathroom,

- use floor coatings that do not get slippery when wet,

- lay down rugs that do not slide,

- exercise regularly to improve leg strength and balance.

Where heating or cooking involves fire, take fire safety precautions—have extinguishing materials such as water, sand, and/or fire extinguishers always at hand. Make it easy to escape quickly from any room to the outside. Remember that those at highest risk of death from smoke and fire are infants, the disabled, and the very old.

## PRESERVING PHYSICAL AND MENTAL FUNCTIONING

For centuries, people believed that the calendar beat the drum in the later years, and that our lives inevitably unraveled into functional decline. Recent social-behavioral studies that follow large groups of older persons over time have clearly changed that belief, however. Now we know that it is we, ourselves, not the calendar, who control the drumbeat and change the rate of our biopsychosocial aging. Any group of people celebrating their 80th birthdays will reveal a range of capacities and functions matching averages for people all the way from ages 65 to 95 years old. Again, the older the group, the greater their range of differences (Rowe and Kahn, 1998).

*All the studies, both of rapid deterioration of health and of successful active aging, can be summarized in a single "prescription": "Use it, or lose it."*

All the studies, both of rapid deterioration of health and of successful active aging, can be summarized in a single "prescription": "Use it, or lose it."

Physical capacity is maintained by regular physical exercise. Hand dexterity and coordination is helped by continually using those skills. Capacity for long walks is retained—as are tennis-playing skills—by doing it. Verbal fluency is helped by reading, doing word puzzles, and discussing new topics. Numeric skills are maintained by doing arithmetic.

Very often, but by no means always, older years bring a slowing of physical and mental performance. With practice, however, people can compensate for the slowing by working longer and with more concentration. Short-term memory also declines (e.g., for names, what one needs from the store, what one did last week), but less rapidly in busy brains than in those left passive.

Rowe and Kahn (1998) cover a list of conditions that strengthen and extend mental capacities in the later years, which are listed below.

## PROTECTIVE FACTORS FOR MENTAL ABILITIES

- Having had longer education as a youth. The effects of longer education persist for more than 50 years in an increased level of mental processing skills, logical thinking, and fund of knowledge as one enters older age; and in a slower decline in mental performance skills during later years.

- Continuing to engage in "cognitive exercise" by tackling complex tasks at the high end of one's capabilities.

- Maintaining a sense of self-efficacy: the belief, faith, and action that "I can do what is necessary or expected"—never giving up without a good try.

- Engaging in regular physical activity that makes one breathe harder and one's heart beat faster.

- Maintaining good lung function through physical exercise. Healthy breathing capacity helps fill blood hemoglobin with oxygen, thus keeping brain cells functioning well.

- Maintaining regular interaction with others. The daily exchange of information and feelings keeps one's sense of reality accurately tuned, exercises social and language skills, modulates the excitatory and inhibitory functions, and probably does much more.

## TREATING PAIN AND SUFFERING

Health promotion and disease prevention aim to increase health and quality of life, as well as to avoid unnecessary suffering, be it mental or physical. Therapeutic medicine aims to relieve pain and restore function—that is, to heal. But

137

inevitably, science-based efforts of human professionals will no longer suffice; pain and suffering take over. But even at that point, many medications are available to effectively relieve almost all kinds of suffering in critical, terminal injury or disease. Modern hospice care has found new levels and timing of dosage of medications that relieve pain, nausea, and other suffering more effectively than most hospital care has achieved in the past. Physicians must learn the newer pain relieving methods and be more willing to use them. Even dying people should not be required to suffer when relief is available. Relieving suffering is the last great gift health professionals can give to those for whom they care.

The major tasks of health professionals who care for persons in the final years of life are to relieve physical and emotional pain, prevent or ameliorate loss of function, and reconnect persons to some kind of "family," so that this part of life's journey need not be traveled alone.

To some professionals reconnecting older persons to other people may seem frivolous, or a luxury for rich nations. Actually, it is both humane and cost-effective no matter what the economic circumstances. People living alone at every age have higher death rates than those who live and interact with others. Research into the health effects of social support is unanimous in showing that positive interpersonal interactions lower older persons' risk of death and postpone their descent into disability, thus generating more healthy life-years. Many older people, especially women, have lost their spouses through death, and their adult children may be geographically scattered or otherwise unable to help them. Communities designed for older people and assisted-living facilities serve to recreate interacting, mutually supportive groups.

Many cultures hold on to the tradition in which adult children's families care for elderly family members. This may well be the most health-promoting system of all for the elderly. There may be some strains on the younger family, but multiple adult children may split the responsibility and the time, and thus lighten the load.

Belonging to groups also enhances health. Religious congregations, shared interest groups, informal gatherings of neighbors—all have been shown to increase healthy years lived. People in such groups tend to look after one another. Feeling needed by others in the group can give an older person, with all his/her former goals now in the past, new reasons to be active, to take better care of oneself, and still to contribute to the well-being of others. In fact, even taking care of infants in the family can have a salutary effect for all three generations.

## COMMUNITY ACTION FOR OLDER CITIZENS

Most of the preventive measures and health screenings recommended above are worded from a clinical perspective. Fortunately, many of the elderly's needs can be partially served by community level activities. Group health education programs, simple screening tests, and referrals can be organized by community agencies, hospital outreach programs, churches, senior citizen groups, retirement homes, and neighborhoods.

The group approach to lifestyle changes has a powerful advantage—a friendly group of people who share similar needs can more effectively teach and motivate each other, better sharpen their skills by imitation and repetition, and reward each other for keeping up a healthier lifestyle. A friendly group achieves this much more subtly, comprehensively, and powerfully than any doctor, nurse, teacher, or expert can, because people often perceive those outsiders from their group as different from them.

These sorts of self-help groups often are started by a health professional and gradually are turned over to group leaders. WHO now recognizes the self-help movement in all its forms as an important vehicle for advancing "health for all." Groups may focus on regular exercise; for example a weight loss club could meet every day to walk a kilometer together. Older persons who have suffered bereavement could meet with others passing through the same "rough seas" to discuss practical and emotional issues involved in adjusting to the death of a loved one. The group would help mourning elders to shift focus from the past, and to plan how to "live forward" and manage a new life on their own. Sharing these experiences can help alleviate depression; it does not make it worse. By walking and talking together or pursuing physically active pastimes, group members help counter depression physiologically.

Social losses and depressive episodes occur with increasing frequency in the older years. The natural antidote is participating in groups that share common interests or hobbies, do active things together, share meals or refreshments, provide a "change of scenery" for people who live alone, and supply a network of social support. The giving and receiving of support is reciprocal; givers and receivers change roles as circumstances fluctuate. Very often the giver is helped even more than the receiver. (Further documentation and "how to" guidance for creating supportive groups is presented in Haber, 1994.)

According to a United States Institute of Medicine report (Rowe and Kahn, 1998), the keys to successful aging are:

- keeping the body active

- keeping the brain active

- maintaining and extending social relationships

The community also can promote health in the elder years by:

- providing, or encouraging others to provide, places where older people can meet and share activities,

- periodically providing simple health promotion and screening where seniors congregate,

- encouraging managers of business and public buildings to make them accessible to disabled or frail persons,

- adopting and enforcing health, safety, and quality-of-care standards for group homes, and

- enlisting the cooperation of organizations, schools, media, churches, and other transmitters of values to make the community's way of life more "elderly-friendly."

# PART III.
# BETTER UNDERSTANDING THE LEADING FORMS OF DEATH AND DISABILITY

# 7. Brain and Behavioral Disorders

Why should the discussion of these disorders precede that of such major killers as cardiovascular disorders and malignant neoplasms? There are several powerful reasons.

- First, because changing thinking, motivations, and behaviors—all of them brain functions—is a gateway to preventing most diseases and disabilities in all organ systems. Genetic makeup and various aspects of the environment also play roles, as later described.

- Second, because these difficult, though low technology, health behavior changes must be sustained over decades and through generations. Societies urgently need to continue updating health beliefs and behaviors to keep in step with a rapidly changing world. Locally and globally, we must continue to adapt or become extinct.

- Third, because a "healthy body" living in the shadows of depression, surrounded by invisible fears, struggling to overcome deep neuroses, captured by addictions to alcohol or drugs, or imprisoned by a brain gone psychotic or demented is condemned to live a diminished, disabled life full of deep personal pain, a life that soaks up more social capital than the afflicted person can ever produce.

- And, fourth, because all the ideals for human life, all prescriptions for a "life well-lived" given by spiritual leaders and philosophers since ancient times, call for the foundation of a healthy mind, and an untroubled spirit housed in a healthy body.

## DISABILITIES OF BRAIN AND BEHAVIOR

The Global Burden of Disease (GBD) Study (Murray and Lopez, 1994, 1996) has developed an index—Disability Adjusted Life Years (DALYs)—that combines years of life lost due to death (as integers) and years of life disabled (as fractions, with larger fractions given to greater degrees of damaged function). Thus, long-lasting disabilities such as blindness, psychiatric disorders, and crippling, can be included in reckoning the burden that nonfatal and fatal conditions place upon individuals, communities, and the world.

The GBD Study reports that neuropsychiatric disorders are responsible for the greatest proportion (22%) of all lost DALYs in the industrially developed world.

These disorders rank fourth in the developing world (9%). The following psychiatric categories, followed by their ranking in parentheses, are among the 30 leading specific diagnoses (considering all causes) for lost DALYs worldwide: unipolar major depression (ranked 4); self-inflicted injuries, including suicide (17); violence or intentional harm to others (19); alcohol abuse (20); bipolar disorder, manic, depressed (22); and schizophrenia and similar psychoses (26).

Mental deficiency should be added to the list. Although the epidemiologic study of mental deficiency is far from complete, according to many studies the reported prevalence of severe mental retardation—an IQ or equivalent below 50—ranges between 3 and 5 per 1,000 population in industrialized countries, and is considerably higher (5–17 per 1,000) in developing countries. Case finding of mild mental retardation (defined as an IQ or local equivalent measure between 50 to 70) is unreliable, unless population-wide testing is performed. Under the conservative assumption that mild deviations from normal occur far more often than extreme deviations, the prevalence of mild retardation is expected to be higher than that of severe retardation. Roeleveld and colleagues (1997) estimated that about 3% (30 per 1,000) of school age children are mentally retarded, and that a "considerable proportion" of these cases is preventable.[1]

> *All prescriptions for a "life well-lived" given by spiritual leaders and philosophers since ancient times call for the foundation of a healthy mind, and an untroubled spirit housed in a healthy body.*

In parallel work using a different indicator—Years of Life with Disability (YLD)—GBD researchers also place neuropsychiatric disorders as the major health problem in developed nations, accounting for 27% of all YLD (although only for 1.4% of deaths), outranking YLD for cardiovascular disorders (17%) and malignant neoplasms (11%) in both sexes and all ages combined. Disability from neuropsychiatric disorders reaches its peak in the age-span 15–44 years and declines in the older ages.

In developing nations neuropsychiatric disorders cause a surprisingly high percentage of a much larger total of YLD. Infections and parasitic diseases, for example, cause 18% of disability, and neuropsychiatric disorders rank second with 15%. Thus, neuropsychiatric disorders are crushing causes of impaired living worldwide, far outdistancing not only cardiovascular disorders and cancers, but also unintentional injuries and musculoskeletal disorders. Even more worrisome, GBD projections for 2020 estimate that unipolar major depression, as a specific diagnosis, will be the greatest cause of lost DALYs in the developing world, and the third greatest in developed regions. Other causes of disability are decreasing, but these clearly are not (Murray and Lopez, 1994, 1997).

---

[1] A review of field studies, contributing causes, and preventive goals for developing regions has been prepared by Hosking G and Murphy G (eds.), *Prevention of Mental Handicap: A World View.* Royal Society of Medicine Services, International Congress and Symposium Series No. 112, 1987.

## WHO IS VULNERABLE?

People of all ages and all cultures can fall prey to disorders of brain and behavior. Nor are these solely the problems of humans. Even higher animals show responses curiously similar to depression (after defeat by another animal), anxiety (when in an unfamiliar place), and even some delinquency and anti-social behavior. In behavioral laboratories, experimental neuroses have been conditioned into many species, and then relieved, which shows that neuropsychiatric disorders are not the fault of the sufferer, nor should parents and family be blamed.

Neuropsychiatric difficulties are liabilities that come most easily to the human brain—the most complicated, most subdivided, and most creative system on earth. The human brain's billions of parts work nobly, most of the time, for about 5.5 to 5.8 billion of the estimated 6.2 billion people in the world. Among adults in the 1990s, however, 6% to 10% had serious, severe, or persistent psychiatric disorders.[2] And estimates are similar for persons aged 9–17 years, with 5% to 9% of this age group affected. According to several references, rates of severe mental disorders are similar in developing and developed countries. When moderate, only partially disabling, psychiatric disorders are included in the prevalence figures, rates about double.[3] The figures from the US *Federal Register* show prevalence rates of severe and moderate disorders combined to be 20% to 24%.

All these estimates are, of course, greatly influenced by which diagnostic definitions or settings of severity threshold are used, by the design of the sampling methods, and by socioeconomic, national, or cultural considerations. But regardless of which estimates are accepted, the impact of neuropsychiatric disorders is far greater than generally realized, with somewhere between 370 million and 660 million persons seriously disabled worldwide. The vast majority of them are never diagnosed professionally and never treated. Can this performance record be improved? The scenario of healthy development detailed below suggests it can.

## A HEALTHY SCENARIO

Like every organ system, the brain and its functions are shaped by genetics, by the biological milieu, and by exposures to protective and damaging forces.

In an ideal world, every new life would begin with two physically and psychologically healthy parents, whose genetically close family is free of mental illness, mental retardation, and social pathology. In the real world, of course, genetically

---

[2] Substance Abuse and Mental Health Services Administration. Estimation methodology for adults with serious mental illness. US *Federal Register:* Vol. 64, No. 121, 24 June, 1999.

[3] Substance Abuse and Mental Health Services Administration. Estimation methodology for adults with serious mental illness. US *Federal Register:* Vol. 62, No. 193, 6 October, 1997.

based disabilities and vulnerabilities may be passed on, with the risk being higher when blood relations have children together.

In order to flourish, the fetus requires a well-nourished intrauterine life that is free of toxins, infections, and metabolic abnormalities. The pregnancy should then culminate in a delivery free of infection, oxygen deficiency, and any forms of permanent damage. The human fetus is very sensitive to toxic and infectious exposures, as well as to oxygen and nutritional deficiencies in utero. All trimesters of pregnancy can be vulnerable, but the first trimester is especially so, because the basic development of the central nervous system is most rapid then. Fetal insults during the second trimester have recently been associated with somewhat higher risk of schizophrenia. **(See the section on improving health in pregnancy in Chapter 3.)** A mother's use of alcohol and illicit drugs during pregnancy, even in small amounts, can cause irreversible neurologic damage in the fetus. Tobacco use leads to low birthweight babies who are at higher risk for brain damage, which, in turn, can lead to behavioral problems, including attention-deficit hyperactivity disorders. Maternal infections or malnutrition can have similar damaging effects.

Before birth the only communication to the baby is through biochemical channels, except for rare instances of physical bruising. Even psychosocial "events" can only reach the baby in the uterus through biochemical, endocrine, and cytokine channels. After birth, all other environmental expressions—sights, sounds, smells, feeding, touching, comforting, people's expressed emotions, recognition of gestures and language—communicate to the infant and influence the brain's synaptic connections, neurotransmitter responses, and endocrine ebb and flow. The products of these processes receive the more familiar names of knowing, feeling, thinking, and expecting.

Nurturing takes several forms: providing milk and food to meet nutritional needs; passing on the mother's antibodies and other immune substances through breast milk to "program" the infant's immunological system; and providing comforting, security, love, relief of discomfort and pain, and stimulation to program the neural and psychological systems. Interestingly, social nurturing can lessen the effects of biological limitations, and learning to cope can protect from social stress. The system is integrated.

New research into the molecular biology of brain function demonstrates that early deprivation of mothering changes the brain chemical levels in both animals and humans. Elevations in cortisol and deficits in serotonin can continue for years in human children. In baby rats, those with environments that have stimulation by peers and objects to manipulate develop 30% more nerve cell connections in their brains than those caged alone. It even appears that a very nurturing mother (at least in rhesus monkeys) can modify the action—and the size—of genes in the infant brain. This finding runs against the long-held assumption that a person's genetic template remains immutable, except for rare damaging mutations (Suomi, 1999).

Positive interpersonal, social, cultural, and ideological environments can teach an infant to trust, love, care for others, and have hope for the future; the converse can instill fear, hurt, despair, suspicion, anger, and the expectation that other people are threatening. A child's immediate family is critical—it should screen and protect the child from damaging stimuli and experiences early in life, guarding the child until basic trust, values, and attitudes have been well-established, before gradually, and in dosages that the child can handle, exposing him or her to more destructive aspects of reality.

Parents can extend their nurturing of mental and physical health by selecting safe, dependable, gentle, and child-centered child care, whether inside or outside the home. A child—in fact, everyone—learns more quickly and enduringly when rewarded for desirable responses, rather than when punished for undesirable ones. And not only are specific behaviors learned, but also attitudes toward others, objects, and themselves that can make individuals and groups eager and able to continue positive learning throughout life.

For older children and adolescents, the family and community can encourage their building peer groups with constructive values and behaviors and discourage their association with harmful groups. Schools and communities, too,

> **A child's immediate family is critical—it should screen and protect the child from damaging stimuli and experiences early in life.**

can work to limit the intrusion of displays of violence, destructive health habits, and antisocial values and behavior into young people's lives, influences that often come through mass media. To their own detriment, people of all ages tend to copy those behaviors that appear to be glamorous or immediately gratifying rather than those that are most beneficial in the long run. Just as good parenting prevents children from eating poisoned food, so it should prevent them from consuming poisoned ideas.

## TEASING OUT THE CAUSES OF BRAIN AND BEHAVIORAL DISORDERS

In the mid-1990s, the United States Institute of Medicine published *Reducing Risks for Mental Disorders: Frontiers for Preventive Intervention Research*. Based on extensive scientific review, the authors recommended preventive programs for mental disorders that relied on the same strategy that has proven so successful with other diseases—the reduction of risk factors and the increase of protective factors on a community-wide scale (Mrazek and Haggerty (eds.), 1994). This publication addresses five illustrative disorders—conduct disorders, depression, alcohol abuse, schizophrenia, and Alzheimer's disease. In addition, three more conditions are responsible for much loss of healthy life years worldwide—self-inflicted injuries, violence, and bipolar disorder (Murray and Lopez, 1996). Because these eight disorders have overlapping risk and protective factors, this chapter will present preventive strategies for their general "contributing causes and partial protectors," rather than trying to deal with each diagnosis separately.

The very nature of behavioral and mental disorders makes it difficult to study them, to identify their specific causes and cures over repeated studies, to treat them successfully, and, certainly, to prevent them. But these research and prevention difficulties are informative in and of themselves, because they help identify the processes that underlie the most common neuropsychiatric disorders: (1) the involvement of multiple contributing causes, no one or two of which are essential for the disease to occur; (2) the interaction of damaging and protective factors such that some protective factors can cancel out the effects of some risk factors, and vice versa; and (3) the common sources of influence for behavioral and neuropsychiatric disorders in most populations. These interacting forces are detailed in the box below.

---

**SOURCES THAT INFLUENCE THE RISK OF BRAIN AND BEHAVIORAL DISORDERS**

- Genetic strengths and vulnerabilities;
- Intrauterine environment;
- Perinatal circumstances;
- Neuropsychological integrity vs. deficits;
- Chronic physical illness or injury disability vs. average health;
- A child's temperament and adaptability (easy vs. difficult);
- A child's ability to learn (intelligence);
- Parental care (quality, quantity, consistency);
- Family environment (including siblings, crowding, housing conditions);
- Social context (average or disadvantaged, including or lacking infrastructure);
- Community stability vs. disorganization (e.g., crime, broken families, transience);
- Quality of schools (e.g., safe, stimulating, responsive to local needs);
- Peer group relationships: nature of supports and values;
- Continuing attachment to parents and others in extended family;
- Social support from caring friends; and
- Cultural-ideological exposures.

---

Another problem inherent to neuropsychiatric research is that any specific, pre-existing deficit that is coupled with any specific immediate trauma or stressor can release different symptom profiles and, hence, different diagnoses. For example, long continuing parent-child conflict is a risk factor for depression, alcohol abuse, and conduct disorder; and low education is reported to be more common in persons who develop alcohol dependence, depression, and, much later, Alzheimer's disease.

While there remain many loose ends and paradoxes in the current state of research knowledge—and all suggestions here deserve more definitive proof—we can still unequivocally say that: *"Deficits and traumas, when not offset by enough of the right protective influences, raise the risk of mental disorders in general; and such disorders can take many forms of expression."*

Although this assertion is scientifically loose and incomplete, it still provides some guidance for interventions. The following analogy perhaps can help to illuminate its utility.

As any small-boat sailor knows, a tropical storm can sink his craft, but he also knows that a good pump to bail out water will help keep the boat afloat. Let's say strong gusty winds and waves come and sink the boat. The sailor may not know exactly which wave made the final difference, which wind gust tipped the boat too far, or what, if anything, was wrong with the pump. Nevertheless, the sailor has learned some important lessons in "sinking prevention and survival promotion," namely: to avoid extremely strong winds (stay in port, stay downwind of a high cliff); avoid extremely high waves (stay in shallower water); keep water out of the boat (install sideboards to keep most water from getting into the hull, get a stronger pump); or resort to a combination of the above.

To date, research into mental disorders is in much the same boat. The details—was it a wave or a wind that sank the boat?—predict almost nothing specific. Moreover, relatively few mental disorder prevention programs with rigorous design have proven such details beyond doubt. Nevertheless, the principles presented here may serve as lighthouses by offering general directions for future research and pilot programs.

Suppose there were a comprehensive prenatal and perinatal program that could reach every population segment in a province—rich and poor, urban and rural, minorities and majorities. If the program reaches 20,000 pregnant women and prevents 1,000 prenatal viral infections, 1,000 toxic exposures to alcohol, tobacco, or drugs, and 500 delivery complications, these 2,500 "preventions" might, in turn, prevent two or three schizophrenias, a handful of conduct disorders, 20 mental deficiencies, and a dozen each of alcohol dependencies and chronic depressive disorders. Such a maternal health program is not the answer to preventing mental disorders or to preventing congenital anomalies, but it is a step in both these directions, and perhaps more. Preventing more mental disorders will take time and many other small steps. Social change advances just that way: many small steps by many people (physicians, nurses, women, men, community officials, teachers, mass media) in many places. Indeed, the whole process of disease prevention and health promotion is one of social and behavioral change.

## ELEVEN CROSSROADS WHERE RISK AND PROTECTIVE FACTORS MEET[4]

Just as an inspiring mosaic can be assembled from shovels-full of small, scattered, colorful stones, a mosaic of improved mental health can be created by many people coming together to share their vision, insight, and flexibility. A review of the research literature identifies eleven circumstances—times or places—in which risk of mental disorders can be changed. By counteracting risk and moving toward protection at each crossroad, family and community mental health can be improved.

### GENETIC STRENGTHS AND VULNERABILITIES

Couples usually have children who look much like themselves and who also share their temperament and mental skills. When people select mates similar to themselves, this can either double the benefit or double the trouble, especially

*A mosaic of improved mental health can be created by many people coming together to share their vision, insight, and flexibility.*

if both mates carry genetic deficiencies (for field study data see Reddy, in Hosking and Murphy (eds.), 1987). The genetic transmission of neuropsychiatric vulnerability raises the chances for developing major depression, bipolar disorder, schizophrenia, alcohol abuse, or severe mental deficiency. Genetic factors are not "simple causes" of these disorders, however; they merely "tilt the table" toward or away from these health outcomes. Self-inflicted injury and suicide usually occur in a context of major depression, and they show some familial aggregation, often via copying the behavior of some other family member. There also is some evidence that criminality may be inheritable as well as learned. Many anatomic and physiologic attributes also are at least partially determined by genetic influences—and these, in turn, shape behavior.

What can be done in terms of prevention? For those already born, programs can attempt to reduce the harmful genetic influence by increasing protective factors in the physical and human environments. It must always be kept in mind that for many conditions that do not involve dominant genes, half or more of offspring will not manifest their parents' condition, especially where the condition is determined by multiple gene locations. Genetic predisposition is neither a

---

[4] Many resources contributed to this section. Of special note were Mrazek and Haggerty (eds.), 1994; Matzen and Lang (eds.), 1993, especially Chapter 10, by Bennetts; and Rutter, 1985.

necessary nor sufficient explanation for the majority of mental disorders in any community. Dealing with this source of risk cannot be the cornerstone of a comprehensive preventive program.

## THE INTRAUTERINE ENVIRONMENT

The uterus is one of the safest environments most persons have ever had, with the mother's body providing an extraordinary degree of protection from physical, chemical, and microbiological insults. The fetus's nutritional needs are, for the most part, well covered. Minor deficiencies in the mother's diet can be compensated for by calling on reserves from the mother's body. Major or protracted deficiencies will exact a price from both the mother and the fetus, so adequate nutrition is essential for both physical and neuropsychological health.

The mother's acquired immunities will be passed on to the fetus, but new infections that the mother's system cannot neutralize will affect the baby. Consequently, a prospective mother must be immunized prior to pregnancy to prevent permanent damage from rubella, tetanus, and STIs (including syphilis, gonorrhea, chlamydia, HIV, and hepatitis B). Guidelines in obstetrical and infectious disease textbooks should be followed for the type and timing of immunizations and antitoxins.

Toxins can pass through the placenta and damage the fetus. The most common toxins are byproducts of tobacco smoking, such as carbon monoxide, nicotine, and other carcinogens. Another is alcohol, which in small amounts causes minor damage to the fetal brain and in large amounts causes the permanently damaging fetal alcohol syndrome. "Recreational" or illegal drugs can be particularly toxic, causing permanent neurological damage to the fetus. And sometimes, therapeutic medications also can be toxic to the fetus. Professionals giving prenatal care should compile a list appropriate to the local situation. Moreover, folk remedies should be scrutinized carefully as some contain toxic metallic salts. Finally, eating non-food substances (i.e., clay or mud) might be harmful, depending on their chemistry.

## THE PERINATAL EXPERIENCE

Carrying pregnancy to its full 40-week duration is important to the health of most of a baby's physiologic systems. Babies born prematurely or at low weight for fetal age are very vulnerable. Low birthweight babies (under 2,500 g) are at risk for congenital anomalies, respiratory distress, and neurobehavioral complications. Low birthweight babies have twice the risk of later behavior problems in school and school failure as do normal weight babies. When combined with a high-risk social environment, low birthweight babies' risk soars to fourfold that of normal weight babies. Low birthweight also has been associated with mental deficiency, cerebral palsy, and higher infant mortality.

Delivery complications include protracted duration of delivery leading to anoxia; toxic or infectious exposures; instrumental deliveries that put excessive pressure on the baby's soft skull; and too early or too heavy use of anesthetics, analgesics, or oxytoxics. An impaired fetus also may complicate delivery. It is easy to see how each of these could damage the brain, a baby's most vulnerable organ.

All the circumstances discussed, as well as other, less common ones, can lead to neuropsychological deficits, but fortunately they do not always do so. When such deficit occurs, however, it becomes a general risk factor for later behavioral and mental problems of various forms (Mrazek and Haggerty, 1994).

## COPING WITH CHRONIC ILLNESS OR INJURY DISABILITY

These conditions weaken overall resilience and adaptive capacity, and expose a young child to the stress of medical care, restricted activity, and hospitalization away from parents and home. This stress has been associated with a double to triple increase in the risk of conduct disorder and with a significant, but perhaps weaker, association with future depression. Childhood is a high-risk time for injuries due to vehicles, falls, poisonings, and child abuse. These frequently leave post-traumatic stress disorders in their wake. If such trauma leaves a baby, child, or youth disfigured or disabled, that, too, will leave enduring psychological, interpersonal, and perhaps occupational limitations.

Repeated blows to the head can be disabling: shaking or banging of the head at any age can cause concussions of varying severity and small hemorrhages in the brain. Moreover, young men who get involved in street fighting or boxing may sustain repeated blows to the head that could cause brain damage ("dementia

---

**HOW TO COPE WITH THE RISKS OF CHRONIC ILLNESS OR DISABILITY**

- Find a child's special skill and encourage it, so the child can build self-esteem based on that talent.
- Stay as close as possible with the child during medical treatments or hospitalizations to minimize separation anxiety.
- Involve the child in activities with other children, so that he does not feel isolated or different.
- Encourage the child fully to use his or her capabilities and skills.
- Maintain behavioral expectations and rules appropriate to the child's limitations and capacities, so as to build self-control and a sense of responsibility.
- Seriously retarded or autistic youngsters who may bang their heads repeatedly should wear protective head coverings, or nearby surfaces should be covered with padding.

pugilistica"), which raises the risk for early Alzheimer's dementia. Obviously, this, too, is preventable.

## TEMPERAMENT AND ADAPTABILITY

The determinants of temperament still live in the caves of the unknown. Neurologic damage is one accepted cause of irritability, shortened attention span, easy loss of emotional control in the face of frustration, and unpredictable loss of temper, yet these problems spread far beyond those persons with any suspicion of neural damage.

Temperament and adaptability are not easily changeable, it seems, but they can help chart the course for successful parenting. Clearly, a difficult child who is less adaptable to change requires more thoughtful, more adaptable, and more persevering parenting. And, because such children's capacities to adapt can vary greatly in the course of the day, parents—and eventually teachers—must stay alert to the child's emotional and coping status at a given moment. They must start at that point, and work incrementally to build, over time, the child's capacity to cope with and master more and different situations, praising the child for calmness, self-control, and problem-solving efforts.

## ABILITY TO LEARN

This capacity refers not only to "book learning," but also to emotional learning, self-management, and social learning in interaction with adults and children. Basic intelligence is, of course, of major importance, but even if cognitive capacity is below average, it may be other factors that limit what is actually learned. Emotional lability, attention deficits, or hyperactivity may be controlled with medication or conditioning procedures, so as to open the child to full use of his/her cognitive capacities.

*Learning means replacing old ideas, feelings, and behaviors with new ones that bring positive rewards or reduce discomforts. Learning is the key to developing into a whole person, to becoming able to adapt more easily to a changing self in a changing world.*

## PARENTAL CARE

Parenting and family relations include the interactions of mother and father with each other and with each child; the relations of brothers and sisters with one another; and the involvement of relatives, other household members, and the extended family; plus the total environment parents provide for the children—physical, biological, interpersonal, socioeconomic, and cultural-ideological.

The United States Institute of Medicine Committee on the Prevention of Mental Disorders in 1994 implicated deficient or disturbed parenting in raising the risk for major depression, conduct disorders (behavioral disorders), and alcohol abuse. Most studies cannot separate the fraction of risk conferred by genetics from the fraction transmitted by experiencing troubled parenting or conflicts in the home; nevertheless, the frequency of more serious disorders in young people who have not had a family history of related problems argues that the psychosocial aspects of family relations by themselves can confer serious risk.

Instructive research conducted mostly in industrialized countries shows that boys who grow up in single-mother families display more aggressive behaviors and more school learning problems than boys from the same neighborhoods who live with both parents. Families headed by a mother, living with a male partner who is neither the child's parent nor the mother's husband, generated even more aggressive behavior, on average, in young boys studied in United States communities. Broken families also are detrimental to girls' adjustment and behavior, but less so. The functional pathways leading to these problems have not been proven, but lower income, parenting distress in the mother, and reduced adult supervision of the children seem likely to be contributing causes (Pearson et al., 1994).

Usually, the breakdowns in family structure cannot be prevented at the individual level, but social and community policies and practices might be changed to reduce their overall frequency in the community. Where broken families are common in a community, the children exposed to this social risk can be supported, in part, by such mentoring programs (usually non-governmental) as community "big brother/big sister" programs, after-school skills and sports programs led by caring adults, and fun programs sponsored by civic clubs or religious groups that provide teaching, social skills training, and practice in behavioral self-control. Such protective factors can often help compensate for unchangeable risk factors.

The protective, health-promoting power of parental care cannot be overstated. Too often, when all other risk factors have been shown inapplicable, parents are blamed as the only remaining "cause" of an offspring's mental problems. Even when true—and often they are not—such explanations are rarely therapeutic. It is more useful instead to try to find ways to build healthier, happier, more stress-resistant people. Workers in this field emphasize three aspects of good parenting, as detailed below.

### Quality

A parent's (and any adult's, for that matter) interaction with a child should be helpful and loving. Parents should be attuned to a child's developmental stage, personal strengths and weaknesses, and likes and dislikes. Adults' gestures should reach out, lift up, and lead along; they should not push forward, put down, disparage, or reject. The parent should provide structure and correction, yet be patient. A parent's role is demanding and requires maturity. All the more reason that anyone who is still physically, mentally, or emotionally immature should be strongly discouraged from having children.

## Quantity

Children require a sufficient amount of personal interaction with friendly, giving, noncompetitive others whom they can trust. These ingredients teach children who they themselves are. An uncertain, malleable mind-body is being shaped into a person every waking and sleeping hour, and this happens by learning, feeling, storing, and processing biopsychosocial memories. By definition, this requires time every day. Please handle with care! Provide enough interaction to fill the child's hunger for contact, meaning, acceptance, guidance, learning, and relearning. Babies and children differ greatly in their hunger for loving contact—give accordingly.

## Consistency

We all function better and save emotional energy if we know what to expect—we can then be ready for what's next. Uncertainty and fear make us feel at risk, tense, and rather ineffective or incompetent. Kids are no different, although they may not be able to put it into words. Provide a predictable social environment in which it is easy for a child to learn what to do.

A child can predict—adapt, even—to a parent who is always emotionally cold, or to a parent who is always too busy to pay attention. But it becomes much tougher when the parent swings unpredictably from warm to cold, from overly attentive to rejecting. Adult situations and feelings can, of course, change day to day, but parents should openly explain this to children in age appropriate ways. For younger children—indeed, for anybody—it is vital to communicate, especially nonverbally, that whatever happens inside or outside the family, the constancy of caring and valuing between parent and children does not change.

*Usually, the breakdowns in family structure cannot be prevented at the individual level, but social and community policies and practices might be changed to reduce their overall frequency in the community.*

Fortunately, parents need not "be cured" of their own problems and weaknesses. It is enough that they be taught—with their motivation being the main limiting factor—to:

* seek help when they or their children can benefit from it—they shouldn't wait until the situation becomes a crisis;

- set aside as much of their weaknesses and turmoil as possible from their interaction with their children;

- seek social support in their parenting and get information, practical help (baby-sitting, doing an errand), emotional support (sharing feelings), and a sense of belonging to a group (of parents or grandparents, of neighbors or friends) who have faced, or are facing, similar family problems.

An advantage of an extended family, or its urban equivalent of close relations among neighboring families, is that if one parent has a problem or weakness, or one child has a special need, other adults can "fill in" to meet those needs. If both parents work outside the home, grandparents, biological or adopted, can fill in needed parenting. The Western "nuclear" family style, with one or two parents and one or more children living alone far from other concerned and caring people, is a particularly vulnerable arrangement.

## FAMILY AND SOCIAL CONTEXT

Parents also are responsible for ensuring that anything that comes in contact with the family is safe and friendly to growth. The home should protect against extreme temperature, rain, or snow and must be filled with clean air; keep out insects, rodents, and vectors of disease; and be free of wastes, poisons, and causes of injury **(also see Chapter 3)**. Each child also needs to be nurtured long enough as "the baby of the family," in order to grow and develop physically, emotionally, and cognitively to adapt adequately to the coming of the next baby. Two or more years is the recommended interval. Siblings need to have parents show them by example how to be caring, loving, and supportive of each other.

The value of the home's cultural-ideological atmosphere cannot be quantified—it is priceless. Things that money can buy, such as modern appliances and televisions—are not part of the family culture. Rather, family culture is made up of attitudes, ways of relating, behaviors, and expectations regarding others' responses—values that can overcome poverty and community chaos, and help build healthy children and adults. If young children are cared for outside the home, these settings, too, should show the same qualities. These outside settings can sometimes even offset deficiencies in the culture of the home by providing a caring consistent experience. The safe and nurturing home or place of care is a stronghold of protection against many sources of risk.

A safe, comfortable neighborhood with a high proportion of friendly interactions clearly provides a protective factor (now called social capital), but poverty by itself need not be a risk factor for mental or physical disorder. This has been shown repeatedly in many poor rural areas or poor ethnic sections in cities, which held onto their community and family integration and promoted health and well being. A community's social capital is composed of a shared sense of responsibility for others, trust in others, willingness to help others, and social participation. High social capital nurtures healthy psychosocial growth at all ages.

## SCHOOL ENVIRONMENT

The transition from home or day-care setting to school is an important step in growing up. Children's distress in making this step can be reduced by caring teachers and by keeping classes relatively small—the pupil-teacher ratio should be lower in the first year than in later years. The teacher—as does the mother—has a labor intensive job, and small classes help ensure every child's successful transition into community-living. Parents and teachers should recognize that a child has much to learn emotionally and interpersonally at ages 5 to 6 years, and that children's readiness varies greatly at these ages.

The school's responsibility goes far beyond imparting information to children. Perhaps its most important task is to teach children how to interact comfortably and cooperate constructively with one another. Studies by personnel departments of large businesses have typically shown that about 80% of those fired from their jobs have been discharged for interpersonal or behavioral reasons; fewer than 20% are dismissed for lack of skills. Clearly, schools must do a better job with social learning. Schools also must teach children how to keep on learning after they finish school. This is more essential than ever if schools are to prepare children for life in a changing world. Good schools have been shown by research to be a positive ingredient for mental health.

A body of research already shows that risk factors can be identified, as early as age 6 years, which foretell higher rates of antisocial behavior, delinquency, and illicit drug and tobacco use. Chief among these risk predictors are aggressive, oppositional behavior and poor school performance, particularly if it is associated with attention deficit or lack of self-control (reviewed in Mrazek and Haggerty, 1994; see also Kellam and Anthony, 1998, regarding several large longitudinal studies on children from major United States cities). This raises the question of whether screening for higher risk of adolescent behavior problems should be done in the first year or two of primary school, at ages 5–7 years. Of course, screening is useless unless follow-up is provided.

A simple teacher-managed intervention—the "Good Behavior Game"—is available, and it shows some promise. The game is described in full in the box on the next page.

## PEER GROUPS

Just before adolescence, a child begins to identify with a group of children about his or her age or slightly older as a preferred reference group—this is the peer

## THE "GOOD BEHAVIOR GAME"

The "Good Behavior Game" was developed in the late 1960s by H. H. Barrish and his colleagues (1969) and further developed by L. J. Dolan and his colleagues (1989). In brief (as described by Kellam and Anthony, 1998), it consists of dividing a classroom's children into small groups, say 6 to 8 children aged 5–8 years old. The groups should have roughly the same number of girls and boys and the same proportion of unruly children, so no one team has an advantage. The teacher posts a list of undesirable classroom behaviors, such as shouting, bullying another child, provoking a fight, damaging property, and talking when silence is requested. Teams are rewarded when no team member lapses into any listed undesirable behavior for the duration of the game. Simple rewards are given to the winning team(s), such as stickers or badges, a pencil, a team banner, or a treat to eat. Teams where children exhibit negative behaviors receive one or two penalty points. None, some, or all teams may win the game.

First the game is played for only 10 minute periods three times per week. Behaviors are rewarded or penalized only during these periods. Gradually, the game should be played more often, and, after more than one team regularly wins the 10-minute game, each game can be extended to 15 and then 20 minutes.

At about this time rewards to winning teams can be shifted gradually away from individual and material rewards to symbolic group rewards, such as being in temporary possession of a banner or having the privilege of being first in a queue. After experiencing prompt rewards for a while, children become ready for longer intervals between success and reward. Scores of all the games played in a week can be totaled, and a weekly prize given, thus teaching the children to work longer and wait longer for a payoff. This makes the game more like real life. Teachers should encourage the children to get involved in the game by adding new or lesser misbehaviors to the forbidden list, making the game more challenging and harder to win.

Do not play the game throughout the school day. Good behavior is a conditioning and learning process, and its effects will naturally spread throughout the whole school day and even outside the school setting. Teachers will observe an important side-benefit of the game—classroom behavior will improve overall.

Kellam and Anthony (1998) followed children in two randomized trials of behavioral interventions given in the first grade (ages 5–6). They found that boys who had participated in either the "Good Behavior Game" or a mastery learning program aimed at improving reading, were significantly less likely to have started smoking tobacco by age 14, compared to boys receiving only the usual classroom teaching. The interventions also produced differences among girls, but these were not adequately measured. It should be noted that neither of the interventions tested made a direct mention of tobacco use. Evaluating the impact of these interventions on other outcomes, such as school dropout or delinquent behavior in adolescence, must await longer follow-up through the high-risk years for each outcome.

This example has been presented in detail here, in order:

* to allow for cross-cultural testing of the approach;
* to stimulate the search early in childhood for risk factors for behavioral and psychosocial problems which can be modified through intervention;
* to test local and cultural adaptations of the game to see if they improve behavior;
* to determine whether such immediate changes actually reduce problems in subsequent years; and
* to show possible ways whereby primary schools can screen and provide corrective learning to reduce the risk and severity of future mental and behavioral health problems.

**This is true primary prevention given to entire classrooms of average children.**

group. The group likes to spend idle time together, with its members absorbing mutual likes and dislikes, learning new vocabulary (not always adult-approved), and trying out behaviors different from those at home. Peers become not only a source for social relationships, but a mirror for the culture and for each child in the group to see him- or herself. Youths try to reshape themselves to be more acceptable in their peers' mirror, and as they do that, they may start to look distorted from an adult's perspective. Peer group influence can lead to conduct disorders, alcohol or drug abuse, and various troubled behaviors.

*The peer-group mirror—much like a carnival or amusement park looking glass—often can distort the child's self-image and even can reflect a grotesque version of the surrounding environments, the school, and the family.*

Thus, parents, teachers, and any others who care about children—as well as the youths themselves—must help develop peer groups that share a pro-community, pro-future set of values and a supportive, affirming style of relating. Fortunately, there are many such groups active in most of the world, usually sponsored by schools, organizations that strive for community improvement, and religious groups. These groups organize appealing activities and provide adult guidance, scheduling, and other elements of structure, but remain flexible enough to adapt the program to the interests of local girls and boys.

Small, informal clusters of young friends are just as important, and perhaps even more so, in developing social and emotional skills, current interests, and future goals. Parents can work with other parents to influence the composition and activities of their children's circle of friends, especially by teaching young people skills, sports, games, or by organizing activities such as hiking, swimming, or agricultural projects (like the 4H Clubs in the United States). Parents can participate jointly in the activities until the young people have acquired enough skills to carry the activities on their own. These experiences build beliefs in self-efficacy ("I can do it") and self-esteem ("I'm OK")—both beliefs are protective against future stressors.

## ATTACHMENT TO PARENTS AND MENTORS

The above suggestion for adults to coach and participate with youth sets the stage for continuing positive relationships between generations—a boon for all involved. We all need helpful, supportive, uplifting people around us. Many epidemiologic studies show that people living in isolation develop more illnesses, both mental and physical, and are more likely to die sooner than people who regularly interact with others. Each generation has special strengths it can offer the others. Each generation has vulnerabilities for which it needs the help of the others.

Each of the eleven critical stages discussed above is a window of opportunity, offering the choice for protection or damage. In each one, health workers, community leaders, and, most of all, local citizens, can overcome the pressures toward poor health or, conversely, build structures to enhance positive health. There is no one magic pill to promote mental health. It will take many people, working on many fronts year by year to construct the delicate mosaic of better health that our children and grandchildren deserve.

## RESTRUCTURING TREATMENT SYSTEMS

When preventive interventions fail, treatment programs are essential, of course. But where prevention has not been seriously tried, the mildly mentally ill have no other recourse than to have their conditions deteriorate until they end up in custodial treatment, often in crowded hospitals. This means that in many countries, nearly the entire mental health budget is spent on mental hospitals. This limited care for severe cases is costly per patient and has a poor prognosis for rehabilitating patients; it also leaves nearly no funds for launching effective preventive programs for a much larger group of people.

With the discovery of more effective psychiatric drugs, more hospitalized patients can live comfortably and safely in halfway houses in the community, usually at a much lower cost. Others can return to live with their families, who make sure the patient takes his/her medications as prescribed. Most relapses of psychiatric patients living in the community are due to failure to take drugs as prescribed. Although many of the newer psychiatric drugs are quite costly, an increasing number of them are coming off-patent after the year 2000. At that time, they can then be made generically by any advanced pharmaceutical laboratory at a lower cost to the consumer. Governmental agencies, too, can negotiate contracts for system-wide use of such drugs in large quantities and at much lower prices.

*Many countries spend nearly all of their mental health budget on mental hospitals. Prevention, early local treatment, and cost-containment are more appropriate paths to the future.*

Neither mental hospitals, nor psychiatric drugs, nor psychotherapy has ever been able to reach even a small fraction of the people who need them, however. And this will worsen as the frequency of behavioral and psychiatric problems balloons as we move toward the year 2020. Prevention, early local treatment, and cost-containment are the appropriate paths to the future.

PAHO has called for a restructuring of mental health services in Latin America and has laid out its technical basis. This reform calls for decentralizing care for incipient and manageable psychiatric disorders by linking these outpatients to local primary health care programs. PAHO recommends a pyramid of mental health services based on self-help groups and social support networks, with referral upwards as needed to health promoters, nurses, primary care facilities, and, finally, to psychologists and psychiatrists if necessary. The goal is to add more resources (non-hospital) to community care, in order to decrease the frequency of hospitalizations. The savings achieved by requiring fewer hospital beds can be used to pay for mental health workers in primary health care clinics and for teachers and social workers to do primary prevention outreach of the types described here.

This approach to psychiatric and behavioral care is worth serious consideration in many parts of the world. It may seem revolutionary, but with traditional tertiary care having woefully failed, only bold new directions hold the hope for containing a rising tide of disorders (Levav, Restrepo, and de Macedo, 1994).

## RECOGNIZING AND DEALING WITH DEPRESSION

In its mild forms depression is the common cold of mental life. In more severe forms, according to the GBD Study, it causes an estimated 50 million life years of disability (YLD) worldwide each year.

Depression is a continuum: it comes in all shades of gray. And depression is truly a biopsychosocial disorder—its signs and symptoms involve biochemistry, emotions, cognitions, and personal interactions. Successful treatment uses all these levels of input. Business leaders should know that depressive symptoms and disorders steal billions of dollars, euros, and pesos from every country's gross national product by forcing workers and managers to take days or weeks off from work, or in milder forms by reducing the quality and quantity of work performed.

Everyone experiences brief episodes of sadness, discouragement, feeling slowed down, or grief after a personal loss. Most people are able to keep on going with their usual responsibilities and activities, although perhaps with less energy and more feeling of burden. Soon, most begin feeling better, more capable, and regain their usual enthusiasm. But some do not.

### RISK FACTORS

Professionals agree about the risk factors for depressive episodes. Here are six major ones (Mrazek and Haggerty, 1994, p. 502):

* having a first-degree biological relative (for example, a parent, grandparent, or sibling) with a depressive mood disorder;

161

- experiencing a severe stressor, such as the death or loss of a close person, marital trouble, job loss, medical crisis, or family or community disaster;

- believing oneself to be incapable, helpless (being a victim), hopeless, unacceptable to others, and unworthy;

- being female (much higher risk for unknown reasons);

- living in poverty or in a powerless social position; and

- having a severe physical illness of a type that may have an impact on brain chemistry.

### SIGNS AND SYMPTOMS

- **Mood:** sad, discouraged, irritable, loss of interest in favorite things, giving up, hopeless, crying spells, and troubled appearance.

- **Physiology:** loss of energy or appetite, slowed movements.

- **Sleep disturbances:** trouble falling asleep, multiple awakenings during the night, waking up far too early, waking up tired and worn out after one's usual amount of sleep. And conversely, regularly sleeping too much (10+ hours), and having trouble staying awake; feeling chronically exhausted.

- **Cognition:** trouble concentrating, slowed decision-making, trouble finishing tasks, feeling everything is going wrong, making more mistakes in work.

- **Thinking about death:** dwelling on family or friends who have died, seeing death as an escape.

- **Social:** person shifts to being more passive, dependent, helpless, sensitive to criticism; feels unloved, lonely, argues and complains more; may increase alcohol use.

- **Co-morbidity:** anxiety symptoms accompany depression in perhaps 70% of episodes (estimates differ greatly by culture). This brings on restlessness, fidgeting, pacing, fearfulness, short attention span, much worrying, inability to relax.

### PREVALENCE

Primary care doctors and clinics can expect that 20% to 40% of patients will carry depression secondary to the physical problem they came to have treated.

Commonly, the depressive physiology: lowers the threshold for reporting body symptoms, aggravates pain, and contributes to the physiological changes behind the presenting problem. In the community, the prevalence of depression is not as high as the percentage among doctors' patients, but many times greater in total numbers. Most depressive signs go unrecognized by health workers. In fact, were it not that way, there would be no time or resources left to deal with other diseases and injuries. This section intends to:

- Alert health workers to the many forms depression can take and its overall prevalence and burden in the community,

- Assess whether the presence of depression in a patient or family is interfering with successful treatment of other conditions (e.g., is a child failing to take her medications regularly because her mother is too depressed to supervise?), and

- Identify more accurately persons with major depression, which can become a fatal condition, and be proactive in treating them.

## THE BRIGHT SIDE: SECONDARY PREVENTION THROUGH EARLY TREATMENT

The good news is that depression is treatable, and sometimes it is preventable. The bad news is that only about 25% to 35% of depressed people in industrialized nations seek help directly for that problem, and the numbers are far lower in rural, poor, or developing areas. Yet, with proper treatment about 80% of persons suffering from depression obtain substantial improvement.

Many classes of antidepressant drugs are available by prescription. If one drug is not effective, it is likely that another class of drug will help, because each class works through different biochemical channels. The newest such drugs are always the most expensive and out of the financial reach of many health care systems, but many older medications no longer have patent protection and can be made and sold more cheaply. They too work well, perhaps nearly as effectively for most patients.

*Socially and clinically important depression occurs:*
- *when symptoms get so troubling as to interfere with normal work and family activities, daily activities, and interactions with others;*
- *when symptoms drag on for weeks or months, either worsening or not improving; or*
- *when a person considers violent action against himself or others.*

And there are other ways to prevent or lessen depression that are easily available. They can be done with groups and they are easily exportable. Inexpensive, successful programs with broad outreach are already going on in some places.

- **Physical Exercise.** Physical exercise for an hour or more daily (several sessions or several hours work better) changes brain endorphins and other neurochemicals—nature's antidepressants. Many psychiatric hospitals now prescribe walking and other activities for depressed patients who are adequately nourished. A brisk physical workout or a longer run can give an adrenaline high, but even a more modest kilometer walk daily can lift sadness, as many people in their later years will attest.

- **More Daylight.** Environments on the polar sides of the temperate zones have longer summer days, but also long winter nights. Extended exposure to darkness changes brain chemistry such that many people develop a higher risk of depression. This is called "Seasonal Affective Disorder." Centers that treat such depressed patients, particularly in Northern Europe and Canada, have them spend hours in brightly-lighted rooms. Increasingly, these treatment centers also employ exercise. Following this example, many factories and offices in higher latitudes are increasing the brightness of illumination in winter as a preventive measure against depression. (Reports of clinical studies can shed light on intensity, wave-length, duration, and safety issues regarding this approach.)

- **Re-thinking One's Situation.** Several cognitive therapies have developed principles and methods for treating depression. In randomized clinical trials evaluating drug therapy and cognitive therapy individually and both together, versus "wait-list" controls (i.e., neither treatment), the two therapies have rather similar results: each is better than no treatment; combined therapy is only a little better than only one modality; and cognitive therapy in some studies has a longer lasting effect than medications. Special training is needed to conduct these therapies effectively, even for psychiatrists and psychologists.

Cognitive therapists argue that most depressive reactions result from the way people think about their problems and themselves. When the therapist can help patients change the way they think about defeat, loss, helplessness, and their own capacities, symptoms of depression are relieved and the person has learned a defense against future stressful events and losses.

Cognitive therapists find that depressed patients commonly have three distorted ways of perceiving their situation. They overgeneralize or inflate their current problems so as to believe:

- that everything is going wrong in their lives;

- that they are to blame (guilt, self-criticism, worthlessness);

- and that things will never get better (no relief ahead, helplessness and hopelessness).

In simple terms, therapy's goal is to reverse all of these presumptions. To extend this therapy to preventive hygiene, children and adults can be taught, through discussion and example:

- that there are always good things remaining in life and about oneself.

- that troubles have multiple causes, and the person is not the cause of all bad things. Next time I can do my part better. I am still accepted. "To err is human."

- that right now is not forever. The person can change and others can change, too—"this (problem), too, will pass" and others can help.[5]

Additional cognitive therapy approaches appear successful in reducing both depressive symptoms and the risk of qualifying for the diagnosis of major depressive disorder (unipolar depression). G. N. Clark and colleagues (1995) randomized 150 high-school teenagers with elevated depression scores to either an untreated group or to group therapy consisting of 15 sessions of 45 minutes each. The goals were to help students identify and challenge negative or irrational thoughts that foster depression, to promote higher self-esteem and better coping skills, and to participate in more pleasurable activities. One-year follow-up showed that only 15% of the treated group incurred episodes of clinical depression, whereas 26% of the untreated adolescents became clinically depressed.

A meta-analysis of 48 high quality randomized controlled trials (765 patients) showed cognitive therapy for depression to be clearly more effective than no treatment (that is, waiting for time to heal) or drug treatment alone. Eight further studies showed that after completion of treatment, patients having only antidepressant drug therapy relapsed sooner than those patients who had cognitive therapy with or without medication (Gloaguen et al., 1998).

A subsequent summary of four additional controlled clinical trials of patients in primary care clinics in the United Kingdom showed similar results (Rowland et al., 2001). Several varieties of cognitive therapies have been found useful in secondary prevention of depression, including cognitive behavioral therapy, family therapies, and non-directive supportive approaches (Kolko et al., 2000).[6] In the case of depression—as well as for many other medical conditions—different individuals respond best to different treatment methods.

It has long been recognized that depressions, as well as more severe disorders such as psychoses, involve important biological changes. Research into brain

---

[5] See also Seligman, 1991.

[6] The following have been some of the leading resources for cognitive therapies: Beck, Rush, Shaw, and Emery, 1979; Seligman, 1991 (more oriented to lay readers). For clinical field trials: Manning and Francis (eds.), 1990.

chemistry and new methods of brain imaging continue to bring forth surprising new information, accompanied by a host of new psychotropic medications for anxiety disorders, schizophrenias, and depressions. Unfortunately, most of these drugs remain too expensive for use among the tens of millions of people who need them. Where clinically appropriate and economically feasible, pharmaceutical treatment should be considered, especially when careful medical supervision is available. Very often the best treatment for individual cases may involve a combination of verbal and drug therapies. Each nation and province must carefully consider what kinds of therapies to make available widely, based on epidemiologic studies of needs and types of resources most feasible to develop.

Depression is expected to become the world's leading cause of disability in 2020. Interested readers are referred to psychiatry textbooks that provide much more thorough coverage of this topic. This section closes with a brief description of four well-defined pieces of the puzzle of depression. While medical practice awaits additional pieces of knowledge, health promoters can perform small, careful field trials based on the suggestions outlined below.

- **Brain Chemistry.** Neurotransmitters, endorphins, and amines are among the organic chemicals whose imbalances may cause or aggravate depression. Antidepressant medications work by various mechanisms to rebalance the system, and behaviors also can change this chemistry. Both drugs and behaviors can affect depression triggered either by neurochemical imbalances or by psychosocial stress.

- **Interpersonal Interaction.** Having someone with whom to share problems, from whom to receive encouragement and acceptance, and who can be the source of new ideas or practical help, has proven to be good therapy for centuries, both to prevent the thinking that encourages depression and to relieve most situationally triggered depressive episodes. For the last 40 years we have called this social support; in prior centuries it was called having good family or having good neighbors. This is an avenue by which families, community groups, and religious organizations can help to prevent and relieve depression, anxiety, and other of the less severe emotional problems.

- **Psychosocial Shock or Stress.** People who have undergone severe stressors or losses (see "Risk Factors," above) are particularly vulnerable to depressive episodes in the 6 to 12 months following the stress. Bereavement often engenders depression from which most people recover over time. Providing support groups or other contact to these people on a routine basis appears to be an effective preventive measure.

- **Loneliness and Depersonalization in a Changing World.** In this age of migration, flow of refugees, shortage of jobs near family homes, family breakup, and troubled, fearful neighborhoods, new ways are needed to provide social

166

support. For example, community volunteer groups or religious gatherings can further this work. Clearly, high technology cannot solve the worldwide epidemic of loneliness. In fact, some forms of technology—television, Internet access, and even the trend toward high-tech, impersonal medical care—actually worsen the epidemic. More face-to-face, hand-to-hand, and heart-to-heart contact is a good starting prescription. Health professionals might help promote this among lay groups in their communities.

> *By far the biggest human and economic costs of alcohol come from physical and psychiatric morbidity, sporadic disability, and the conflict and breakup of families.*

## ALCOHOL ABUSE AND DEPENDENCE

The Global Burden of Disease Study ranks disability due to abuse of or dependence upon alcohol as second only to major depression as a top psychiatric cause of disability worldwide. There is a 14-fold difference in the rate of disability (DALYs) attributed to alcohol across regions of the world, ranging from a low of 0.6 per 1,000 population in the Middle East Crescent to a high of 8.5 per 1,000 in Latin America and the Caribbean. Market economies (at 5.9 per 1,000) and former socialist economies (at 5.2) are the next highest for alcohol-induced disability. Worldwide, men bring 7.5 times as much alcohol disability (in DALYs) upon themselves as do women. Of course, these data must be treated with care, especially where reported rates are low. Individuals, clinics, and ministries of health all tend to underestimate alcohol consumption and its sequellae; for example, for many years the former Soviet Union did not even list cirrhosis of the liver as a possible cause of death in its mortality reports to WHO.

Alcohol abuse actually accounts for a relatively small proportion of deaths directly. When injuries while under the influence of alcohol, cirrhosis and cancer of the liver, alcoholic cardiomyopathy and hypertension, some stomach cancers, and other alcohol-accentuated diseases are counted, however, the total becomes a matter of public health concern. J.M. Last lists 76 medical diagnoses in 13 systemic categories, all of which are associated with excess alcohol consumption (Last, 1987, p. 234). By far the biggest human and economic costs of alcohol come from physical and psychiatric morbidity, sporadic disability, and the conflict and breakup of families. Crimes committed while drunk are responsible for a substantial fraction of persons incarcerated in prisons around the world—a societal pathology often not added to the total bill.

The greatest international variability in prevalence of alcohol-caused problems is due to social and cultural forces. In regions that have the strongest religious and legal restrictions against alcohol (Islamic nations), reported problems are fewest. In places where the culture accepts alcohol and it is readily available, the prevalence of alcohol abuse and its medical and psychosocial sequellae are very high. Even in these places, however, most people who use alcohol are able to limit their use. There seems to be a roughly equivalent proportion of people (about 10%) in most populations who, if exposed to alcohol, become addicted to it. Community control of alcohol abuse and dependence can, therefore, use two strategies: reduce the number of people who can gain access to alcohol (thus putting the 10% over a smaller denominator) and educate and screen the community so they can identify themselves or friends who show signs of early alcohol misuse and can be enrolled in group treatment or community alcohol cessation programs, such as Alcoholics Anonymous.

## RISK FACTORS[7]

- Having a parent or other close biological relative who has alcohol problems. Transmission can be both genetic and through environmental exposure.

- Having biological markers that show an altered metabolism of alcohol and decreased sensitivity to it.

- Childhood expression of aggressive behaviors or "oppositional" (rebellious) conduct disorders.

- Having limited coping mechanisms for dealing with emotional or interpersonal problems, or to adjust to stresses, life changes, or family problems.

- Being in an environment that encourages unwise alcohol use, whether by direct example or a lack of teaching the advantages of abstinence or strictly limited use.

- Having alcohol easily available—in the home, at low cost, at many stores, bars, etc.

- Having other neuropsychiatric co-morbidities, such as antisocial personality, difficulty in expressing feelings, or repeated depressive periods. These may lead to self-medication with alcohol.

## PROTECTIVE FACTORS AND INTERVENTIONS

Alcohol abuse is but one way that generalized neuropsychiatric and psychosocial vulnerabilities may express themselves. Preventive efforts covered in the "Eleven

---

[7] Adapted from Mrazek and Haggerty, 1994.

Crossroads where Risk and Protective Factors Meet" (earlier in this chapter) help reduce prevalence of alcohol abuse as well as of other community-wide mental health problems.

Alcohol abuse interventions include:

- Control of availability of alcohol. Without access, this channel of abuse dries up, although true alcohol addicts will find ways to obtain it, even brewing or distilling it themselves. Reduced availability has its effect "upstream," where young people are beginning to experiment with alcohol and others are building up the habit. This approach continues to be effective in many places.

- Positive parental example and casual teaching, such as whenever alcohol products are advertised, when drunkenness is observed, and providing information or direct contact with persons at the end stages of alcoholism. (In some European countries up to 25% of hospital beds are occupied by persons with alcoholic morbidity or co-morbidity.)

- Effective anti-alcohol education in the schools. Many studies have shown that merely teaching the facts about alcohol or other drugs of abuse does not change actual behavior of youth. However, those teachings which change norms, values, attitudes, and beliefs about substances including alcohol, marijuana (cannabis), and cigarette smoking do substantially reduce the rate of starting such usage over the next few years. Teaching children how to resist peer influence to try harmful substances—how, in fact, to say "No"—also can have significant positive effects (Hansen, 1992; Hansen and Graham, 1991).

- Parental and community support for those youth peer groups, such as sports teams, that exclude alcohol from their activities and consider it "a problem" rather than an accepted part of their culture.

- Children and adolescents maintaining a continuing close relationship to parents and mentors (youth leaders, teachers, athletic coaches), relatives and adult friends who model safe behaviors regarding alcohol, drugs, and other risks.

- Participation in a social milieu, such as ethical and religious organizations that embrace a pro-social, pro-health lifestyle.

The goal of these interventions not only is to prevent alcoholism, but also to prevent unintentional injuries. Alcohol raises risk of pedestrian and motor vehicle injuries and deaths—about half of all fatalities caused by motor vehicles in the United States involve alcohol. And alcohol is also judged to be involved in the following estimated percentages of the following traumatic deaths (in the

U.S.): fires, 50%; falls, 50%; drownings, 30% to 40%; suicides, 30% (Mrazek and Haggerty, 1994). These percentages will vary by nation, depending on economics and alcohol consumption habits.

Intentional injuries and homicide are often inflicted by or upon intoxicated persons. Alcohol reduces one's normal self-control and dims foresight as to the consequences of violence. A serious proportion of spouse and child abuse is committed when men are intoxicated. Many men are in prison because of acts committed under the influence of alcohol or other drugs. The alcohol habit costs money, reduces productivity, and increases the chances of job loss. These three economic drains on a family's resources usually create conflict and poorer psychosocial health for all family members. All these points argue for more active community involvement in the prevention of alcohol abuse and dependence.

Treatment of alcohol abuse is difficult, however. For extreme cases it often must involve hospitalization or institutionalization in a restricted place where the patient has no access to alcohol; such places also treat withdrawal symptoms medically. Group therapy should begin in the hospital and continue after discharge. The 12 step program developed by Alcoholics Anonymous (AA) has been the most widely used internationally. There is little controlled research as to its efficacy, but many medical experts in alcoholism are now including it in treatment plans. Individual therapy usually fails, group therapy works better, and groups of the AA style may be less expensive and possibly more effective than other group approaches.[8]

## CONDUCT DISORDERS/DELINQUENCY

Child mental health clinics treat more conduct disorders than any other diagnosis. These behaviors start in childhood as behavior problems, often growing into delinquency and illegal activity by the teen years. At that point they are recognized as legal and police problems. Then, the criminal justice sector takes charge of the problem person. This sector usually lacks a developmental or therapeutic perspective and proposes to solve the problem by putting more people in prisons—90% of them men—for long periods of time. In some parts of the United States, for example, privately built, corporately managed prisons have come to be valued as an economic resource. Such for-profit organizations tend not to make rehabilitation a priority.

These broken lives are much like the fractured victims that emergency rescue squads pick up after an accident, say a fall down a river's steep waterfall. Rather than enlarging the rescue squad, it would be far wiser and more effective to ask

---

[8] This non-profit organization may be reached at Alcoholics Anonymous, World Wide Services, P.O. Box 459, Grand Central Station, New York, NY 10163.

what is happening "upstream" to make all these people land broken at the base of the fall. What in fact is happening is that the same neuropsychiatric impairments that are implanted from conception through childhood—and which raise the general risk of mental deficiency, schizophrenia, major depression, and the rest—also raise the risk of conduct disorders. These, in turn, later promote school drop-out, juvenile delinquency, fighting, thieving, alcohol and drug abuse, failed marriages, births outside of marriage, and the recycling of these problems through another generation. This metaphor of "upstream prevention" applies to all public health problems.

The overall risk and protective factors for the mix of neuropsychiatric vulnerabilities were discussed earlier, in the section entitled "Eleven Crossroads where Risk and Protective Factors Meet." What follows is a discussion of some diagnostic signs and risk factors specific to conduct disorders.

## EMERGENCE OF SIGNS

The onset of uncontrolled behavior may occur as early as ages 4–6 years, with another wave coming in mid-childhood, and a final wave in adolescence. Boys start problems earlier than girls; their high-risk time is the teen years. All conduct disorders are judged by the adult culture's criteria for right and wrong. Children so judged do not share the value systems and behavioral controls deemed necessary for their stage of development.

*The onset of uncontrolled behavior may occur as early as ages 4–6 years, with another wave coming in mid-childhood, and a final wave in adolescence.*

In general, children who develop conduct disorders experience less than normal anxiety about the possible outcomes of their aggressive or intrusive deeds, and they do not feel guilt afterward. The lessons that punishment is supposed to teach them are quickly forgotten. This deficit has been attributed to a blunting of autonomic nervous system responsiveness and alterations in hormonal and neurotransmitter metabolism.

## RISK FACTORS

- A temperament that is chronically irritable, difficult to manage.

- A child overly troubled by changes in schedule, environment, or caretakers.

- Presence of attention deficit hyperactivity disorder (ADHD) or approximations to it.

- A child who is a target of parental irritation or anger, deserved or not.

- A child that displays oppositional behavior—a tendency to object to most requests and often to do the opposite of what others request.

- Delays in cognitive and language development, and reading disorders, go hand-in-hand with conduct disorder, sometimes preceding it, sometimes following it.

- Parents with behavioral or mental disorders who continually fight with each other and abuse the children or reject them. According to some longitudinal studies, about 25% of abused or neglected children later become delinquent (Mrazek and Haggerty, 1994, pp. 171–182).

- Children with disabling chronic illness, injuries, or limitations.

- Children who show a combination of aggressiveness with peer rejection.

- Children living in overcrowded neighborhoods with substandard housing, poverty, broken families, crime—where negative role models abound.

- Children subjected to harsh, erratic punishment that is inappropriate for the offense or the child's age, or confusing to the child.

### PROTECTIVE FACTORS

These interventions include all the positive factors, as detailed in this chapter and as implied in the "Checklist for Ages 5–14 Years" in Chapter 3 and the "Checklist for Ages 15–24 Years" in Chapter 4 of this Handbook. The following are especially important life-lines to lift children who may be starting to show signs of conduct disorder:

1. **Improving and supplementing parenting skills.** This can be accomplished by teaching youth and prospective parents the basics. Another strategy may involve enlisting part-time, volunteer parent surrogates to provide a respite for children and natural parents experiencing distress (surrogates may be grandparents or community adults who love children, including childless couples). (Mrazek and Haggerty, 1994, have reviewed community programs to enhance child development.)

2. **Enabling schools to teach healthy human-relating skills.** In high-risk neighborhoods, classes may have to become smaller and social workers, school nurses, or counselors may need to be added. (See also the section on the "Good Behavior Game," presented earlier in this chapter.)

3. **Teaching skills and preventing the harmful use of idle hours through after-school programs for children of working parents.** These are oppor-

tunities to teach non-academic skills, including sports and vocational abilities. These skills are another protective resource, because they teach children how to cooperate with others, to increase their self-efficacy and self-esteem, and to prepare for leadership roles.

4. **Developing and maintaining positive relationships between children and youths and their parents, uncles, aunts, grandparents, older siblings, neighbors, schoolteachers, athletic coaches, and youth group leaders.** Adults will need to have patience, and perhaps firmness, to maintain these relationships. Scientific evidence now shows that having a special adult close to the life of a child reduces the risk of delinquency; a position corroborated by many adult model citizens who attribute their healthy lives to a special person who turned them away from a troubled adolescence.

Social and behavioral therapies to slow and even to halt the development of delinquent behavior have become sufficiently advanced to be tested in randomized controlled clinical trials. The group treatments are variously based on social learning, cognitive conditioning, and/or family therapy models. Because of the overwhelming prevalence of conduct disorder, delinquency, and their precursors, these therapies are almost always given to groups.

S. R. Woolfenden and colleagues (2002) in New Zealand qualitatively reviewed eight high-quality controlled trials involving 749 youths ages 10–14 years, all of whom already showed antisocial conduct disorders. A variety of family and parenting interventions reduced chances of re-arrest by 34% on average, and significantly reduced the time spent in correctional institutions, as compared to similar untreated youths.

The Conduct Problems Prevention Research Group (1999) reports a major controlled study in which 378 classrooms of students were randomized to usual teaching versus the "fast track" conduct disorder prevention curriculum. The latter comprises 57 lessons focusing on self-control, emotional awareness, peer relations, and problem solving. The "fast track" curriculum was associated prospectively with reduced hyperactive, disruptive behavior and improved classroom atmosphere. The research team argues for greater use of school-based programs for reducing behavioral problems. This position also is supported by Rones and Hoagwood (2000) in their extensive review of school-based mental health services.

These programs may not apply in the same way in different social and cultural environments. They are reviewed here to alert public health, mental health, and school health professionals to the great potential social value of such prevention efforts. The extensive reference lists contained in each cited report can provide blueprints and building blocks for local professionals worldwide.[9]

---

[9] Key references include Kendall (ed.), 1991, chapters by Feindler and Lochman, and Hersen et al. (eds.), 1996, Volume 25 and later volumes.

# POSITIVE BEHAVIORAL AND MENTAL HEALTH

Health promoters—and that should include every reader who can make a difference in another person's life—should not just try to rescue persons already suffering from a disorder. Health promoters also should seek to help average folks become better, to develop more of their positive potentials. Once again, the discussion returns to the "population approach," discussed in Chapter 2, which argues that by raising the capabilities and functions of the entire community, one age cohort at a time, the number and proportion of the population functioning below the threshold of disorder can be decreased—and the number of high achievers can be increased.

Might such a program help create a community where everyone is above average? Statisticians may vehemently shout "No!" If we reshape this aspiration, however, and ask whether it is possible to have communities where the vast majority of persons function above the average (of past generations), the resounding chorus may well be, "Yes!"

Positive behavioral and mental health have been variously defined. Sigmund Freud's assertion that good mental health is the ability to love and to work is a good starting place. More specifically, persons or groups with positive behavioral and mental health share certain qualities, such as are described in the following sections.

## AT THE INDIVIDUAL LEVEL[10]

### Within the Self

**Self-acceptance.** Self-accepting persons feel comfortable with themselves—not necessarily always satisfied, and certainly not prideful or uncritical, but accepting of their value to those around them. Basically, they believe they're OK.

**Self-esteem.** Persons with self-esteem feel that their lives are of value, that they are worthy of being respected and loved by themselves and by others.

**Realistic perceptions.** People with realistic perceptions have a reasonably accurate understanding of the world around them and of their own abilities and limitations. Psychiatrists refer to this as "good reality testing."

---

[10] The following points have been abridged and modified from materials by the National Mental Health Association (U.S.A.).

**Self-efficacy.** Persons with this quality have the skills to take care of the usual tasks of life and the ability to deal with new problems. They have a realistic amount of faith in their own abilities and planning.

**Emotional self-management.** This quality enables people not only to deal with everyday tasks and problems, but also with the psychological processes inside them, such as strong emotions, fears, uncertainty, and interpersonal conflicts. These people do not get swept away by their own strong feelings or those of others. They can rise above disappointments.

## In Relationships with Others

Persons endowed with superior mental and behavioral health are able to maintain ongoing relationships that are satisfying to all involved. They are able to develop trust in others and, in turn, to earn others' trust and respect.

They do not cheat or hurt others and refuse to accept such behaviors from others. They also are able to love and care deeply for those close to them, whether family or friends, and put these persons' well-being above their own.

## Living Productively

Life's daily responsibilities differ greatly throughout the life cycle. Extreme dependency is the norm for infants and the seriously disabled, while responsibility, fulfillment of roles, and social productivity is expected of those functioning with greater capability. Sometimes, however, circumstances and demand must be modified to fit personal limitations. Conversely, education, job training, preparation for parenting, and improving self-efficacy are all intended to increase personal capabilities to cope, overcome negative circumstances if necessary, and fulfill life's demands.

*Health promoters should not just try to rescue persons already suffering from a disorder, they also should help average folks become better.*

Persons with positive health accept and fulfill appropriate responsibilities, often achieving beyond them. They think and plan realistically, unburdened by undue fears or unrealistic expectations. These persons are open to new experiences and challenges and work to resolve problems for the betterment of those around them and of their communities.

These same qualities that go into an individual's positive mental health can easily be extrapolated to the family and to the community at large. In fact, they can be expanded to apply to more complex units such as health institutions or even national organizations. The same basic principles remain easily recognizable.

The following two sections summarize how these principles can be applied to the family and the community.

## AT THE FAMILY LEVEL

### Self-acceptance, Self-esteem, Realism, Efficacy

Does the family feel accepting about all its members? About itself as a family? Can it work on those issues about which it is dissatisfied? Does it look forward to its own future as a caring group? Does it generate pleasure and mutual support for all its members most of the time?

### Continuity of Satisfying, Trusting, and Caring Relationships

Does the family and its members feel comfortable relating with others outside the family—with neighbors, people at their schools, shops, workplaces? Are there close family friends that link it to the rest of the community? Are there community conflicts that make the family dislike or hate other families or groups, or fear those whom they suspect may hate them?

### Coping with Life Responsibly and Productively

Can the family take care of itself and the needs of its members? Do adults provide food, shelter, support, and care for dependent members? Do adults provide a healthy social-emotional environment? Do they show and teach children to follow healthy life habits? Do they nurture children's talents? Do they help them mature? Do they help them to respect and help others? Does the family plan ahead? Does it deal with its problems promptly, taking into consideration everyone's needs?

## AT THE COMMUNITY LEVEL

### Self-acceptance, Self-esteem, Effectiveness

Does the community believe that it and its purposes are valuable? Does it accept its members? Does it acknowledge its members' full diversity, accepting their diverse needs, qualities, and gifts? Do the community's members work cohesively? Is the community realistic in its perceptions of itself and its environment?

### Relations with Other Groups

Does the community or organization maintain constructive, mutually beneficial relations with individuals and organizations outside itself? Does it promote positive ethical values and respect for others?

## Responsible Productivity

Is the community responsible, productive, and flexible? Does it plan ahead for the good of all? Can it manage its collective needs?

In evaluating a community's health, a sanitary engineer will check drinking water quality, sewage and waste disposal systems, and air pollution controls. A public health planner might count the number of health providers and health facilities in the community. Now health promoters, too, can systematically evaluate family and community behavioral health. Starting from the three criteria discussed above, and selecting specific indicators to measure each, they will be able to evaluate far more than mental health.

> *Where behavioral and mental health are high, physical health also is likely to be good, and social well-being will flourish.*

The next leap forward in improving world health depends on teaching, enabling, and practicing those behaviors that prevent disease and advance health. These behaviors, the science that supports them, and the motivations that energize them are presented in this Handbook, as well as in many other sources. That is why this chapter on behavioral and mental health is placed first in this part of the Handbook. Taking care of one's lungs, liver, limbs, and heart must begin with behavioral and mental health, and so must taking care of one's family and community.

# 8. Diseases of the Heart and Blood Vessels

## CARDIOVASCULAR DISORDERS

Collectively, cardiovascular disorders are the leading cause of death worldwide, responsible for more than 14 million fatalities each year (Murray and Lopez, 1996). The most common heart diseases emerge later in life, often disabling people for some years before killing them. These disorders are the fourth leading contributor to worldwide loss of healthy life years (DALYs) over the entire life span, following infections and parasitic diseases, injuries, and neuropsychiatric disorders. From ages 45 to 59 years in both women and men, however, cardiovascular disorders rank first as the cause of lost DALYs. After age 60, these disorders are responsible for twice to three times the amount of lost healthy years as the next ranking major pathology. Hence, the reduction of cardiovascular disorders yields a three-point advantage: less disease, less disability, less premature death.

Cardiovascular disorders are very costly to treat and place a major burden on the health care system. They are far less costly to prevent, however, and fortunately some nations have made remarkable strides in reducing some forms of cardiovascular disorders.

While both developing and developed nations experience high mortality and disability due to diseases of the heart and blood vessels, the underlying nature of the diseases differs in each group. Canada, the United States, and Scandinavian and Western European nations have long suffered primarily from atherosclerosis, which results in such diseases as ischemic heart disease or coronary heart disease (heart attack), and cerebrovascular infarction (stroke). Most sudden cardiac deaths and true angina pectoris cases have the same atherosclerotic origins. This epidemic peaked in the 1960s and 1970s in Western countries. Since then, both the incidence and mortality from ischemic heart disease (coronary heart disease) have been declining by about 2% to 3% per year. The causes of this dramatic, continuous reduction are not fully understood, but intensive risk reduction programs and the populations' positive responses have played a major role in substantially reducing the major risk factors.

Meanwhile, in Eastern Europe, economically transitional countries in the Middle and Far East, and in Central and South America, the incidence and mortality of ischemic heart disease are rising each year. In these regions, populations are increasing their cigarette smoking, eating more fatty foods, getting less physical exercise, and experiencing more competition and stress that increase blood pressure and serum cholesterol levels. Unfortunately, these nations have many serious epidemics to confront all at once, including controlling infectious diseases and the inflammatory and parasitic diseases remaining from earlier in their economic development. All epidemics are created by the culture in which they appear. With cultures now changing more rapidly than ever, health experts are challenged both to vanquish old epidemics and forestall or weaken new ones.

There is no reason why developing and transitional countries must repeat the painful history that more industrialized countries are now leaving behind. It requires only limited resources to begin primary prevention—by informing the public about the risk behaviors and risk factors for ischemic heart disease and related diseases—to chart a different, healthier route for the future. **(Also see the section "Tobacco Use" in Chapter 13.)**

For developing countries, the major cardiovascular killers today are inflammatory heart diseases, cardiomyopathies, and pulmonary heart disease (cor pulmonale). Hypertension has a high prevalence in the tropics, and, in the absence of effective control, develops into hypertensive heart disease, variously leading to congestive heart failure, stroke, pulmonary heart disease, or kidney failure. Distinguishing between "developed" and "developing" nations is clear at the extremes of the range, but what about countries in the middle?

The International Classification of Diseases (ICD) attributes most of the non-atherosclerotic cardiovascular deaths to ICD entries 415–429—diseases of pulmonary circulation and other forms of heart disease (including pericarditis, endocarditis, myocarditis, cardiomyopathy, dysrhythmias, and heart failure due to edema; this category excludes rheumatic heart disease, cardiac valve diseases, sequellae of hypertensive heart disease, myocardial infarction, atherosclerosis, cerebrovascular disease, and "other and unspecified").

Table 8.1 shows the percentages of all cardiovascular deaths that have been attributed to ischemic heart disease and atherosclerosis (combined) in contrast to diseases of pulmonary circulation and other forms of heart diseases for 13 countries in the Americas. Caution must be utilized in interpreting the data, because various countries use different diagnostic criteria and have different levels of reliability. For countries in other areas of the world, rough comparisons can be made to tabulated countries of similar climate and economic development, until such time as local data are obtained.

The first surprise to North American and Western European health professionals is the size of the problem of non-atherosclerotic heart diseases. In 8 of the 13 countries in the table, deaths due to pulmonary heart disease and inflammatory

**TABLE 8.1.** Percentage of cardiovascular deaths attributed to ischemic heart disease and atherosclerosis, compared to percentages of cardiovascular disease deaths due to diseases of pulmonary circulation, inflammations of the heart, and heart failure, selected countries in the Americas.[a]

| Country | Cardiovascular deaths due to ischemic heart disease and atherosclerosis (%)[b] | Cardiovascular deaths due to diseases of pulmonary circulation, inflammations of the heart, and heart failure (%)[c] |
|---|---|---|
| Canada | 59.7 | 14.2 |
| United States | 54.6 | 22.3 |
| Costa Rica | 49.4 | 15.1 |
| Cuba | 49.0 | 6.8 |
| Trinidad and Tobago | 45.5 | 10.4 |
| Chile | 41.5 | 15.3 |
| Mexico | 39.0 | 23.5 |
| Colombia | 38.1 | 25.9 |
| Peru | 33.0 | 29.9 |
| Brazil | 31.5 | 24.8 |
| Paraguay | 26.3 | 32.8 |
| Argentina | 25.4 | 45.8 |
| El Salvador | 24.4 | 45.6 |

*Source:* PAHO, 1995.
[a] The same trends are seen in countries in Northern Africa, the Middle East, and Asia. China, India, and Egypt, for example, have higher mortality from the pulmonary circulation and inflammation category than from the atherosclerosis categories.
[b] ICD-9, 410–416 and 440.
[c] ICD-9, 415–429.
**Note:** Percentages do not add to 100% because some categories have been omitted.

heart disease exceed 20% of total cardiovascular deaths; in three countries, the values exceed the ischemic heart disease total. Another notable finding is that the strength of the negative correlation between the rankings of the percentages goes well beyond the mathematical expectation. This chapter will first examine the forms of cardiovascular disease still awaiting prevention in less developed areas.

> *For developing countries, the major cardiovascular killers today are inflammatory heart diseases, cardiomyopathies, and pulmonary heart disease*

## INFLAMMATORY HEART DISEASES

Congestive (or dilated) cardiomyopathy and restrictive cardiomyopathy (also called endomyocardial fibrosis) are rampant in Sub-Saharan Africa, where autopsy series attribute 25% to 40% of all cardiac deaths to these conditions. Congestive cardiomyopathy occurs in many parts of the world, with concentration in the tropics. Congestive cardiomyopathy often impairs the pumping action of both sides of the heart, and leads to heart failure. Some experts classify this disease as an autoimmune disorder set up by repeated viral infections (for example, from echo and Cocksackie), rheumatic fever, or toxoplasmosis. It can also result from thiamin deficiency or alcoholism. When these agents or other chronic bacterial or parasitic infections set up a chronic inflammation of the myocardium, pericardium, or endocardium, the autoimmune battle is engaged, and cardiomyopathies often emerge.

Epidemiologic risk factors include living in tropical or poor countries or in poor conditions in affluent countries, inadequacy of environmental control of these infections and their vectors, lack of medical care, and lack of balanced nutrition. The road to prevention lies in environmental and behavioral changes that prevent and treat these infections, and in provision of healthy foods that will raise host resistance.

Congestive cardiomyopathy is no stranger in tropical America, but there a major cause is Chagas' disease (American trypanosomiasis). Chagas' disease is heavily endemic in Venezuela and Brazil, with lesser prevalence from the southern United States to the South America's Southern Cone. Other congestive cardiomyopathies operate there, too, through the final common path of myocarditis or chronic inflammations of other heart tissues. Chagas' disease, now found only in the Western Hemisphere, is spread by a crawling insect, a triatomid (a cone-nosed bug), which itself is infected by a parasite, *Trypanosoma cruzi*. When the triatomid bites a human, seeking a blood meal, the bug's feces containing a form of the trypanosome pass through breaks in the skin, enter the bloodstream, and multiply. Trypanosomes mainly seek out the heart, followed by the gastrointestinal tract. The cardiac inflammation caused by the parasite can develop into cardiomyopathy and/or other conditions elsewhere in the body.

---

**PRIMARY PREVENTION OF CHAGAS' DISEASE**
- making homes "bug tight," by filling holes and cracks and by setting up screening;
- applying residual insecticides in all buildings or shelters where humans or animals live;
- establishing community programs to help residents cover rough inside walls (especially of thatch, mud, or rough wood) and crevices in walls and floors with smooth inorganic plaster—this seals off the living and hiding places of triatomids;
- cleaning beds and furniture that may have plant coverings or stuffing (such as mattresses) and carefully using residual insecticides on bedding surfaces that do not touch people for further protection; and
- using fine mesh bed nets to prevent triatomid attacks while in bed.

---

Treatment measures are currently based on two types of antibiotic drugs that quickly lead to remission of symptoms, including fever and inflammation. The antibiotics halt the acute disease episode, but do not lessen the damage already done by the chronic disease (Last, 1986; Cheng, 1986, Chapter 52).

## RHEUMATIC HEART DISEASE

This disease also is of infectious origin: it begins with repeated infections with Group A beta-hemolytic streptococci (strep throat, for example), which may be followed by an autoimmune process in one to five weeks—resulting in acute rheumatic fever. Usually occurring in school-aged children, acute rheumatic fever may affect the heart, central nervous system, kidneys, and/or joints. Once children have had one attack of acute rheumatic fever, they appear to be more susceptible to recurrent streptococcal infections and acute rheumatic fever reactions. Nearly half of acute rheumatic fever cases incur a cardiac inflammation, usually without immediate symptoms. Progression of the rheumatic process often causes mitral stenosis and mitral valve prolapse, especially in young women. Rheumatic fever inflammations also may lead to cardiomyopathy.

Rheumatic heart disease is associated with poverty in every climate. Overcrowding, poor housing, and inadequate sanitation encourage the spread of streptococcal infections. The lack of medical care associated with poverty reduces the chances that infections will be treated either acutely or by a long-term regimen of prophylactic penicillin in children with acute rheumatic fever episodes. Because ethnic and racial minority groups are often much poorer than the rest of a community, they also have higher acute rheumatic fever and rheumatic heart disease rates.

Rates of rheumatic heart disease have been declining in Westernized nations since about 1890. In the Region of the Americas, mortality data from 20 nations show that the percentage of all deaths due to rheumatic heart disease ranges from 0.1% to 1.3% in men and 0.3% to 2.4% in women. This is one of the few diseases that disables and kills more women than men. In the Americas, the countries with the highest percentages of rheumatic heart disease mortality are Belize, Chile, and Mexico for men, and Belize, Chile, Costa Rica, Ecuador, Mexico, and Panama for women (PAHO, 1995, 1989–1990 data). Developing nations in the Eastern Hemisphere (especially if tropical) also experience much rheumatic heart disease.

## PULMONARY HEART DISEASE

Pulmonary heart disease—often referred to as cor pulmonale—affects the right side of the heart and the vessels carrying blood to and from the lungs; it can follow any of 37 known causes (Cheng, 1986, Chapter 54). This disease often starts with pulmonary hypertension—high blood pressure from the right side of the heart, through the pulmonary arteries, the lungs, and then back to the heart. This puts a load on the right ventricle to keep pumping blood through the lungs against a greater pressure than the heart is prepared to handle. This results in hypertrophy of the heart muscle, thickening of blood vessel walls, and poorer exchange of carbon dioxide for fresh oxygen. In turn, this demands that the heart pump harder to get adequate oxygen, thus worsening the pathology.

Pulmonary heart disease also can originate in the lungs from chronic obstructive pulmonary disease or emphysema. In post-industrial populations, cigarette smoking is the most frequent cause of chronic obstructive pulmonary disease. Industrial exposures also are important instigators and promoters of this disease, including exposure to asbestos, coal dust, dusts from mining, cotton fiber dust, beryllium, toxic gases and vapors, carbon monoxide, smoke, and radiation. Diseases causing chronic obstructive pulmonary disease include tuberculosis, lung infections, lupus erythematosis, sickle cell disease, pulmonary granulomas, thromboses, emboli, and Chagas' disease.

Populations in developing and transitional nations experience excessive pulmonary heart disease mortality, as do populations where hypertension is endemic. In the 1990s pulmonary heart disease was increasing in the former Soviet Union, Japan, and, especially, in some parts of China.

In warm-climate countries where schistosomiasis is endemic, this parasite is a major cause of pulmonary hypertension and pulmonary heart disease. The chance of serious cardiopulmonary disease is small among persons having schistosomiasis, only about 5%. Nevertheless, the estimated 200 million infected persons in the world can be expected to generate up to 10 million cases of pulmonary hypertension and, in time, pulmonary heart disease. Schistosomiasis causes other pathologies in the liver, gastrointestinal tract, and bladder, so cardiovascular impairment is just one more reason to eradicate it. Eradication must be done on a community-wide basis.

In some areas, the prime cause of pulmonary heart disease is chronic pulmonary hypertension; in others, the prime cause is chronic obstructive pulmonary disease. Preventive programs may attack either or both these causes, depending on the presence of local risk factors and local feasibility of programs.

### Risk Factors

**Respiratory.** Exposure to primary or second-hand cigarette smoke; exposure to particulate air pollutants (e.g., dusts, quarrying and mining particulates, beryllium); exposure to caustic chemical air pollution (e.g., carbon monoxide, organophosphates in pesticides, nitrates, smoke, some gases); repeated chest radiation; asthma; fibrosis in lungs; or chronic obstructive pulmonary disease.

**Cardiovascular.** Pulmonary hypertension; thromboses or emboli in the lungs; sickle cell disease; diseases of blood vessels in the pulmonary circulation.

**Parasitic Infections.** Schistosomiasis; chronic bronchitis; tuberculosis; Chagas' disease; other chronic infections or parasitic damage to small airways or lung alveoli.

**Other Diseases.** Lupus erythematosis; cystic disease; granulomas or fibrosis in the lungs.

### Protective Factors

* Never starting tobacco smoking and stopping once started;

* Protecting families and workers from second-hand smoke;

* The community or government insisting on protecting workers in dusty, smoky workplaces (e.g., by distributing filter breathing masks, controlling dust by electrostatic precipitation or by water sprays);

* Making clean air a community priority (just like clean water to drink);

* Promptly controlling infections and parasitic diseases affecting the lungs, especially tuberculosis;

* Eliminating Chagas' disease from homes;

- Preventing and/or treating chronic obstructive pulmonary disease;

- Medically monitoring and treating sickle cell disease, lupus, cystic disease of lungs to postpone development of chronic obstructive pulmonary disease and pulmonary heart disease;

- Screening for and controlling pulmonary hypertension with periodic follow-up.

## NUTRITIONAL HEART DISEASES

Programs to reverse the epidemic of ischemic (coronary) heart disease in North America and Western Europe have made a strong case that ischemic heart disease is, in large part, a nutritional disease—specifically, an overconsumption of saturated fats, salt, and excess calories, leading to overweight. Excess calories means that fats are stored, not metabolized. Saturated fats, along with dietary cholesterol, recycle through the digestive system, blood vessels, liver, intestine and back to the bloodstream, thus having the opportunity to paint a thin layer of fatty streak (and later atherosclerotic plaque) on arterial walls several times over. Finally, salt raises blood pressure, as does obesity. Hence, most of the ischemic heart disease risk factors are clearly present in this dietary pattern.

*Protein-energy malnutrition sometimes follows crop failures or famine. Far more frequently, however, it follows breakdowns in commerce, the fall of governments, war, or the forced movement of people from their homes and lands.*

Alcohol consumption also can contribute to heart diseases in several ways. Especially when consumption exceeds one or two alcoholic drinks per day, it adds "empty calories," leading to a bulging abdomen. Furthermore, it hurts liver function, thus raising low-density (harmful) lipids. Over time it raises blood pressure. In excess, it causes alcoholic cardiomyopathy. Simply put, overnutrition and wrong nutrition raise major risk factors for ischemic heart disease.

Meanwhile, on the other side of the globe, health authorities confront those cardiovascular diseases due to undernutrition. They are becoming less prevalent, but warrant public attention until they disappear. There are two major types: protein energy malnutrition and thiamin deficiency.

Protein-energy malnutrition sometimes follows crop failures or famine. Far more frequently, however, it follows breakdowns in commerce, the fall of governments, war, or the forced movement of people from their homes and lands. The final common result of all these disruptions is semi- or total starvation of vast groups of people. The common solution of such problems is the provision of enough foods to reverse, as much as possible, the diseases of starvation.

Protein-energy malnutrition continues to be endemic in areas of Southeast Asia and Sub-Saharan Africa, but it also should be suspected in pockets of deep poverty anywhere in the world. Health authorities who assume it cannot happen in their countries, usually have not screened susceptible subgroups. According to Charithiraphan (Cheng, 1986, Chapter 50), ". . . whenever it is screened for, its prevalence is higher than expected." The longer this deficiency goes uncorrected, the more severe and chronic cardiac damage becomes. In most circumstances, the protein deficiency is worse than calorie deficiency; hence, protein supplementation (including vegetable sources) might require higher priority. **(Also see the section on "Malnutrition" in Chapter 9.)**

Thiamin deficiency can strike malnourished infants and children acutely with a range of severe symptoms, including beri beri heart disease. The acute stage of this disease can be fatal in the very young, but will be quickly reversed by the administration of thiamin, intravenously if urgent, or by mouth for longer follow-up care. Thiamin deficiency often also manifests in abnormal neurological signs. Where beri beri has become chronic, permanent defects in the heart will remain.

In infants, children, and adults, beri beri and its cardiac components can result either from inadequate consumption of thiamin-containing protein foods, or from acute physical stresses that deplete body stores of amino acids. Strenuous exertion, fever, parasitic loads, and other illnesses can precipitate this deficiency. Certain raw fermented fish eaten in Southeast Asia can destroy thiamin stored in the body.

Thiamin-deficiency heart disease also occurs in Western nations, but not among adequately nourished people. In these countries it is often found as a result of chronic alcoholism. Again, depletion of the body's storage of amino acids by acute diseases, malabsorption syndromes, or heavy labor can precipitate beri beri with its cardiac sequellae. In adults beri beri progresses more slowly than in children and is often accompanied by neuropathies.

In industrialized nations another subgroup at risk of nutritional heart diseases are young women who put themselves on starvation diets, by bingeing and purging or by extreme weight loss. This should be kept in mind by health professionals working with young women.

## HYPERTENSION AND HYPERTENSIVE HEART DISEASE

Clinicians apply the term "hypertension" when they find that a person's blood pressure remains higher than an arbitrary critical value, even while that person sits quietly. That observation needs to be found consistently on several occasions weeks apart to confirm the diagnosis. Hypertension—chronic high blood pressure—is undesirable because:

- it raises the risk of heart attack (ischemic heart disease);

- it raises the risk of stroke (cerebrovascular disease);

- over time, it causes structural changes in the heart (the muscles of the left ventricle grow bigger, affecting pumping ability), thus causing hypertensive heart disease; and

- the observed blood pressure elevation may be the start of a larger increase, which would accelerate the problems in all of the above, as well as create a risk for damage to the kidneys.

Everyone's blood pressure changes minute to minute. It is higher when we work hard physically or mentally, and when we are angry or frightened. It is lower when we are resting, and lowest of all when we are deeply asleep. A study of more than 400 air traffic controllers measured blood pressure every 20 minutes for 5 consecutive hours. All readings were made while the air traffic controller was seated; no measures were taken during physical exertion. The average man's range (high minus low) of systolic blood pressure under these controlled conditions was 35 mmHg (+/− 12); the average diastolic range was 27 mmHg (+/− 8). Thus, about one-sixth of these healthy men had a fluctuation of 49 mmHg in systolic blood pressure, or 35 mmHg in diastolic blood pressure while seated in the five hour period (Rose, Jenkins, and Hurst, 1978).

Such profound rises and falls in blood pressures are the ways healthy people's bodies adjust to daily activities. The problem of hypertension arises when the body loses the ability to drop pressure to a low healthy baseline. Forces determining blood pressure level at any time include:

- how much fluid volume is in the system of blood vessels;

- how much blood the heart pushes out at any one beat;

- how rapidly the heart beats;

- how much the peripheral arteries and arterioles have contracted to squeeze smaller the space the blood has available to it;

- how much elasticity ("compliance") the major arteries have that spreads out the peaks of cardiac output pressure, so that more distal vessels incur lower, spread-out peaks and less deep drops in pressure between heart contractions.

The risk factors for hypertension, as well as the methods for treating it, involve these five mechanisms.

**Family Aggregation.** Hypertension runs in families, primarily due to genetics and secondarily to shared lifestyle.

**Age.** Blood pressure tends to rise with age in industrialized societies. Diastolic blood pressure rises in populations until about age 55 years, then levels off. Average systolic blood pressure rises to the end of the lifespan. The amount of increase with age is often very small in simple agrarian cultures, but most people have a marked increase in blood pressure if they move from a rural place to an urban one, with the stress of rapid modernization of daily life that it brings. According to cross-sectional studies, blood pressure rises more steeply in urban settings, but longitudinal studies of the same persons over a decade or more show that a sizeable minority (about 40% in one 14-year study) do not have a rising slope of annually measured blood pressure. The remaining people have large enough increases to make the group averages rise.

> *Being too heavy for one's skeletal size raises blood pressure, and obesity does so even more dramatically. The more fat, the harder the heart must work.*

**Overweight.** Being too heavy for one's skeletal size raises blood pressure, and obesity does so even more dramatically. Each pound of fat is filled with miles of capillaries that require pressure for blood to move through. The more fat, the harder the heart must work. Of course, many forces affect blood pressure, and depending on these other forces, some "skinny" people may have high blood pressure and some obese people may have normal blood pressure. But as with many other generalizations in the risk factor literature, the averages for groups of people more than overcome the individual exceptions. Preventive medicine programs are generally addressed to large groups.

**Sodium in the Diet.** Some people's blood pressure level is sensitive to sodium. In general, populations with high salt intake have higher blood pressures. Such people can lower their blood pressures without medications, simply by cutting out naturally salty foods, and not adding salt or monosodium glutamate to bland foods. Instead, herbal spices can be used to enhance flavor. Sodium holds water within the blood vessels, increasing their fluid volume—thereby raising blood pressure. Physicians sometimes prescribe diuretics to treat hypertension. They stimulate the kidneys to excrete water and sodium more quickly, thus reducing fluid volume.

**Alcohol Consumption.** Regularly drinking more than two alcoholic drinks each day raises blood pressure chronically in groups, and some individuals may be adversely influenced by less alcohol than this. This is one of many reasons to minimize alcohol consumption.

**Other Diseases.** Some acute and chronic diseases raise blood pressure to dangerous levels. This is called secondary hypertension. Obtain a medical diagnosis and treatment for any such diseases.

**Some Environmental Stressors.** Both animal and human research has shown that some environmental stressors can raise blood pressure not only acutely, but also chronically. Ostfeld and Shekelle identified five conditions that increase the chances that long-sustained psychosocial stress is most likely to elevate blood pressure chronically:

- an uncertain life situation;

- lack of experience to learn which behavioral response will solve a given problem;

- the possibility of serious harm;

- the fact that fight or flight are unlikely to help; and

- the need for sustained mental vigilance.

Air traffic controllers experience four of the five stressors detailed above—all except lack of experience. Air traffic controllers have a very high incidence of hypertension (Stamler (ed.), 1967).[1]

**Temperament.** Studies from several industrialized areas suggest that people experiencing stressful circumstances who complain, feel upset, and show their emotions are *less* likely to develop sustained high blood pressure. They may, however, have acute rises in blood pressure only while they express their feelings. Those who deny that they face any problems, who show below average anxiety, and don't complain about tough circumstances tend to have higher risk of gradually raising the baseline of their resting blood pressure.

**Social or Economic Disadvantage.** People who have low education, low income, or who are subject to racism or discrimination run clearly higher blood pressures as a group. Numerous studies of neighborhoods, patient groups, and factory workers in several nations have supported this finding.

People who are discriminated against or who are poor face an uncertain life situation; lack enough experience to solve their current problems; are threatened with the possibility of serious harm; don't have the option of escaping or fighting their circumstances; and must be constantly and continually vigilant. In short, all five of the Ostfeld and Shekelle criteria are fulfilled.

---

[1] This work has withstood 30 years of subsequent research.

**Receive treatment.** Seek treatment for any disease or condition that may be causing high blood pressure.

**Maintain a normal weight for height and body frame.** If overweight, reduce caloric intake and increase moderate exercise—there is a direct correlation between pounds of body fat *lost* and reduction of resting blood pressure.

**Reduce sodium intake.** The cheapest way to determine whether people are sodium-sensitive is to make a sharp reduction in sodium intake and see whether blood pressure goes down. Simply reducing salt from 10 times the body's needs to 7 times may not help much; one may have to decrease perhaps to 3 or 4 times the daily requirement. Be careful to replenish the body's need for potassium and calcium. Also be cautious when sweating profusely in hot weather.

**Reduce or stop drinking alcohol.**

**Increase the level of daily physical activity.** Engaging in walking or sports will lower most people's blood pressure over time.

**Try to avoid the environmental stressors listed under "Risk Factors."** This may be approached either by changing circumstances, changing the way you perceive and think about them, or discharging tension by finding ways to express to friends how you really feel.

**Practice relaxation exercises daily.** It has been established for a century that the central and autonomic nervous systems are the main regulators of blood pressure, so the last three risk factors listed above should come as no surprise. Various relaxation exercises and yogic practices have been shown to lower blood pressure both acutely and chronically, modestly on average for groups, but more effectively in some individuals. Studies have shown that relaxation practices in some persons taking anti-hypertensive medication, allow the drug dosage to be reduced without their blood pressure rising. More attention should be paid to natural, psycho-neural means of lowering blood pressure in groups of moderate hypertensives who lack the traditional biologic risk factors.

*In places where hypertension (and stroke) are epidemic and the population very large—such as Northern China, with hundreds of millions of people—individual or family treatment with drugs is futile for solving the public health problem. Population-wide programs to lower the modifiable risk factors and increase protective factors, however, should make a population impact over time.*

**Use physician-prescribed medication to lower blood pressure.** Advise the physician if you are also using any of the protective factors above. There are now many anti-hypertensive drugs available with different modes of action and at different prices.

## ISCHEMIC HEART DISEASE

Ischemic heart disease, also known as coronary artery or coronary heart disease—and by the general public as "heart attack"—has been the leading cause of cardiovascular mortality for most of the 20th century in Western and Northern Europe and in Canada and the United States. In the 21st century it is expected to become the top cause of cardiac death in the rest of the world. Ischemic heart disease, although not an infectious disease, spreads like an epidemic, propelled by cultural change.

Atherosclerosis is the main underlying pathological process leading to ischemic heart disease, including myocardial infarction (heart attack), sudden coronary death, angina pectoris, stroke (cerebrovascular infarction or hemorrhage), and peripheral vascular disease. Atherosclerosis consists of fat deposits along susceptible surfaces of arteries; the fat forms plaques that enlarge and harden, narrowing the artery channel. When this occurs in coronary arteries, the now smaller passages can get blocked by little blood clots (thrombi) or other debris in the bloodstream (emboli), thus shutting off blood flow to parts of the heart (ischemia).

Lack of oxygen causes the severe chest pain of a "heart attack" (acute myocardial infarction), myocardial (heart muscle) cells die, and if the heart can no longer deliver enough blood, the patient dies, too. About 25% of first attacks are quickly fatal. The remaining stricken patients survive—the time of survival relates to the amount and placement of the dead heart muscle, and to the speed, adequacy, and continuity of medical care received. The science of acute care and rehabilitation after myocardial infarction has advanced greatly, and most patients return to normal functioning.

The rise (starting about 1930) and fall (starting around 1970) of the ischemic heart disease epidemic in industrialized nations holds forth the possibility that other nations can abort this epidemic rising within their borders, and start their decline even now by reducing the risk factors for atherosclerosis. They should begin this primary prevention now, before the epidemic peaks.

### Risk Factors

**Sedentary lifestyle.** In industrialized countries lack of physical exercise has contributed to more ischemic heart disease deaths than any other single risk factor.

That is because more people are doing more sitting than are engaging in any other risk behavior. As farm and factory work becomes more automated, society has benefited from extraordinary gains in productivity. Most people, however, did not replace the physical work they used to do—which exercised their heart, lungs, and limbs all day—with even a daily hour of challenging activity. Too many of us are taking "the chair lift" to the peak of cardiac risk, and the downfall afterwards is rapid, indeed. Sedentary life is a risk factor at every age.

**High blood pressure.** The pounding of high blood pressure into arterial walls, especially head-on at curves of the arteries, appears to damage their inner linings (intima) and build up atherosclerosis. The high pressure also raises risk of vessels tearing (hemorrhage) or ballooning outward (aneurysm). High blood pressure raises the risk for many disorders. This too is a risk factor at every age.

*Ischemic heart disease, although not an infectious disease, spreads like an epidemic, propelled by cultural change.*

**Cigarette smoking.** In this we have a "quadruple threat" aggressor. Cigarette smoking delivers nicotine to the bloodstream, irritating the intima and adding to plaque. It delivers carbon monoxide, which stops red blood cells from delivering oxygen the body needs. Cigarette smoke delivers carcinogens to other organs through the lungs and to all the body's organs through the bloodstream. It damages small blood vessels in arms and legs, causing or worsening peripheral vascular disease.

Ultrasound studies in Finland have shown cigarette smoking causes distinctive small vascular lesions of its own (other than sclerotic plaque), which can be detected in carotid arteries. They may also be found in other parts of the body once the techniques can be applied.

**Low density serum lipids.** Research has advanced well beyond its concern about "cholesterol" to the point of identifying different kinds of cholesterol, different types of lipoproteins that carry them, and numerous interacting biochemicals. The "bottom line" for preventive medicine remains much the same: limit the consumption of meat, dairy products, or any other foods rich in fats that are solid or pasty at room temperature (liquid oils, in moderation, are better); engage in regular exercise to burn calories and help convert some of the body's harmful, low density cholesterol into protective, high density cholesterol; avoid weight gain—adding fat to the body pumps fats into the bloodstream and onto the vessel walls.

**Diabetes mellitus.** Diabetes is a very strong risk factor for ischemic heart disease and all atherosclerotic diseases. The degree of its contribution to cardiovascular mortality in a population depends on its prevalence in the population and on how well blood sugar levels are controlled in patients.

**Obesity.** Obesity is a precursor and contributor to many of the mentioned risk factors—it raises blood pressure, it raises low density serum lipids. It sits in the same lounge chair as sedentary lifestyle. It helps cause adult-onset diabetes. Some overweight smokers even say that they don't want to give up cigarettes lest they gain more weight! Obesity can be reversed effectively, and smoking can be stopped, too.

**Psychosocial and behavioral factors.** The power of emotions and behaviors, other than the risk behaviors discussed above, to contribute to ischemic heart disease/coronary heart disease risk continues to be debated. This is a difficult area for research measurement, and there are many reasons why studies may not agree. Yet over the past 35 years, enough large studies have been reported to allow some general statements.

*Anxiety and neuroticism* seem to be related primarily to angina pectoris, usually not to myocardial infarction.

*Depression* is a powerful risk factor for poor recovery and fatal outcome of ischemic heart disease and other diseases; it also relates to a progression of atherosclerosis in living patients and other harmful physiological changes.

*Anger, hostility, and aggression* have been associated with ischemic heart disease endpoints, according to many studies conducted in the 1980s and the 1990s. Hostility shares with the Type A Behavior Pattern (discussed below) the element of frequent arousal of the autonomic nervous system. Such arousals raise blood pressure briefly but acutely, and also cause bursts of noradrenaline secretion which irritate arterial intima making it more susceptible to atherosclerotic plaque.

*Chronic sleep disturbance* also has been implicated. Whether it involves trouble falling asleep, multiple awakenings in the night, awaking far too early and being unable to return to sleep, or awakening feeling tired and worn out after one's usual amount of sleep, these signs, when long lasting, raise the risk of ischemic heart disease. Prolonged sleep-deprivation can cause many negative impacts on health, including a higher mortality rate.

*Certain occupational conditions* sometimes place high demands on workers but leave them little or no flexibility as to how to meet those demands. Workers on assembly lines that move too rapidly are an example, and here, it is the psychological strain, rather than the physical one, that seems to be responsible for raising risk of disease.

*A behavioral style of continual intense activation* also seems to put people at higher risk of ischemic heart disease. This style of behavior describes people who are "always on the go" and always in a hurry, who are competitive, aggressive, and have difficulty relaxing—the Type A Behavior Pattern. Research has shown prospective associations between chronic hyperarousal and ischemic heart disease, and also has identified pathophysiological pathways that link them. The Type A risk factor appears to have reduced its predictive strength in some developed nations, but it has become a predictive factor for ischemic heart disease in transitional nations where people of higher social status still have greater ischemic heart disease rates than persons with lower education and job prestige.

**Socioeconomic status.** The natural history of the rise and fall of the ischemic heart disease epidemic in a society is that it begins as a disease of the upper classes, then, over the course of several decades, moves into the working class. This seems to happen as the working classes take on lifestyle habits of more prestigious people—smoking cigarettes, eating more fatty foods, becoming more sedentary. Innovation begins in more educated and cosmopolitan groups—both in the onset of risk factors and in the acquisition of protective factors. Hence, the widespread adoption of healthier behaviors also begins higher on the social ladder. This leaves persons at middle and lower socioeconomic levels in Western and Northern Europe, Australia, Canada, and the United States the victims of the first (unhealthy) risk factors and not yet the beneficiaries of a "health revolution." This world phenomenon is not something health professionals can "treat," but the information can be used to identify higher risk groups and prepare primary prevention outreach. **(Specific approaches for tobacco, dietary, and screening programs will be dealt with in Chapter 12.)**

**Older age.** Rates of ischemic heart disease and most other chronic diseases advance sharply with age. Obviously, this risk factor cannot be changed directly, but it need not be a measure of "exposure" to risk, if changeable risk factors are corrected earlier in life. The calendar does not count one's age as truly as does one's body and behavior. Healthy living, not the years behind one, predicts the quality and quantity of years ahead.

## Protective Factors

Briefly stated, eliminating the risk factors listed above is a community's and an individual's best protection against ischemic heart disease and its costs. People can increase physical activity, stop smoking, eat a healthier diet, lose weight, control blood pressure, and find ways to escape stress. These six tasks are not all separate, they interact and promote each other. Some epidemiologic data suggest that persons who consume about one alcoholic drink per day (usually one glass of wine or beer) are better protected from heart attack and possibly stroke than those people who never consume alcohol or those who consume two or more drinks per day. It is not yet fully established whether this effect is due to the alcohol itself, other components of the beverages, or to other characteristics of lifestyle or temperament of this distinct group. Given the tendency for alcohol to become abused and lead to many other pathologies, we recommend safer ways to reduce heart disease risk.

Another protective factor is female gender until the age of menopause. After that, women experience the rising gradient of risk that men went through ten years earlier. In industrialized areas, ischemic heart disease becomes the leading specific cause of death in women after about age 55. In developing and transitional nations stroke and cancers usually lead women's causes of death until age 65.

International studies have shown that reducing consumption of animal protein and increasing proteins from plants (especially soy beans) lowers levels of low density (unhealthy) cholesterol. Other legume plants (from the family of peas and beans) are also protective (Blaufox and Langford, 1987, pp. 246ff).

## CEREBROVASCULAR DISEASES—"STROKE"

Cerebrovascular diseases are caused by pathology in the blood vessels to the brain. When these vessels get blocked by atherosclerosis, a thrombus, or an embolus, the blood supply to the brain is cut off, and many neurons die. When an aneurysm (bulging of a weak area of the blood vessel) occurs, pressure squeezes the brain and pathways malfunction. If a vessel tears or bursts, a hemorrhage occurs; the blood spilled into the space of the neurons also destroys their normal activity. The result in each case is neurological damage extending to the parts of the body controlled by the damaged or dead nerves. Depending on the location and size of the brain damage, permanent disability or death may follow.

The incidence of stroke is low in younger adults. The GBD Study estimates worldwide death rates to be about 12.6 per 100,000 for persons ages 30–44 years old (Murray and Lopez, 1996). By age 70 and older, the rate has multiplied more than 100 times—to 1,334 per 100,000! Men tend to be at higher risk than women, up until the late 60s. Cerebrovascular diseases rank second only to ischemic heart disease as the leading cause of disability and death combined (DALYs) in the world for both women and men from age 45 to the end of the lifespan.

The regions with the highest prevalence of hypertension, China and Sub-Saharan Africa, also have the highest rates of cerebrovascular deaths as a percentage of total cardiovascular mortality. This is not surprising, since high blood pressure is by far the most potent risk factor for stroke.

Incidence of and mortality from cerebrovascular diseases have fluctuated during much of the 20th century, with unmistakable declines apparent in the post-industrialized countries since about 1970. This has been credited largely to the programs of blood pressure screening and treatment by pharmaceuticals and now also by lifestyle changes.

Randomized clinical trials in several nations have shown that the incidence of strokes can be reduced sharply and cost-effectively by lowering blood pressure. Most such trials have used antihypertensive drugs, especially diuretics, to achieve this goal. The consensus of findings is that for every 6 mmHg reduction in diastolic blood pressure maintained over five years, there is about a 40% reduction in the incidence of strokes (Yusuf et al., 1993; MacMahon, 1996). This is a remarkably large saving of lives for a small reduction in blood pressure.

*Cerebrovascular diseases rank second only to ischemic heart disease as the leading cause of disability and death combined (DALYs) in the world for both women and men from age 45 to the end of the lifespan.*

These findings apply to groups of mild to moderate hypertensives and greater reductions might be achieved in severe hypertensives or other maximal risk groups.

### Risk Factors

**Hypertension.** High blood pressure raises the risk of stroke three to four times that of people with normal blood pressure. Both systolic and diastolic elevations raise risk in proportion to their elevations at all ages. It is claimed that up to 70% of strokes can be prevented by reduction of blood pressure (Gorelick, 1995).

**Age.** Stroke risk increases with age, rising especially rapidly after age 60. Reducing blood pressure reduces stroke risk even in people over 80 years old, however (Cheng (ed.), 1986, Chapter 43).

**Dietary factors.** Too much salt and other sources of sodium; inadequate dietary potassium and calcium.

**Cardiac diseases.** These include atherosclerosis (ischemic heart disease), left ventricular hypertrophy, congestive failure, atrial fibrillation, or mitral stenosis caused by rheumatic fever.

**Diabetes mellitus.** Diabetes leads to adverse changes in blood vessels throughout the body, and to stroke.

**Cigarette smoking.** This is an independent risk factor for stroke; its impact follows a dose-response curve.

**Sickle cell disease.** By reducing the ease of blood flow, this disease raises the probability of blockage of smaller arteries and, thus, of stroke.

**Depression.** This condition influences both the incidence and severity of strokes. In some studies, hypertensives with serious depression had about 2.5 times the rate of strokes as non-depressed hypertensives. As with many other conditions, depressed persons have an elevated risk of their stroke being fatal or of their recovery being delayed (Simonsick et al., 1995).

**All other risk factors for hypertension.** Obesity, alcohol consumption, lack of exercise. See the section on high blood pressure earlier in this chapter.

Some have proposed race as a risk factor, too. In the United States, for example, African Americans have about twice the rates of hypertension, hypertensive heart disease, and stroke as White Americans. This fact has been seen as a cornerstone for the belief that racial genetics is an important determinant of risk, intensity, and sequellae of hypertension. Recent international epidemiologic studies, however, show that White Americans have more hypertension than West Africans, who have similar genetic heritage as African Americans. Further, it was found that Africans living in rural areas have lower blood pressures than those living in cities. As people migrate to urban areas their blood pressures and rate of hypertension go up. Studies of Pacific Islanders concur that urbanization into Western lifestyles raises blood pressure. These international findings allow genetics, in the form of family aggregation of hypertension, as a risk factor, but suggest that the interaction of genetics with environment, particularly a rapidly changing environment or a stressful or punitive environment, is the more pow-

---

**WARNING SIGNALS OF TRANSIENT ISCHEMIC ATTACKS**

Transient ischemic attacks (TIAs) are beyond the state of a risk factor. They are a sign of emerging cerebrovascular disease that often occurs shortly before a serious stroke. A TIA consists of brief neurological symptoms such as:

- sudden weakness or numbness on one side of body—face, arm, leg;
- sudden darkening or loss of vision, usually in one eye;
- difficulty in talking or understanding others;
- unexplained dizziness or sudden falling.

Most TIAs clear up in five minutes to an hour, and the person feels well again. If such symptoms persist beyond 24 hours, they are diagnosed as a cerebrovascular accident—a stroke. The public should recognize the importance of the above signs, especially if more than one occur together. Since a TIA is a warning announcing the likely arrival of a vascular crisis in the brain, it is to be used as a signal to seek prompt medical attention. People who experience TIAs have a tenfold increased risk for a stroke coming soon than others. Hence, health professionals at all levels of background should arrange for prompt care. Blood pressure should be measured and, if too high, reduced immediately. Clotting factors in the blood should be assessed and treated. A period of medical observation or further diagnosis may be indicated. The patient should be cautioned to avoid behaviors or circumstances likely to raise blood pressure acutely. Strokes cannot be "cured," but most—maybe even 70%—can be prevented.

---

erful (and more modifiable) cause of elevated hypertension and stroke rates in population groups.

Asian races, such as Chinese and Japanese, also manifest high prevalence of hypertension and its pathological outcomes. Dietary factors (high sodium, low potassium, low calcium) may play a more important role than race. Witness the geographic gradient of twice as much hypertension and stroke fatality in northern China compared to southern China. In both areas 95% of people are of Han ancestry, but diet and aspects of the culture are quite different.

### Protective Factors

Since hypertension is a stepping stone on the path to cerebrovascular disease, all the protective factors for that condition apply here also. Removing the risk factors above confers much protection.

Reinforcing the protective factors person-by-person is the usual approach in a clinical setting, but this will make little overall impact in the community. To do that, the population approach, not the high risk approach, must be pursued. This can be achieved throughout the life cycle, wherever groups eat together or live together. From childhood to old age, schools, group housing, the military, factory lunch rooms, hospitals, and meal services for the elderly can reduce sodium and increase potassium and calcium in foods served. Institutions also can discourage cigarette smoking, drinking more than two alcoholic drinks per day, and obesity. They also can encourage regular exercise and stress reduction techniques when indicated.

## PROTECTION SUMMARY

In summary, the key to reducing diseases of the heart and blood vessels is to reduce risk factors and promote protective factors in whatever group one serves. Someone might only be able to help his or her family: then that's what should be done. A smaller target group can provide more focus, intensity, and success. For those with influence on factories, offices, or schools, there is much that can be achieved in these settings. The next step is to influence communities and larger groups using proven population approaches to enhance health.

# 9. Cancers

In all cancers, cell nuclei lose their ability to control cell growth and multiplication. As a result, primitive kinds of cells rapidly proliferate. When these "wild cells" invade nearby tissues—damaging organs and systems—the process is considered malignant. If these growing cell clusters are not removed or stopped, the "host" will die.

For cells to become "cancerous," they usually must sustain often-repeated physical or chemical damage. In fact, most persons sustain this sort of damage rather frequently, but fortunately most also have a well-functioning immune system that finds and destroys such cells continually. However, if the damage proves to be greater than the body's ability to fight it, a malignant neoplasm—cancer—will develop. Cancers also can occur in blood-forming tissues and in the blood. Some abnormal growths may not invade other tissues and may not be life-threatening; these are called benign tumors.

*Cancers rank among the leading causes of death in every nation, although there are vast differences across cultures and environments in the rates at specific sites.*

Cancers rank among the leading causes of death in every nation. Nevertheless, there are great differences across cultures and environments in the rates of cancer at specific sites. Neoplasms of the lung, breast, and colon, for example, lead the list in industrialized nations. In developing countries, on the other hand, cancers of the stomach, liver, and cervix uteri are the major cancer killers. Data estimate that between 80% and 85% of all cancers are determined by lifestyle and environmental factors (McGinnis and Foege, 1993). In developed countries, industrial exposure accounts for only about 5% of malignancies (Higginson, 1980). In developing countries, the percentage is higher, given the fact that in these countries' health and safety regulations are generally fewer and less consistently enforced. Not surprisingly, many industrialists in regulated, developed countries are moving carcinogenic manufacturing to developing countries. While some cancer risks are passed on partly by genetic processes, environmental or lifestyle factors still must release, or suppress, their expression. That means that environmental and behavioral changes are vital components of all cancer prevention programs.

These huge geographic differences prove that specific cancers are not inevitable. And, no nation has to accept high incidence and mortality rates. If only every nation could adopt both the lifestyle that keeps lung, breast, and colon cancers rare in developing countries *and* the lifestyle that keeps cancers of the stomach, liver, and uterine cervix infrequent in industrialized countries, this planet's overall population would have much lower mortality from these diseases.

The development of a malignant neoplasm is not as simple as that of an infectious disease. Research into causes (etiology) and processes (pathogenesis) of cancers indicates that at least two exposure events are necessary for the malignancy to develop—an initiating event and a promoting event. The "causes" of any malignancy are multiple, and it often takes many years for the process to advance far enough to be clinically apparent. All the while, the body's

**Both an initiating event and a promoting event are necessary for a malignancy to develop.**

biochemical and immunological systems are fighting to destroy the mutated cells that might replicate themselves to become tumors. Much research is underway to spell out the full story behind this over-simplified outline. Meanwhile, our preliminary information tells us that we can prevent many cases of cancer with a three-pronged approach:

- Reduce contact with the "initiator carcinogens,"

- Reduce contact with the "promoter carcinogens," and

- Strengthen the body's natural defenses.

## DIGESTIVE SYSTEM CANCERS

Based on data from 1992 to 1995 for 19 of the most populous countries of the Americas, digestive system cancers—cancers of the esophagus, stomach, small intestine, colon, rectum, liver, pancreas, other digestive organs, and peritoneum[1]—cause more deaths than cancers of the trachea, bronchus, and lung[2] combined (PAHO, 1995).

This holds for women in all 19 countries in the Region of the Americas, among whom digestive system cancers are responsible for 21% to 48% of all cancer deaths. In men in all countries except Canada, Cuba, and the United States, those cancers also inflict the most cancer deaths.[3] Digestive cancers in men range from 24% to 50% of total cancer deaths, whereas trachea, bronchus, and lung cancers range from 8% in El Salvador and Nicaragua to 34% in the United

---

[1] ICD-9, 150–159.

[2] ICD-9, 162.

[3] This pattern is changing: trachea, bronchus, and lung cancers are rapidly increasing for both women and men. Moreover, the excess in gastrointestinal mortality is greatest in the oldest age groups. As these cohorts die and middle-aged smokers become the oldest generations, respiratory cancers will become the most common cancers.

States (PAHO, 1992, 1995). Clearly, high priority should be given to the prevention of digestive cancers in most countries.

Digestive system cancers ranked high as a cause of death all over the world in the early 20th century, but have been declining for at least 50 years. This decline parallels the process of industrialization. And while the sociobiological mechanisms involved are still incompletely understood, the decline in stomach cancers tends to coincide with the implementation of more hygienic food processing and storage by preservation in air-tight containers, freezing, or other means that use minimal salt and halt microbial growth. Esophageal, colorectal, and liver cancers follow from other contributing causes, and will be dealt with individually.


## STOMACH CANCER

Industrialized nations experience the lowest rates for stomach cancer, while at the same time having higher rates of colon cancer. Developing and transitioning nations have high rates of stomach neoplasms (and their deaths), whilst generally having infrequent cancer of the colon. WHO estimates that annually there are about 575,000 deaths in the world due to stomach cancer, with 300,000 occurring in developing countries (Hansluwka, 1986). Geographical high-risk areas include Japan, Korea, South and Central America, Eastern and Northern Europe, East and South Asia, and Sub-Saharan Africa. The huge national differences in stomach neoplasm mortality are explained largely by the currently known risk factors and protective factors. Men typically generate two to three times the incidence compared to women.


### Risk Factors

- **Consuming diets high in salty foods and those to which sodium chloride or monosodium glutamate have been added.** These include foods preserved by salt or brine (Riboli, 1996; Trichopoulos and Willett, 1996).

- **Eating foods containing nitrites (often used as a preservative) or nitrates that stomach bacteria can convert easily into nitrites or nitrosamines.** Preliminary evidence also points to the fact that N-nitroso compounds may raise the risk of malignancies in other sites such as the esophagus, colon, or bladder.

- **Smoking cigarettes.** Smoking has been associated, on average, with a 50% excess in stomach cancers in eight cohort studies.

- **Chronic infection with *Helicobacter pylori*.** Infection with this bacteria greatly raises the risk for peptic ulcers, which may, in time, lay the foundation for gastric cancer. Whether uncomplicated peptic ulcer itself is a risk factor is still debated. It appears that *H. pylori* infection might require co-carcinogens or deficiencies in protective factors in order to result in cancer. Because *H. pylori* bacteria are transmitted primarily via the fecal-oral route, improved sanitation could reduce both its transmission and the frequency of reinfection.

- **Atrophic gastritis.** This condition often is a forerunner to gastric carcinoma. The atrophic state may follow from pernicious anemia, reflux of bile acids through the pyloris, or from ingested irritants such as salt and, especially, alcohol.

### Protective Factors

- **Eating vegetables, salads, and fruits every day.** These have been shown the strongest and most consistent protective factor supported by studies all over the world. Green and yellow vegetables and those of the broccoli-cabbage family seem particularly protective against cancers of several sites. Fruits with vitamin C are also valuable (Riboli, 1996; Trichopoulos and Willett, 1996, entire issue).

- **Including animal proteins in the diet.** Some studies have shown dairy products to be protective. This may be due both to the presence of calcium and fat-soluble vitamins.

- **Including foods containing antioxidants, such as vitamin C (water soluble), vitamins E and A (fat soluble), and vitamin A's close relative, beta carotene, in the diet.** Several clinical studies have supplemented participants' diets with these nutrients in the form of pills, but results have generally been disappointing. Ingesting these nutrients in their natural chemical milieu in vegetables, fruits, and other whole foods is not only more protective, but far cheaper.

To prevent gastric cancers, it may be more efficient to add protective factors than to try and remove non-dietary risk factors. For example, changing eating habits to include more of the protective foods—vegetables, salads, and fruits—need not await national policies or economic development. Formal or informal local groups can encourage families to plant vegetable and fruit gardens that include protective foods appropriate to local climate and soil conditions. Even in climates with long, cold winters, warm productive summers can yield produce that can be "home canned" without salt or preservatives and used throughout the year. Local schools can lead the way with demonstration gardens, with the added bonus of teaching children and youth how to teach their families.

Low levels of salt and sodium consumption seem likely to reduce a group's risk of gastric cancers and hypertension. And there are no adverse side effects. The human body's need for sodium is only a small fraction of the amount usually consumed. Salt restriction in adults may create a craving or hunger for it, but this disappears in about a month as the body adapts to a lower intake. Meanwhile non-mineral herbs and spices can give traditional foods new appealing flavors.

## CANCERS OF THE COLON AND RECTUM

Colon cancer ranks as the third leading cause of cancer incidence and mortality for both men and women in the United States; it also takes a heavy toll in Western Europe. It is much less frequent in developing countries, especially in Africa, India, and China. The incidence of colon cancer is low in most of Central and South America, except Uruguay. Economically transitioning areas are seeing an increase in rates, however. Twenty-fold differences in colon cancer mortality are seen across nations, arguing for strong environmental differences in the risk factors. The gut's microenvironment, of course, is shaped by the ingested food passing through, and hence research into dietary practices has been rewarding.

Cancers of the colon and rectum are often first discovered clinically when they cause intestinal blockage or after they have spread. Earlier detection can be achieved by regular check-ups for occult blood in the stool (but the test generates many false positive results) and by colonoscopy. These procedures are too expensive for widespread community use, and so the population-wide strategy of prevention stands out as the one best hope. Fortunately, several strong risk factors are known and can be changed.

### Risk Factors

- **Having close relatives who have had colon cancer.** How much of the risk is genetic and how much is due to a common lifestyle has not been apportioned. A person's family history and the presence of ulcerative colitis or adenomatous polyps point to the need for more frequent follow-up for early detection. Colorectal adenomatous polyps are considered to be a frequent precursor to cancerous growth. They are commonly removed during colonoscopy as a prophylactic measure. Ulcerative colitis should be actively treated to reduce its chances of initiating neoplastic growth.

- **Excessive consumption of red meat and animal fat.**

- **Excessive alcohol consumption.** This has a stronger impact on rectal than on colon cancer.

- **Obesity.** This is a weaker risk (Trichopoulos and Willett, 1996).

- **Tobacco smoking.** This is a risk factor especially for adenomatous polyps (Schottenfeld and Fraumeni, 1996).

### Protective Factors

- **Physical exercise.** Exercise, especially walking, is the best proven risk reducer.

- **A diet rich in vegetables and fruits, and other sources of fiber.**

- **Eating foods rich in calcium and folate.** (Limited evidence.)

- **Consuming fish and seafood.** (Limited evidence.)

- **Regular use of aspirin.** The protective effect of aspirin strengthens with more years of regular use.

Reducing risk factors and increasing protective factors for colon cancer fit into a single lifestyle package. The preventive power of regular physical exercise—be it occupational, recreational, and/or leisure-related—may come as a surprise to many. Consider this, however: walking, walking and running as part of a sport, or doing work that requires total body exertion move the intestines into peristaltic activity, shortening the time that digested and decomposed food—and various naturally toxic, mutagenic, or carcinogenic chemicals—remain in contact with the lining of the small intestines, colon, and rectum. Hence, the exposure both to cancer-initiating and promoting chemicals is reduced. However, neither slowed transit time nor constipation has been linked directly to colorectal cancer. Exercise has a stronger protective effect for colon cancer than for rectal cancer.

The risk and protective mechanisms of diet on colon cancer have not been fully proven yet. Many chemical interactions and the physical impact of fiber are being examined. Fortunately, the preventive messages are already well defined. The protective power of vegetables has been strongly documented (Potter, 1996, 23 of 28 studies reviewed), as has the protective effect of fiber, whether from vegetables, fruit, or whole grain sources. The risk-raising effects of meat protein and fat also have been repeatedly confirmed (15 of the 19 studies).

The effect of regular use of aspirin as a protector against colon cancers has been replicated in several nations. It may also reduce risk of esophageal and stomach cancers. Aspirin also inhibits the growth of colonic and rectal polyps, perhaps by means of inhibiting prostaglandin synthesis. Given the known tendency for aspirin to irritate the stomach and help induce gastric bleeding, aspirin should be taken in a buffered compound to reduce its acidity. Taking aspirin with a meal also protects the stomach lining. There is limited evidence that other nonsteroidal anti-inflammatory drugs (NSAIDs) also may have a protective effect on parts of the gastrointestinal tract (Thun, 1996).

The population strategy of prevention, as outlined in Chapter 2, calls for programs to change culture and lifestyle. These programs should emphasize stomach and colon cancer prevention, as well as the prevention of ischemic heart disease and diabetes. Moreover, programs should emphasize how these changes can make a person feel better immediately, and have more vitality and endurance. The drama of victory over digestive cancers has the same plot as many of the preventive dramas in this book. More exercise. More vegetables, fruits, and whole grains. Less red meat and fats. Reduce overweight. Reduce or quit use of alcohol and tobacco (Potter, 1996; Colditz, 1997).

## CANCERS OF THE ORAL CAVITY, ESOPHAGUS, LARYNX, AND PHARYNX

These cancers are discussed together because they have adjacent locations and share similar risk and protective factors. Moreover, cancers of neighboring sites are sometimes difficult to distinguish clinically, especially after the growth has spread.

These head and neck cancers generally have a high mortality rate. People living in poverty and poorly nourished persons are at higher risk. Southeast Asia and the Middle East experience the greatest incidence of these malignancies, although they are of some concern everywhere. N.C. Madan and colleagues (1986) report that of all diagnosed cancers in India's provinces, 30% to 45% are cancers of the mouth and throat. Elsewhere in the world, the proportion can dip as low as 5%. There are about 300,000 new cases of esophageal cancer in the world each year, 80% of which are in developing countries. France has the highest incidence of cancers of the pharynx and surrounding tissues. Epstein-Barr viral infection appears to be involved in many cancers of the pharynx, and the human papilloma virus has been linked to some oral cancers.

> *Combining excessive alcohol consumption with tobacco use multiplies the risk for cancers of the oral cavity, esophagus, and pharynx.*

### Risk Factors

The major risk factors are heavy tobacco use, including smoking, chewing, or holding tobacco between the gums and cheek, as "snuff" users do. In Asia, the habit of chewing mixtures of betel nut (areca), lime, or tobacco is responsible for tens of thousands of these malignancies each year. Cigar- and pipe-smoking can trigger lip and tongue cancers. Drinking alcohol also causes head and neck cancers, and combining excessive alcohol consumption with tobacco use multiplies the risk. In the Far East, routine consumption of aged, pickled, and molded foods is a major risk.

Poor oral hygiene and lack of dental care are commonly cited as contributing causes to cancers in the mouth. The chronic irritation from long-term use of poorly fitted dentures has been blamed for some cases. Drinking extremely hot beverages has been implicated in raising the risk of esophageal cancer in China, India, and Latin America. The repeated scorching of oral and esophageal mucosa appears to promote such lesions.

### Protective Factors

Once again, protective factors include the generous consumption of vegetables and fruits. Studies of laryngeal and pharyngeal neoplasms add fish and vegetable oils (polyunsaturated) to the list of protective foods. Prevention of this class of cancers should focus on reducing the use of the most potent carcinogens: tobacco, alcohol, and, where indicated, betel nut and the like. The effort will require education and a cultural shift to accomplish this in highly endemic areas.

## CANCER OF THE LIVER

Also called hepatocellular carcinoma, cancer of the liver varies widely by region. It is relatively infrequent in Latin America, but it is a major killer in Asia, China, Thailand and Japan, and Sub-Saharan Africa. Overall, liver carcinoma is one of the top ten causes of cancer deaths in the world (Parkin et al., 1997).

In areas with high rates of liver cancer, most cases are secondary consequences of infection with hepatitis B virus (HBV) or the presence of aflatoxin in foods. Aflatoxin, produced by certain fungi that spread through grains and other crops in warm, moist climates, is particularly destructive to liver cells. As the name implies, hepatitis viruses can cause disabling or fatal liver damage; types B and C are more likely to precipitate neoplasms.

These infections, toxic exposures, and the excessive drinking of alcohol can cause cirrhosis of the liver, and this can be an intermediary to liver cancer. In 1976, Shikata estimated that 60% to 90% of liver cancers, depending on region, emerge from livers that are already cirrhotic (cited by London and McGlynn, 1996). In regions relatively free of aflatoxin, excess alcohol use is the major risk factor, followed by hepatitis B. Hepatitis C virus also is a potent cause of hepatic cancers. As hepatitis C spreads more widely, it will be responsible for an increasing proportion of liver cancers.

Because of the major geographic disparities in the causes of liver cancer, prevention efforts must be tailored to local conditions. A sampling of programs follows:

- Vaccinating infants against hepatitis B. In high prevalence areas, this would mean universal vaccination.

- Improving hygiene to reduce perinatal and person-to-person contact with body fluids and blood products that may carry the hepatitis B virus.

- Reducing the number of sexual partners, encouraging sexual hygiene, and disseminating "safer sex" guidelines to reduce the spread of hepatitis B and human papilloma virus.

- Reducing intravenous drug use, especially sharing or reusing needles.

- Testing blood donations for hepatitis B (and for HIV and other infections) and establishing measures to stop transmission in hospitals and clinics.

- Vaccinating adults at high risk for hepatitis B, such as hospital workers and close contacts of hepatitis B cases and carriers.

- Reducing alcohol use, especially among heavy drinkers.

- Preventing occupational exposure to liver-damaging chemicals.

- Setting up systems for storing and drying grains and bulk foods that protect against aflatoxin-generating fungi.

## CANCERS OF THE TRACHEA, BRONCHUS, AND LUNG

These cancers are treated together because they share similar risk factors and protective mechanisms. After all, they all depend on the air we breathe. Moreover, these cancers are treated as a combined category in international mortality reporting.

The trachea (windpipe), bronchus, and lung are the cancer sites which contribute most to cancer mortality in the majority of industrialized nations. Countries undergoing a transition into full economic development also are experiencing the developed world's epidemic of tobacco use. As a result, trachea, bronchus, and lung cancers will rise in the latter countries, soon to surpass every other cancer.

> *Cancers of the trachea, bronchus, and lung share similar factors and protective mechanisms—after all, they all depend on the air we breathe.*

Occupations that put workers in contact with airborne dust—such as coal mining, ore mining, and quarrying—or industrial emissions of smoke, gases, and chemicals also raise the rates of these cancers among persons exposed. It should be noted, however, that the contribution of these factors to these cancers' rates in the total population is much smaller that that of tobacco. Underground miners exposed to the radioactive gas radon have more trachea, bronchus, and lung cancers, but efforts to link household radon levels to these cancers have been mostly unsuccessful. The effect of industrial exposure is compounded if workers also smoke tobacco. Conversely, rates for these cancers are very low in countries where tobacco is rarely used.

*In every country the world over, the rates of trachea, bronchus, and lung cancers in men are higher than those in women.*

As of the 1990s, the world's highest mortality rates from trachea, bronchus, and lung cancers were among African-American men, New Zealand Maori men, and men living in coal mining areas of Poland, the Netherlands, and Scotland (Parkin et al., 1997).

Air pollution—from smoke, auto exhaust, improperly vented home heating systems, or industrial emissions—has long been implicated in lung cancer and chronic pulmonary disease. In post-industrialized nations, the direct impact of air pollution on cancer is usually overestimated, until tobacco-smoking is properly considered. In industrializing areas that have extremely high pollutant loads, especially inside buildings, cancer rates can rise by 20% to 50% (Blot and Fraumeni, 1996).

In every country the world over, the rates of trachea, bronchus, and lung cancers in men are higher than those in women. In urban areas where tobacco advertising targets women, however, these cancers are rising to become the leading cause of cancer mortality among women.

There is about a 20-year incubation period for lung cancer. In what might be called "a natural cultural experiment" in the United States, cigarette smoking became common among men early in the 1900s, rising sharply in popularity during World War I and through the 1920s. Men's lung cancer mortality, which already was rising in the 1930s, increased dramatically since about 1945. For women in the United states, smoking became not only acceptable but also chic during World War II. Trachea, bronchus, and lung cancer mortality in women, which had been the lowest of all cancers in women, began rising rapidly in the early 1960s, and continued its sharp increase until it became the leading cause of cancer death in women in the United States in the late 1980s—surpassing breast cancer and cancers in any other sites.

Cigarette smoking became hyperendemic among men in China starting in the 1980s, with 60% to 70% of Chinese men smoking in the 1990s. The epidemic

BUILDING BETTER HEALTH

of trachea, bronchus, and lung cancers can be expected to reach alarming proportions in the first decade of the 21st century, with estimated deaths reaching 500,000 per year in that country. These deaths will be in addition to the current annual burden of approximately three million deaths due to tobacco-related diseases worldwide—about one tobacco-related death every 10 seconds (World Health Organization, 1997). Other nations lured into the "tobacco epidemic" will contribute proportionally to this increase in mortality over the next half-century. Of the world's 1.1 billion smokers around the year 2000, 800 million live in less developed countries. The sooner these countries act to stop the marketing and use of tobacco, the sooner their now unavoidable epidemics will subside.

Recent studies agree that a person need not be a tobacco user to suffer from tobacco diseases and death. Several international studies have shown that second-hand smoke or "environmental tobacco smoke" damages fetuses, infants, children, spouses, and co-workers who breathe the same air as smokers.

A prospective population study which followed 256,118 Japanese men and women aged 40 years and older for 17 years generated the following findings: the risk of lung cancer for nonsmoking women living with husbands who smoked more than 20 cigarettes each day was 91% higher than that of nonsmoking women who lived with nonsmoking husbands. The former also developed considerably more cases of breast cancer and brain tumor (Hirayama, 1986). Since about 1980, 30 additional epidemiologic studies have been reported that generally support this finding. Heavily smoking husbands raise their nonsmoking wives' risks of trachea, bronchus, and lung cancers from 30% to more than 100% (London and McGlynn, 1996, p. 643).

Other sections in this handbook that deal with pregnancy, infancy, childhood, and youth, as well as with cardiovascular and respiratory diseases, further document the damage that tobacco use inflicts on families. **(The section "Tobacco Use" in Chapter 13 discusses interventions to prevent and help stop tobacco usage.)**

### Risk Factors

- **Smoking cigarettes and, to a lesser degree, cigars, pipes, and other forms of tobacco.** This accounts for at least 80% of cases of lung cancer.

- **Exposure to radon.** Radon is a radioactive gas emerging from uranium and soils containing this element. Uranium workers and miners for coal or ore who work underground in the vicinity of uranium deposits are at highest risk. Radon gas attaches to dust and aerosol surfaces, entering the body as one breathes. Radon is odorless, tasteless, and colorless. Smoking multiplies its effect (Matzen and Lang, 1993, pp. 922–923). Radon is of little concern in most parts of the world.

- **Asbestos exposure.** This mineral has a long history for causing asbestosis and laryngeal and gastrointestinal cancers, as well as having a major impact on lung cancer. Persons who work with insulation materials, in shipyards, railway yards, and brake factories are at highest risk of encountering this mineral. Concerted efforts are under way in many countries to eliminate asbestos from products and from public buildings.

- **Exposure to other industrial dusts and gases.** Exposure to such compounds as arsenic, chromium processing compounds, coal tar, diesel exhaust, and soot causes additional malignancies of the respiratory apparatus. Various mining, smelting, and refining processes contribute risk, unless their airborne effluents are safely contained.

### Protective Factors

- **Breathing the cleanest air possible.** Avoid tobacco smoke and steer clear of places that have cigarette smoke or smoke from stoves, heaters, or other sources. Industries that generate smoke, fumes, and dust should protect workers by providing adequate venting, filters, precipitators, and the like, or by distributing breathing masks that effectively remove all airborne pathogens.

- **Dietary habits emphasizing vegetables and fruits.** Vegetables and fruits containing vitamin A and beta-carotene are particularly protective. It should be noted, however, that some clinical trials with beta-carotene in pill form have been unsuccessful and others were stopped prematurely because the supplement either raised the incidence of lung cancer or strokes (Riboli, 1996). The protective effect of vegetables and fruits has been supported by ecologic, case-control, and other study designs in several countries. Therefore, these foods can safely be incorporated into community programs.

### Social Influences

Although cigarette smoking is a habit of individuals, it invades communities under the umbrella of a social norm. Tobacco advertising targeted towards young people shows rich and attractive people smoking, and portrays smoking as a "cool" habit. Once the habit takes hold, nicotine's addictive properties make it difficult to get rid of the habit.

Prevention and control of tobacco use are best achieved by policy actions at the sociopolitical level and by cultural change, reaching children and young people through schools, youth groups, the mass media, religious groups, health professionals, and families. This is a moment of opportunity for nations to make a preemptive strike against smoking before smoking becomes socially acceptable and their societies fall prey to its addiction. Primary schools are the ideal place to start implanting anti-tobacco attitudes and feelings as well as disseminating knowledge about its ill effects. This is the time to teach refusal skills to children and youth— to teach them how to refuse the offer of free tobacco. Children thus taught will then become teachers to their families and the community at large. Adding import restrictions, imposing higher taxes, barring the sale of tobacco products to persons under age 17 or 18, and making health facilities and public buildings smoke free also will reduce cigarette usage.

> **Primary schools are the ideal place to start implanting anti-tobacco attitudes and feelings as well as disseminating knowledge about its ill effects.**

Traditional cultures and communities also must impress upon their women and girls that they do not have to copy the ignorance and weakness of those men and boys who have allowed themselves to be victimized by tobacco habits. Girls and women, the great majority of whom are still non-smokers, can remain wiser, stronger, and healthier than male smokers by resisting what is obviously a self-destructive addiction, one that has dire health and economic consequences even for the tobacco-free members of the family. **(See further preventive efforts in the section "Tobacco Use" in Chapter 13.)**

## CANCER OF THE BLADDER

Cancer of the bladder is relatively infrequent in North America and Western Europe, more common in South America and the Caribbean, and a major cause of cancer death in the Middle East, Asia, and Africa. Where schistosomiasis is prevalent, cancer of the bladder is endemic. The parasitic flukes and eggs circulate throughout the body's systems, including blood and lymph vessels, heart, digestive system, and bladder. Relatively few of the thousands of cases of schistosomiasis finally initiate a cancer in the bladder, but enough do to make it a common malignancy in some countries.

Elsewhere, the main established risk factor is cigarette smoking. Some of the inhaled carcinogens are stored in the bladder until discharged. Many chemicals used in the rubber, shoe, and crude oil refining industries also target the bladder.

Protective actions include avoiding the above exposures, plus eating vegetables and fruits every day. No other dietary associations have been demonstrated yet. Individuals and families can quit smoking or never start, as well as incorporate healthy eating habits. However, it requires continued governmental action to deal with the exposures to schistosomiasis and industrial chemicals.

## SKIN CANCERS

Skin cancers are the most prevalent form of carcinoma in fair-skinned populations. Fortunately, although they present themselves in several pathological types, most are easily detected, easily removed, and rarely cause death. The most common types are basal cell and squamous cell carcinomas. About 99% are treated successfully by local physicians. The main agent is exposure to the sun's ultraviolet rays. The vulnerability factor is fair complexion, or blonde or red hair. Anatomically, about 80% occur on the face, head, and neck.

The most lethal type of skin cancer is malignant melanoma. It is increasing at an alarming rate (about 3% to 7% per year) among fair-skinned people, many of whom are overly dedicated to getting "a healthy tan" every summer or who are exposed to ultraviolet light in winter. It is mostly a cancer that affects younger adults. The incidence of malignant melanoma in the populations of northern European origins ranges from 3 to 20 per 100,000 population worldwide. Persons having Asian, Mediterranean, African, or Indigenous American descendents are much more protected from skin cancers. Fortunately, most lesions are discovered and treated early enough to prevent death. Thanks to earlier detection, the five-year survival rate of diagnosed melanoma has risen from only 40% in the 1940s to 80% in the late 1980s. Early lesions are flat and thin, less than 0.76 mm penetration from the epidermis inward. Prompt surgical removal of such early lesions assures survival. Melanomas usually appear in skin areas with the most sun exposure, but some forms also occur in unexposed areas. This calls for personal as well as health worker vigilance.

The primary risk factor for skin cancers generally is exposure of unprotected white skin for many years to direct sunlight or repeated severe sunburn over a shorter period. The shorter wavelengths (less than 400 nm) of ultraviolet-B radiation are most damaging because they penetrate the skin more deeply. Ozone in the atmosphere absorbs ultraviolet rays, but as ozone continues to be depleted by certain air pollutants, sunburn problems will become more severe and more widespread. Ultraviolet-A rays contribute to retinal damage and cataracts, ultraviolet-B rays contribute to skin cancers, and both contribute to premature aging of the skin and the lens of the eye. Most people are protected indoors, in that window glass blocks most ultraviolet-B and up to half of ultraviolet-A rays. It should be pointed out that total avoidance of exposure to the sun also is unhealthy. Sunshine helps generate vitamin D, which works with calcium to develop strong bones and teeth. Some sunshine is essential to life and health. It is the extremes that should be avoided.

Occupational exposure can also cause skin cancers. Contact with coal tar, pitch, creosote, arsenic, and radium can be carcinogenic.

## Risk Factors

The risk and protective factors are quite similar for all cell-types of skin cancer. The list here emphasizes those that have been best documented for malignant melanoma.

- **History of melanoma in a first-degree relative.**

- **Blonde or red hair.**

- **Marked freckling on upper back.**

- **History of three or more sunburns with blisters before age 20.**

- **History of three or more summers working at an outdoor job before age 20.**

- **Presence of actinic keratoses (skin lesions).**

According to R.J. Friedman and colleagues (1991), persons with three or more of the above risk factors have a 20-fold increased risk of developing malignant melanoma.

In addition, the following factors also identify high-risk persons:

- **Eye color not brown.**

- **Inability of skin to tan; skin that gets red, then peels.**

- **Skin that has many moles.**

Environmental risks include:

- **Living in tropical latitudes.**

- **Exposure to the sun in the middle of the day.**

- **Exposure to the sun at high altitudes.**

- **Exposure to bright reflections off water or snow.**

Attention should be paid during cloudy bright days. Clouds do not block ultraviolet-B rays and because the air feels cooler, people can get severely sunburnt before they realize it.

- **Covering the skin with light-blocking clothing.**

- **Using umbrellas or wide-brimmed hats to protect the face and neck.**

- **Constantly protecting babies and young children, whose skin is extremely vulnerable to sun damage.**

- **Using sunscreens.** Lotions and creams should have enough sun protective factor—labeled as "SPF." An SPF value higher than 15 blocks about 90% of ultraviolet-B rays. For people with sensitive skin, SPF of 30 or more is recommended. Sunscreen creams work best when applied 45 minutes before going into the sun. Water-resistant sun creams "hold on" somewhat better through perspiration and water contact while swimming, but do need reapplication to regain their initial strength. After a base tan is established, lower SPF values may be tried. Turning tan is the skin's own effort to block UV rays from penetrating.

- **Teaching people to work out their own balance between sun exposure and sun protection.** Any burn that hurts or stings for more than an hour or two is your body's way of saying: "You've had too much sun. I'm hurting you to remind you not to do this again."

- **Parents and those working with children "taking control" of children's sun exposure.** Children get so involved in play and fun that they may resist coming out of the sun in time to avoid a burn. Prudent adult supervision has immediate value, and also can reduce the far future risks of malignant melanoma.

### Secondary Prevention

People of all ages should be taught to check the skin over their entire body periodically, looking for spots of changed color, rashes, raised growths on the skin, and, especially, dark moles. Suspicious changes or lesions should be brought to a health professional familiar with dermatology for more expert evaluation. Changes in congenital birthmarks anywhere on the body are also a reason for referral. The key word here is *changes*. Any of the following changes in the spot or surrounding skin warrants a medical evaluation: color, size, shape, elevation from skin surface, sensation (tenderness, itching) (Friedman et al., 1991).

Teachers, athletic coaches, and lifeguards, as well as health professionals, already are in good positions to be observant for skin lesions. Pre-cancerous changes usually appear on parts of the body frequently exposed to the sun.

Thorisdottir and colleagues (1993) present a simple algorithm for estimating the risk that a mole, a "skin sore," or pigmented skin spots may be, or may become, a malignant melanoma. It is as easy as A, B, C, D.

**A**symmetry—one-half of the sore is not shaped like the other.

**B**order of the lesion is irregular—may have a scalloped or leafy edge or irregular points, perhaps irregular thickness.

**C**olor that varies across the lesion, possibly including two or three shades of tan, brown, black, blue, red, or white.

**D**iameter—usually greater than 6 mm (or about ¼ of an inch)—the diameter of an average pencil.

If more than one of these features are present, the person should be brought to a physician familiar with dermatology for a definite diagnosis. Such active case finding and diagnosis is mandatory because of the necessity of early diagnosis to prevent a melanoma from becoming fatal. Professional and public education and early detection and referral can reverse this steadily rising death rate.

## CANCERS OF THE UTERINE CERVIX

Cervical cancer is reported to be the second most common cancer in women in many parts of the world. Most nations of the world report cervical cancer incidence ranging between 5 to 20 per 100,000 population per year. Again, differences between countries based on economic development are large and troubling, and they can be overcome. Many Latin American nations have incidence rates between 50 and 60 per 100,000 population. In Peru, for example, the capital, Lima, has an incidence rate of 27 per 100,000, while the city of Trujillo has a rate of 54 per 100,000 (Parkin, 1997, pp. 803–1053). Jamaica and Mexico had the highest cervical cancer mortality rates in the Americas in the late 1980s. In the United States, there are ethnic differences, with Hispanic, Korean, and African-American women having the highest cervical cancer rates in the country. Economic status seems to be one of the strongest determinants. For example, before reunification, East Germany had about twice the rate of these cancers as West Germany (21 and 11 per 100,000 population, respectively).

*Studies of cervical cancer repeatedly show that this malignancy behaves like an infectious disease. It appears to begin as a sexually transmitted viral infection, and over time develops into a neoplasm with uncontrolled cellular multiplication and spread.*

A country's economic development is a potent determinant for the kind of female cancer that is most prevalent and causes most deaths. In developing countries, for instance, women have more cervical cancer, whereas in industrialized countries with fully developed infrastructure, breast cancer far outnumbers cervical cancers, both in incidence and number of deaths. As economic and health service development proceeds, an area's uterine cancer rates fall and breast cancer rates increase simultaneously—clear evidence that cultural changes affect the population's way of living and its way of dying.

Epidemiologic and clinical studies of cervical cancer repeatedly show that this malignancy behaves like an infectious disease. It appears to begin as a sexually transmitted viral infection, and over time develops into a neoplasm with uncontrolled cellular multiplication and spread. Several viruses have been intensively studied in this connection, including herpes simplex 2, but most experts now attribute most cases of this cancer to prior infections with the human papilloma virus (HPV). More than 60 types of HPV have been identified thus far: some have been shown to spark neoplasms and additional ones are being identified. Among sexually active, healthy women, 20% to 50% (depending on the sample examined) have evidence of HPV infection, past or present. It is not known whether they harbor a "safe" variant of HPV, or if they will develop cervical cancers in the future. The similarity of cervical cancers to late stage sexually transmitted infections (STIs) is demonstrated by the risk factors.

### Risk Factors

As the following list shows, risk factors for cervical cancer include both women's sexual behavior and other lifestyle factors (Matzen and Lang (eds.), 1993, Chapter 30; Peters et al., 1986; Chin, 2000).

- **Starting sexual intercourse soon after menarche.** Compared to later starters, girls who start sexual relations before one year after menarche have 26 times the risk; girls who become sexually active within one to five years after menarche only have seven times the risk.

- **Women who become sexually active before age 16.** These women have 16 times the risk.

- **Women who have had four or more sexual partners.** These women have 3.6 times the risk of those who had none or one partner until the time of exam.

- **Women with a history of genital warts caused by HPV.** These women have 3.2 times the risk.

- **Being married to a man who was previously married to a woman having cervical cancer.**

- **Being married to a man who has penile or prostate cancer.**

- **Smoking cigarettes.** This factor may be secondary to the above factors, however.

## Protective Factors

Actions that reduce risk of STIs also reduce risk of HPV infections and, thus, of cervical cancer. Protection can be had by:

- **Using condoms or other barrier protection.**

- **Both partners practicing monogamy.** Both partners must have tested negative for STIs, including HPV and HIV.

- **Testing for all STIs and getting prompt treatment as necessary. (**Also see the section "Unsafe Sex" in Chapter 13.**)**

All the above relate to primary prevention. These should be given a greater priority by health services, many of which rely only on screening for changes in cervical tissue. All women testing positive on a Pap smear should be taught these primary risk and protective factors, to help them reduce risks of repeated infection leading to more malignant tissue changes.

## Secondary Prevention

The Papanicolaou (Pap) smear has become the primary weapon in the campaign to discover cervical tissue changes early enough to treat surgically and prevent death. The sharp reductions in cervical cancer in economically advanced nations have been attributed to effective screening of adult female populations with this test. It is essential to note, however, that the downward trend in cervical cancer mortality in the United States began more than a decade before the Pap smear was widely available. Given this, one might conclude that something inherent in economic development helps to reduce mortality from this cause, perhaps educational improvements, fewer sexual partners, greater self-care among women, better hygiene, and better STI control.

*Women over 65 years of age account for nearly half of cervical cancer deaths. The first priority should be to get every woman screened at least once, starting with older women and progressing to younger ones.*

The effectiveness of cervical screening in reducing uterine cancer mortality is no longer debated. Canada's well-organized British Columbia Cervical Cancer Screening Program between 1955 and 1990 produced a 78% decrease in the incidence of invasive cancer and a 72% decrease in mortality (Matzen and Lang, 1993). Two similar screening programs in the United States have shown a 40% and a 50% decline in mortality, respectively.

The International Agency for Research in Cancer (IARC) recommends that every woman be given a Pap smear every three years. The Agency estimates that this would reduce invasive cervical cancers by up to 90%. Other official agencies recommend screening shortly after a woman becomes sexually active, with a second test one year later. After two negative smears, move to a schedule of once every three years. Women over 65 years of age account for nearly half of cervical cancer deaths. The first priority should be to get every woman screened at least once, starting with older women and progressing to younger ones.

Women who have never been screened, over time generate four times the rate of cervical cancers than those coming to screening. There seems to be a positive correlation between some life habits and adverse social environments that contribute both to cervical cancer and failure to participate in screening programs. Sponsors of screening need to persevere, aware of the reward that the higher percentage of lives saved will occur among the last persons screened. **(Also see Chapter 11.)**

Cancers of the body of the uterus (corpus uteri) also are also relatively common in the United States, but are less frequent elsewhere. They are often called endometrial cancers, because it is the endometrial lining of the uterus in which the carcinoma develops. Mortality from cancer at this site has declined dramatically since 1950, and it is not a major public health threat. Its risk factors differ from those for cervical carcinoma. Further information on this cancer can be found in gynecologic textbooks.

## BREAST CANCER

With economic development come rising levels of education, increasing attention to personal hygiene, better sanitary facilities in homes, and greater availability of health services. Greater education gives people a sense of responsibility for themselves—greater ability to make decisions and to do what is necessary to implement them. These changes in social development, including women's greater participation in paid work outside the home, tend to delay the age of marriage, reduce the average number of pregnancies, and shorten the duration of breast feeding. And all these raise the risk for developing breast cancer. Breast cancer occurs more often in women of middle to upper socioeconomic status.

The risk of getting breast cancer does not correlate highly with the risk of dying from it. And again, socioeconomic development plays the critical role. Women with access to, and participation in, early detection have a much greater chance of surviving breast cancer and returning to a fully active life. Advanced tertiary interventions, despite their high costs, have contributed relatively little in the past to reducing a community's mortality from breast cancer, but early detection and prompt treatment have.

The highest incidence of breast cancer occurs in the United States. White, non-Hispanic women in large California cities have rates that exceed 100 cases per

100,000 population per year. Western Europe and Scandinavia have incidence rates that range between 40 and 90 per 100,000. Developing countries in South America report rates of 20 to 40 per 100,000, except for Westernized countries such as Uruguay, which has a rate of 93 per 100,000. A striking example of the power of lifestyle and ethnicity over environment comes from Zimbabwe, where the incidence of breast cancer is 128 per 100,000 among residents of European descent, compared to only 20 among those of African ethnicity. Clearly, less developed countries and localities have a much lower incidence of new breast cancer, although they collectively still experience about 125,000 deaths per year. That is about the same total generated by all developed countries—for a world total of about 250,000 deaths annually (Hansluwka, 1986).

On the bright side:

- some of the risk factors for incidence are known,

- early detection and treatment can greatly reduce the risks of death per 1,000 cases, and

- breast examinations and mammography have proven to be effective in many studies.

On the dark side:

- Breast cancer incidence rates in the United States increased by about 3% per year during the 1980s. While many experts believe this was largely due to more effective screening outreach, how much was due to a true surge in malignancies is not known. This apparent increase leveled off in the 1990s. One might therefore expect that as other nations intensify breast examination and mammography outreach, they too will discover many more cases that require advanced diagnosis and treatment services. These services will reduce mortality rates, however.

- Known risk factors account for only 20% to 30% of the diagnosed breast cancer cases. This means that by far most new cases will continue to be found in women who have no established risk factors. A "total population" approach may need to be used for screening efforts. The risk factors below can be used to set priorities for the people with whom to start programs, but not for when to consider stopping.

### Risk Factors

- **Age.** Breast cancer mortality rises sharply with age. One source considers that high risk starts at age 40, another at age 65. Women over 65 years old have four times the risk of breast cancer compared to those under 40, with intermediate risk applying to ages 40–64. The gradient of risk with increasing age goes up moderately in developing countries, but rises sharply in industrialized ones.

- **Personal history.** A prior breast cancer or biopsy evidence of atypical hyperplasia raises the risk.

- **Family history.** A close relative having premenopausal or bilateral breast cancer raises the risk.

- **Early menarche and late menopause compared to local population.**

- **Being a Caucasian woman born in North America or Northern Europe.** There is some genetic effect, especially for cancers emerging before age 50.

- **Higher socioeconomic status.**

- **Never having a completed pregnancy, or late age at first pregnancy.**

- **History of ionizing radiation or radiation therapy to the chest or mid-back, especially before age 20.**

And for some risk factors that are easier to change:

- **Obesity, and possibly excess dietary fat, especially after menopause.**

- **Diet too low in vegetables and fruits.**

- **Alcohol intake of two or more drinks per day.**

While research has identified many risk factors, public health planners and clinicians must remember that most women who develop breast cancer may show none of the above risk factors.

### Protective Factors

- **Avoid drinking alcohol regularly.**

- **Maintain appropriate weight, keeping the percent of body weight in fat low.**

- **Avoid unnecessary exposure to X-rays, especially under age 20.**

- **Eat vegetables and fruits regularly.**

- **A low-fat diet.** (The benefits of a low-fat diet are still being debated.)

## Secondary Prevention

The goal of secondary prevention is to discover a disease early and treat it promptly. This allows for simpler, more effective elimination of the problems before suffering, disability, or death occurs. There are three approaches to screening, at three levels of "technology." The first is the cheapest, but requires the most effort to make it function in a community.

- **Breast self-examination.** Breast self-examination (BSE) can be taught to groups of women by a woman health professional. In many places nurses have become the experts for such teaching. The teaching goal is for women over age 40 to know how to do a proper self-examination and to repeat it every month, one week after the end of their menstrual period, and monthly after menopause. Instruction manuals are available in many languages. In places where breast self-examination is widely practiced, 70% to 80% of breast cancers are discovered by the patients themselves. Suspicious small lumps or hard spots should be brought to a health professional for further diagnosis. Women can do this knowing that 80% of lumps are not cancerous, and the ones that are dangerous can be removed or treated in ways to make them harmless.

Despite public health's years of teaching and reinforcing proper and regular breast self-examination, large scale follow-up studies to date have been unable to document its effectiveness at the community level. Recent breast self-examination training programs based on social cognitive learning models have demonstrated positive results lasting six months or more (Clark and Becker, 1996). It will take more trainees and more time to determine whether there are positive results in terms of stages at which cancers are discovered.

- **Clinical examination by a trained professional.** This second level of screening should be done each year by a health professional who has had focused training in breast examination. This clinical exam should detect more subtle changes missed in the self-exam. This is also an opportunity for the health professional (of any discipline) to check on the woman's techniques for breast self-examination, reteach if needed, and remotivate the patient to continue self-examination faithfully until the next clinical examination.

> *Large-scale mammographic screening programs should receive a higher priority in localities where risk of breast cancer is high.*

- **Mammography.** The most sensitive method for detecting early breast lesions is the mammogram. The United States Preventive Services Task Force recommends that this radiologic exam be done in all women without symptoms every one to two years, starting at age 50. Of course, it or a biopsy should be used to make definite diagnoses when breast self-examination or clinical examination are questionable. In large field studies, routine mammography has been shown to lower mortality effectively only in women over age 50. The value of routine mammography in young women without signs or symptoms has not been established (Fletcher et al., 1993). In many parts of the world mammography is not yet available. Fortunately in most such developing areas, breast cancer risk is relatively low.

Large-scale mammographic screening programs should receive a higher priority in localities where risk of breast cancer is high. As with all other preventive expenditures, priorities should be determined based on local burdens of disease, using some measure of quality-adjusted life years (QALYs) saved per 100,000 units of currency expended.

Despite the costs of mammography, it is one of the few screening tests (along with Pap smears for cervical cancer) that has actually been shown to save many lives, even after adjusting for biases. It catches malignancies earlier than other methods, when treatment can be less radical and more successful (Budd and Bhatia, 1993; Thomas, 1986; Schottenfeld and Fraumeni, 1996).

## PROSTATE CANCER

As men's life expectancy increases in most parts of the world, the prevalence of diagnosed prostate cancer will continue to rise. Differences in incidence are huge worldwide, ranging from 0.8 per 100,000 in a screening center in China to more than 100 per 100,000 among urban men in the United States. In the United States, African-American men have higher rates compared to European-Americans, with Asian-Americans having the lowest incidence of all. Around 1990, cancer of the prostate became the most prevalent malignancy in men in the United States, excluding skin cancers.

*Prostate cancer can be called "the iceberg" of all malignancies, because such a small fraction of it is ever discovered clinically.*

Men in Australia, Iceland, Scandinavia, and Switzerland have incidence rates of 40–60 per 100,000. In Central and South America, prostate cancer is less frequent, except in Westernized industrialized areas. Cancer registries and standardized screening programs are few in Central and South America, so estimates are based on mortality figures. Reported rates might be underestimated by a low index of suspicion for this cancer site among persons completing death certificates.

Prostate cancer can be called "the iceberg" of all malignancies, because such a small fraction of it is ever discovered clinically. Studies in the United States show that in a large series of male deaths between ages 80 and 89 years, 70% of men showed evidence of undiscovered prostate cancer at autopsy. Most prostate malignancies begin later in life and progress so slowly that far fewer prevalence cases die because of that diagnosis, and instead die of other unrelated causes. The few men developing this cancer in their 50s or younger often have a more rapidly growing cell type of malignancy, and the benefit-to-cost ratio for screening and treatment is much more advantageous for these younger men than for men older than 70 or 75 years.

The risk factors and causes of prostate cancer remain poorly understood, despite its high frequency. A genetic component is involved, with a man's risk rising sharply according to the number of close relatives who have had the disease. It is still being debated whether enlargement of the prostate gland that comes with age is an independent risk factor. Several findings point to the likelihood that androgens and testosterone might be involved, either in terms of their quantity or in their balance with other hormones. There is some evidence that high dietary intake of animal fat and red meat may be associated with increased risk, and that regular consumption of vegetables and fruits may reduce risk. Regular physical activity may also have some protective effect. Nevertheless, public health has few clues firm enough to aid primary prevention.

### Secondary Prevention

Men over 50 years old who come in for periodic health examinations will benefit from having a digital rectal exam (DRE) by the clinician. This will detect benign prostatic hypertrophy—enlargement of the gland—and will also reveal any lesions on the surface of the prostate gland. Many men, usually in their older years, will report the symptoms of benign prostatic hypertrophy: difficulty in starting and stopping urine flow; increased frequency of urination, especially at night; and reduced pressure in the urine flow (dribbling). Prostatic cancer also can cause such signs and symptoms, yet may not do so until the lesion is far advanced. All such signs warrant a more thorough search for a malignancy.

The United States Preventive Services Task Force does not recommend routine prostatic screening for men without signs or symptoms. The prostate specific antigen (PSA) blood test is fairly sensitive in identifying cancers, but since PSA values rise with age and in men with enlarged prostates, the test generates excessive "false positives." Other current screening techniques also tend to generate too many "false positives." This means that many men are told that they might have cancer—a frightening thought—only to have the disease ruled out later through more invasive and expensive diagnostic tests. Current screens, especially the DRE, also fail to identify many true cases. In addition, current treatment options are difficult or painful, and too often unsuccessful.

This section is included to describe the current status of this increasingly prevalent cancer, and to argue for more research into its etiology, prevention, improved screening, and treatment.

# 10. Chronic Lung Disorders

Each day, the average adult inhales between 10,000 and 20,000 liters of air. Given this huge quantity, even minute amounts of airborne toxins can accumulate to a serious body burden of damaging substances. Even with air pollution as dilute as one part per million, a sedentary adult will take in about 10 cm$^3$ of concentrated toxic burden, and a person actively working or exercising will take in about 20 cm$^3$. (Some of this may be quickly exhaled or coughed out.) Since the bronchial and lung surfaces adsorb much of the airborne pollutants, the body burden builds each day of exposure, accumulating over the years. In the case of a commonly used class of pesticides, the organophosphates, this could become deadly.

This section deals with chronic obstructive pulmonary diseases (COPD), emphysema, asthma, respiratory allergies, and other chronic diseases of the lungs, including tuberculosis. It does not include acute infections of the upper and lower respiratory tracts, influenza, and pneumonia. While these acute respiratory infections reap their mortality mostly among infants and children, chronic lung diseases disable and kill mostly older persons, with worldwide death rates doubling every decade from age 50 to 80 years.

> *... respiratory disease, perhaps more than any other type of disease, can be prevented more easily than cured. Emphysema and all the respiratory cancers (nasal, laryngeal, bronchial, alveolar, and pleural) could all be rare if only society applied the knowledge that it already has to prevent them.*
>
> —Sir Richard Doll (1993)
> Pioneer researcher in the
> epidemiology of cancer

Chronic lung disorders are the third leading cause of lost years of health—disability adjusted life years (DALYs)—for both women and men over age 60 (Murray and Lopez (eds.), 1996, pp. 573–576). On average worldwide, men over 60 years old lose 47 healthy years per 1,000 population annually, whereas women these ages lose 31 healthy years per 1,000. Death rates for respiratory cancers in these ages are much higher than for chronic lung diseases, but the longer duration of the latter accumulate more years of disabled living.

## CHRONIC OBSTRUCTIVE LUNG DISEASES

The pathology of chronic obstructive lung diseases involves irreversible loss of elasticity of lung airway tissue and partial obstruction of large and small airways. Subsequently, the walls of the lung air sacs (alveoli) become damaged and lose their efficiency in transporting oxygen and carbon dioxide between the lungs and bloodstream. Cigarette smoke especially damages the moist surfaces where exchange of these gases takes place. This, in turn, reduces a person's capacity for exercise, increases shortness of breath and the frequency of coughing, and renders breathing difficult, rather than "being automatic."

Chronic obstructive lung diseases constitute an accelerated aging of the lungs. The same dysfunctional changes occur gradually over time, such that people 80 years old may show the same symptoms as do smokers 50 years old. Earlier cases are mostly due to years of "bad air"—in most patients, air polluted by tobacco smoke, and in others, exposure to industrial smoke, irritating fumes, dust from mines, quarries, road-building, cotton processing, farming dusts and molds, and metal smelting and processing. Family differences in lung vulnerability have been occasionally documented, but such influence is small and plays no part in prevention.

> *"Cure" is not an option for chronic obstructive lung diseases or emphysema. Primary prevention—"clean air for all"—is the cheapest and best option for the community.*

"Cure" is not an option for chronic obstructive lung diseases or emphysema, because the tissue damage is irreversible. Moreover, treatment and rehabilitation are costly and often unsuccessful. Clearly, primary prevention is the cheapest and best option for the community. And primary prevention in this instance means "clean air for all."

The disease agents for chronic obstructive lung diseases include many kinds of chemical vapors and fumes, and suspended particulates of certain sizes and shapes. Preventive efforts can succeed even when based on a more simplistic model.

### INDOOR AIR POLLUTION

By far the most prevalent indoor air pollutant worldwide is tobacco smoke. As a result, primary prevention falls along two tracks: reducing the smoke burden in the air and effectively preventing nonsmokers from having contact with such polluted air. Over time, open cooking or heating fires in the home can create serious lung damage if they are not adequately vented to remove smoke and fumes out of the home.

Other indoor pollutants occur mostly in the workplace. **(The best documented harmful chemicals and dusts are listed in the section "Occupational Health Hazards" in Chapter 13.)** For example, cotton dusts in processing plants cause byssinosis, a form of chronic obstructive pulmonary disease. It has been shown that forced expiratory volume in one second (FEV-1)—a measure of lung function—can decrease from 5% to 10% in the course of one

228

work shift in a cotton processing plant, although most of this function returns after exposure ceases. Further, the longer one works as a spinner or weaver in a typical cotton textile plant, the higher the prevalence of clinical byssinosis and its associated reduced respiratory function. Studies in developing nations have recorded byssinosis prevalence ranging from 18% to 30%. Prevalence is much lower where factories have successfully reduced airborne particles (Mur, 1993, pp. 18–19). Similar chronic, but less lethal, problems have been reported for airborne flour dust in flour milling and commercial baking industries. As with most pollutants, the risk of disease is directly correlated with the amount of acute and accumulated body burdens.

Isocyanate exposure also has been linked to chronic obstructive pulmonary disease. These chemicals are used in paints, varnishes, and polyurethane foam. Painters in factories or working alone are at higher risk; workmen using spray-painters are at particular risk. Again, smoking tobacco multiplies the lung damage these chemicals inflict (Mur, 1993).

## OUTDOOR AIR POLLUTION

Farming also can expose persons to risks for serious lung diseases. Working with grain, hay, and straw can raise great amounts of dust, and both farmers and grain storage workers are at risk. In addition, grain, hay, and straw may contain mold and other micro-organisms. These particles can cause acute or chronic lung problems, including allergic reactions. Some of these lung problems include:

- Toxic syndrome due to organic dust. Symptoms begin a few hours after exposure, and may include coughing, trouble breathing, fever, muscle pains, and headaches. Although symptoms typically last only a few days, repeated bouts with this syndrome can lead to chronic bronchitis.

- Farmer's lung. This condition occurs only after repeated exposure to grain, hay, and straw dust. It shows the same symptoms as the above syndrome, lasting from a few days to a few weeks. After exposure stops, farmer's lung improves more rapidly than does toxic syndrome.

- Chronic obstructive bronchopneumopathies. These conditions are marked by the same symptoms as the two conditions above, plus productive cough (i.e., spitting up phlegm), shortness of breath, and wheezing from the chest (not bronchi). This condition does not go away after exposure ceases, and is associated with reduced lung function, as measured by forced vital capacity and FEV-1.

Other outdoor exposures include polluted air in cities and surrounding populated places. Sites downwind from factories or power generation plants that emit smoke are particularly dangerous. If prevailing winds blow smoke or fumes to an area, the risk for chronic and acute respiratory disorders increases for people living or working there.

Fumes and smoke from motor vehicles carry odorless and colorless—and lethal—carbon monoxide, as well as smelly, smoky byproducts of combustion, such as fuel vapors and suspended smoke particles. Trucks and buses contribute far more pollution per vehicle than do automobiles and motorcycles, but the greater number of smaller vehicles makes them collectively the greatest source of city air pollution. Auto repair shops become dangerous unless doors and windows are left open, and places in which gasoline or diesel motors are running also need to have exhaust fans. Particularly damaging substances are carbon monoxide, sulphur dioxide, nitrogen oxides, lead fumes, ozone, polycyclic hydrocarbons, and suspended particles of carbon, carbon ash, and mineral dusts.

*Millions of people live in cities where vehicle fumes cause them to cough acutely or even to choke on the air. Local or regional governments can reduce such health threats by establishing and enforcing emission standards on fuel burning motor vehicles.*

Millions of people live in cities where vehicle fumes cause them to cough acutely or even to choke on the air. This may well be an unscientific measure, but nature clearly is saying that human health is endangered. Local or regional governments can reduce such health threats by establishing and enforcing emission standards on fuel burning motor vehicles. It may be more politically feasible to begin by regulating trucks and buses, because of their obvious smoke, and later proceed to regulate automobiles and motorcycles.

## ASTHMA

Asthma afflicts people of all ages. In the past, the clinical focus was on childhood asthma, but in the last few decades, asthma has become much more prevalent in older persons in market economies. The reasons for this are unclear, and may include longer histories of smoke exposure, better treatment that prevents death but does not cure the disease, and a higher index of suspicion for this diagnosis causing it to be made more often. The same causes that create chronic obstructive pulmonary disease are responsible for activating full-blown asthma attacks and making acute episodes more frequent.

Asthma is a disease involving reversible episodes of airway obstruction caused by muscular constriction of the trachea and bronchi. Excessive reactivity of the air passages is involved along with inflammation. Asthma episodes may be caused by inhaling irritants or may be an allergic reaction, such that both external irri-

230

tants and allergic responses to those irritants may combine to cause symptoms. The usual sequence of asthma development involves initial exposures to airborne irritants, a period of bodily sensitization, and then the development of abnormal airway hyper-reactivity. The primary symptoms are shortness of breath, coughing, wheezing from bronchi, tightness in the chest, and fatigue due to the increased effort to breathe. Severe acute asthma can cause death if not promptly and properly treated. Lung function tests done with a simple spirometer are good field screening methods both for seriousness of asthma and for degree of chronic obstructive pulmonary disease.

Asthma is the most common occupational respiratory disorder in the United States, Canada, and other developed nations. It is increasing rapidly in developing nations, as certain industries increase. About 200 different agents are estimated to cause occupational asthma in exposed sensitized persons. The list of specific agents is quite similar to that for chronic obstructive pulmonary disease, but also includes exposure to animals, especially cats, and furry laboratory animals.

The economic costs of progressive asthma are considerable, because disability after long exposure to irritants and a long history of symptoms will persist after exposure stops. Many workers are forced to seek other kinds of work, or require some social assistance for partial disability.

### Prevention

Primary prevention includes:

- Stop tobacco smoking.

- Remove environmental tobacco smoke left by smokers.

- Use newer technologies to precipitate industrial air pollutants before they reach human air space.

- Screen workers for hypersensitivity to lung irritants and counsel them to avoid jobs where they are exposed to irritants that affect them.

Secondary prevention includes performing lung function tests, such as spirometry, every year or two (depending on level of exposure). For persons with reduced lung function, total cessation of tobacco smoking is mandatory and job reassignment to work in cleaner air is strongly recommended. The respiratory system cannot repair itself from chronic damage, and as of now there are no medications that will heal it. Act accordingly.

## FIRST STEPS TO CONTROL ENVIRONMENTAL AIR POLLUTION

It would be a daunting task, indeed, to set up a program to measure and cleanse community or worksite air from the dozens of chemicals, dusts, and combustion end-products identified here. Nations and provinces would be delayed for years by pursuing the goal of cleaner air via such an "itemized" approach.

Fortunately, a quicker, cheaper strategy is available. The United Kingdom since 1956 has focused its clean air programs on smoke control. The effort consisted of measuring the darkness and density of smoke using a standardized chart which rates the shades of gray from black to white. Black smoke contains more pollutants and suspended particles than light, gray smoke. The object is to work with factories and vehicle owners to make their smoke as light and transparent as possible. This simple system was evaluated in a U.K. smoke control area using air sampling techniques. Tests found that both suspended particulates and sulphur dioxide were greatly reduced (Samet and Spengler, 1993). This is a good beginning to pollution reduction. After this is rigorously implemented, environmental scientists can determine whether further higher technology programs are needed to deal with invisible gases.

A similar system might be developed to measure dust levels. A focused light beam (or several) could be projected across a textile factory, flour mill, quarry, or mine, with a light meter at the other side. The loss of lumens between projector and meter should be directly related to the density of pollution.

Another approach to evaluate the need for air cleansing is to have workers wear breathing masks with effective filters, then measure the nature and amount of pollutants caught by the filters. Will it make a health difference if every worker breathes properly filtered air? Does use of such filters reduce the loss of lung function measured over the course of a work day?

## SECONDARY PREVENTION OF CHRONIC OBSTRUCTIVE PULMONARY DISEASE

Secondary prevention involves screening of workers and subpopulations. For persons showing partial airway obstruction or decreased airflow, it is necessary to intervene aggressively to halt their exposure before they become seriously disabled.

Respiratory screening usually is done with a hand-held spirometer. This simple, inexpensive device (about US$ 10) measures the total volume exhaled in one second (FEV-1) and the total volume exhaled in one breath (FVC) when the subject blows into the spirometer's tube. Spirometers are supplied with disposable paper mouthpieces—a new clean one for each user. (The task is forced exhaling only.

To prevent infections, caution subjects against inhaling.) According to T.L. Petty (1993) these two simple indicators are adequate for most screening and clinical purposes. Spirometers are to respiratory function what blood pressure instruments are to cardiovascular function. Petty urges that they be available and used regularly in all clinics and medical practices. FEV-1 and FVC should be measured and recorded annually, especially in occupational settings, so that downward trends can be detected and stopped. They are also important for mass screening.

Chronic pulmonary diseases have been one of the plagues of the 20th century. There is no need for them to continue in the 21st century. We know how to stop this plague. A young "clean air generation" should not gasp for breath, lose mobility, and die from chronic obstructive pulmonary disease as their grandparents did.

## TUBERCULOSIS

Tuberculosis is covered in this chapter because it is a chronic disease of the lungs. Clinical disease usually first emerges long after the initial infection. Active cases are usually discovered by tuberculin skin tests, which reveal a history of infection, or by chest X-ray. Tuberculosis occasionally attacks organs of the body other than the lungs. After treatment the disease can remain dormant in patients for many years, always with the risk of reactivating into advanced disease and spreading infection to other people.

Tuberculosis is becoming epidemic again, especially in developing countries. People of all ages are susceptible to the infections, but the highest death rates occur between ages 30 and 59, accounting for nearly half (46%) of the nearly two million total tuberculosis deaths each year (Murray and Lopez (eds.), 1996). While the tubercle bacillus is necessary for diagnosing the disease, it is by no means a sufficient cause. In some economically advantaged areas, only 1% or 2% of infected people (by PPD skin test) become clinically ill in the next decade. In some disadvantaged areas more than 50% of infected persons may become clinically ill.

*Tuberculosis as a cause of disability and death comes to full force in localities without adequate sanitation and public health programs, where people live in crowded, poor housing with substandard working and living conditions and poor nutrition.*

Tuberculosis as a cause of disability and death comes to full force in localities without adequate sanitation and public health programs, where people live in crowded, poor housing with substandard working and living conditions and poor nutrition. Professor George Comstock (in J.M. Last, 1986) calls tuberculosis "to some degree a barometer of social welfare." In industrialized nations, tuberculosis also is increasing again, especially among the poor, the homeless, the poorly nourished, and those with impaired immune systems, such as persons with HIV. About one-third of HIV cases in the world are expected to have tuberculosis listed as their final cause of death.

Tuberculosis takes a greater toll on men. Because it strikes early in life, with elevated death rates from age 15 onward, the disease has a greater economic impact on developing communities than do those chronic diseases whose impact becomes serious only after about age 50. Tuberculosis ranked as the sixth leading cause of loss of healthy life-years (DALYs) in the developing world in 1990 (18.5 million per year for ages 15–59 years). Nearly 40 million healthy years of functioning were lost for the entire age span. No improvement is projected through 2010.

The tuberculosis bacillus is transmitted by airborne droplet nuclei put into the air by actively infected persons who cough, sneeze, or otherwise suddenly exhale. Their sputum also is infective. In areas where cattle are not tuberculin tested and dairy products are not pasteurized, tuberculosis can be passed on to humans.

In low-incidence groups, such as middle-class populations in developed areas, most clinical cases of tuberculosis are caused by the reactivation of dormant (latent) encasements of bacilli in the patients' lungs. Tuberculosis can be kept from spreading by continuing treatment with antibiotics, such as isoniazid, rifampin, and in instances of drug resistance, newer antibiotics. Proper dosages and combinations of antibiotics can make the patient non-infectious usually in one to three months. This also stops progression of the disease in the original patient. Dormant, encased pockets of the bacillus can reactivate under stressors such as malnutrition, exhaustion, extended exposure to silica dusts, or another serious infectious disease.

Treatment failure in patients is usually due to an incorrect combination or dosage of antibiotic drugs or to inadequate adherence to the prescribed drugs by patients. Some treatment centers are using a technique called Directly Observed Treatment Short Course (DOTS), whereby the patient is directly observed taking each medication dose by a health worker or trusted relative or work supervisor. This speeds the transition of sputum and aerosols to non-infectivity and stops the advance of the disease in the patient.

Primary prevention of tuberculosis involves several concurrent actions: teaching everyone, especially infected persons, always to cover their mouths and noses while coughing or sneezing, use of aerosol blocking masks by caretakers when in the presence of persons with uncontrolled coughing or sneezing, hand washing and general cleanliness, finding and testing close contacts of the patient to determine whether they also are infected, and improving social and living conditions for families (Chin, 2000).

The overwhelming importance of behavior, social conditions, and environment in the rise, fall, and resurgence of the tuberculosis pandemic has been highlighted by a United Kingdom study. Around 1848, death certification became adequate enough in geographic spread and reliability to assess annual tuberculosis mortality per 100,000 population in England. The death rate from tuberculosis declined without antibiotics by 97% between 1848 and 1948, the year that streptomycin, the first antibiotic for tuberculosis, became widely available in England. The use of antibiotics between 1948 and 1971 reduced tuberculosis mortality by only an additional 1.5% from the 1848 rate (McKeown, 1976). McKeown attributed the pre-1948 decline to concerted social action against poverty.

Treating tuberculosis with antibiotics is one of the most cost-effective of all public health interventions, costing only US$ 3 to US$ 7 for each year of disability prevented. Given the cost of the disease, starting with two million lives per year, plus uncounted disability, lost production, broken families, etc., a much higher priority should be given to its prevention.

# 11. Injuries and Violence

This chapter deals with acute damaging events—motor vehicle crashes, falls, injuries from machinery, drownings, poisonings, gun shots, fires, smoke inhalation, lacerations, head trauma, suffocation, and other intentional or unintentional traumata. Injuries typically involve a transfer of energy to an organism in a quantity or form that the organism is not prepared to receive. The impact is usually sudden, but also may be subliminal and cumulative, as in repetitive movement injuries or radon exposure. **(Also see the section "Reducing Rates of Unintentional Injuries" in Chapter 3.)**

Worldwide, injuries and violence account for 19% of years of lost health (DALYs) in men and 11% in women of all ages. Hardest hit, however, are men and women 5 to 44 years old. Table 11.1 shows "externally caused" deaths as a percentage of total mortality by sex and age.

Men's death rates from injuries are double to triple those in women for most specific trauma categories. The total estimated numbers of deaths due to intentional and unintentional injuries for all ages were 834,000 in developed regions, compared to 4,250,000 in developing areas. (These are estimated death counts and do not take population sizes into consideration.) These numbers lay to rest the long-held belief that injuries are primarily a problem of the industrialized world (Murray and Lopez, 1996). **(See also Chapters 12 and 13 for further discussion.)**

Two ways of thinking help the pandemic of injuries and violence continue at full throttle. These false assumptions are:

- that such events occur randomly, that they are "accidental";

- that this is "just the way life is around here"—that it has always been this way and the community has learned to accept it.

> *There were an estimated 834,000 deaths due to intentional and unintentional injuries for all ages in the developed world, compared to 4,250,000 in developing areas. These numbers lay to rest the long-held belief that injuries are primarily a problem of the industrialized world.*

Those false assumptions are easily replaced by the following two scientific axioms, which already have saved many thousands of lives in all regions of the world:

- Trauma and injuries are not "accidents." They have causes and risk factors. We may not be able to predict the exact time and persons to be involved in any one injury situation, but some useful truths are known about higher risk times, places, and persons. For example, intoxicated persons sustain more injuries than sober ones; the chance of a motorcycle injury becoming fatal is directly proportional to the bike's speed and the rider's lack of helmet; medicine bottles with child-proof closures are less likely to be involved in childhood poisonings than open medicine bottles—and the list goes on.

Furthermore, many injuries are intentionally caused (see Table 11.1), and, clearly, these are not accidents, either. In many instances, intentional injuries can be prevented by keeping the aggressor, the weapon, and the victim separated. **(Table 2.1 in Chapter 2 illustrates a broadly applicable epidemiologic strategy, using auto injuries as an example. Chapter 7 offers suggestions for reducing the intensity of intent which lies behind intentional injuries.)**

- "People who do not learn the lessons of the past are forced to re-live it." But we have learned that the future need not be like the past, as attested by some of the success stories in the battle against diseases.

For example, yellow fever and neonatal tetanus have been eradicated from many places, but this only happened after people believed that they did not have to accept these diseases as part of their geography or culture. People learned that they could help eliminate troubles from their lives—and so they did.

**TABLE 11.1.** **Mortality due to injuries and violence, reported as a percentage of all deaths within each age and gender subgroup, worldwide, 1990.**

| Age | Males | | Females | |
|---|---|---|---|---|
| | Unintentional | Intentional | Unintentional | Intentional |
| 0–4 | 4.6% | 1.1 | 3.9% | 1.3 |
| 5–14 | 26.6 | 5.4 | 17.9 | 3.7 |
| 15–29 | 31.9 | 26.9 | 14.8 | 17.9 |
| 30–44 | 20.8 | 14.8 | 8.9 | 9.3 |
| 45–59 | 7.8 | 4.4 | 4.6 | 3.3 |
| 60–69 | 2.9 | 1.7 | 2.3 | 1.5 |
| 70+ | 2.0 | 0.9 | 1.9 | 0.6 |
| Total (in thousands) | (2,137) | (1,186)[a] | (1,096) | (665)[a] |

**Source:** Calculated from data in Murray and Lopez, 1996.

[a] Among the intentional deaths, self-inflicted deaths (suicides) were estimated at 456,000 for men (38% of the "Intentional" total), and at 330,000 for women (50% of their "Intentional" total). About 502,000 deaths were attributed to war in 1990. This total includes 211,000 men, 141,000 women, and 150,000 children under age 15 years. Over half—58%—were women and children.

The same can be done for many forms of child and adult injury. Health promoters can start working to reduce risks, increase protections, and lower disability step-by-step. And, like any journey, it will take time. Dramatic reductions in injuries and traumatic deaths can be achieved in the same ways as the conquests of many diseases: after the systematic population study of risk and protective factors, and field trials of the efficacy of intervention programs.

## MOTOR VEHICLE INJURIES

Road traffic collisions were estimated to have caused almost one million deaths worldwide in 1990. Counting both years lost to premature death and years lost from disabilities, the GBD Study estimates a burden of more than 34 million years of healthy life lost (DALYs). Worldwide, motor vehicle accidents are the single largest cause of death and disability due to external causes. Nearly half (45%) of these lost DALYs and 40% of these deaths occur among males 15–44 years old. Motor vehicle deaths are increasing most rapidly in developing nations.

### THE CULTURAL HISTORY OF VEHICLE INJURIES

Nations follow a natural history in the rate and nature of vehicular injuries. It goes something like this. First, motorbikes, trucks, and cars begin to enter the environment; then they increase in numbers; then roadways are improved, going from pathways, to roads, to superhighways; then average speeds and the disparity in speeds increase. The increase in numbers of vehicles per 1,000 km (or miles) of roadways is referred to as a nation's motorization.

Early in the process of motorization, the number of injuries relates more closely to the number of vehicles, rather than to the size of the population. At this stage, political decisions must be made and updated to protect the rights and safety of the unmotorized majority versus the motorized minority. One example is the paving of "speed bumps" on streets where many people live or walk and vehicles go too fast for safety. Speed bumps can be designed to allow different speeds depending on the location. Drivers hate speed bumps, but the lives of many pedestrians and bicyclers can be saved. Another example involves cutting parallel grooves a few centimeters apart across a concrete roadway. This creates a vibration in cars that warns drivers of excess speed or other reasons for caution. As the density of motorization rises, limitations on the nonmotorized population increase, as pedestrians are told to cross the street or road only at marked crosswalks, and bicycle

> *Worldwide, motor vehicle accidents are the single largest cause of death and disability due to external causes. And motor vehicle deaths are increasing most rapidly in developing nations.*

and cart traffic is limited to the outside lane of the right-of-way, or even to special lanes separated by lines or barriers from lanes used for motor vehicles.

Roadway traumata are of two types: injuries to persons inside vehicles and injuries to persons outside vehicles (nonmotorized). The relative proportion of these in a given area depends on the number of moving vehicles . . . sometimes. Early in a nation's motorization, most injuries and fatalities occur to people who are walking or riding bicycles, to children and others who run out into streets and roadways, and to people in carts pulled by animals. As more motor vehicles take to the road the frequency of collision between them rises, and the balance of injury shifts more to vehicle occupants. There are well proven procedures which can safeguard each group (Trianca et al., 1988).

The traffic injury epidemic in every nation results from three interacting components: roadways, vehicles, and roadway users (drivers, bikers, walkers). In the past, traffic safety programs focused mainly on getting "bad drivers" off the roads, but actually, the majority of all crashes involve "average drivers." Hence, traffic safety needs to deal with all three factors.

To address each of the three interacting components of traffic injuries, communities should apply the three Es of intervention—Education, Engineering, and Enforcement. For the public, these interventions can be *active*, when a person must do something to be safe (e.g., keep from driving across the median into oncoming traffic or buckle a seat belt); or *passive*, when the safety measure is "built in" (e.g., concrete barriers separating two traffic directions or roll-over bars built into vehicles). Passive interventions usually are far more effective in preventing injuries.

## THE EDUCATIONAL CHALLENGE

It often takes a full generation of experience with "motorization" (widespread use of motor vehicles) for a cultural group to learn to live safely with motor vehicles. The route to safety can be analyzed in terms of four broad stages.

**First,** the community must overcome the fallacious thinking that injuries are "accidents," that they must be accepted rather than prevented (see earlier discussion).

**Second,** there must be intense education of everyone from young children through the elderly—but especially of males prior to ages 15–44—about the proper use of roadways and vehicles and their dangers. Such teaching can take place within families and at child-care centers and schools (elementary, secondary, and technical). Maternal and child health clinics, workplaces, agricultural agents, the police, and the media all can play important roles.

What is to be taught? Respect, even fear, of motor vehicles. How to cross roads safely. How to walk along roadways (at the edge, facing oncoming traffic). Bicycle safety.

What should be taught to drivers? Safe driving skills and attitudes. Obedience of the rules of the road. Limitations of speed. Hazards in roadways. Sharp attention to the road ahead (many crashes occur just after brief lapses in the driver's attention). Proper care of vehicle, especially brakes, steering, lights, tires. When children are passengers, they should sit in the rear seats of cars. When small, they should sit in properly attached safety seats; when larger, they should use seat belts. Children should not ride in the back of open trucks because of danger of falling into the roadway.

> *Maternal and child health clinics, workplaces, agricultural agents, the police, and the media all can play critical roles in teaching roadway and vehicle safety.*

Forjuoh and Li (1996) rate the efficacy, affordability, feasibility, and sustainability of 19 interventions aimed at reducing transport injuries. Educational interventions rank highly on the last three criteria, but do not rank well in terms of efficacy in reducing injuries and deaths. Historically, the introduction of new engineering and better enforcement has proven to be more effective.

Local media, such as town and district radio stations and newspapers, can render an important educational service by reporting traumatic deaths and severe injuries (due to motor vehicles, for example), including the place of crash and name of the victim. Studies of infectious diseases have shown that members of the public who know a person with a given disease (a "case") are more likely to take preventive action (a vaccine). The same principle should operate for trauma, and should increase safe behaviors. People one knows mean much, much more than statistics.

**Third,** communities must improve the quality of drivers of vehicles, be they mopeds, autos, farm trucks, or 18-wheel tractor trailers. Training in operating skills is the simple part, and often the only part formally taught. Riding as a passenger with a careful driver provides a model for how to perform these tasks safely. More important is training in judgment of speeds, distance, times and places for overtaking other vehicles, and the likelihood of having persons entering the roadway. Perhaps most important is learning and practicing rules of the road and driving ethics, as well as exercising emotional control when frustrated or angered. Even persons who are otherwise psychiatrically normal can so identify themselves with the power of a motor vehicle as its driver, that they claim for themselves a driver's "divine right," ignoring the rights of all others. Aggressive driving, in men or women, creates the same dangers. Psychologically speaking, being in a vehicle permits expression of aggression from within a cloak of anonymity (Professor B.J. Campbell, personal communication). Drivers must accept that their rightful goal is not to subdue or defeat all other vehicles, only to pass through traffic safely. A culture tends to learn driver ethics through 20 to 30 years of painful experience. Can proper teaching and role modeling make this learning happen faster?

**Fourth,** pedestrians also need training, especially in localities where motor vehicle traffic has traditionally been light. Everyone needs to keep children from running out into roadways, and to make sure that children keep their wagons, tricycles, and other wheeled toys from carrying them into danger. **(Also see text on reducing rates of unintentional injuries in the section "From Birth Through Age 4 Years" and in "Screening Checklist from Ages 5 through 14 years in Chapter 3.)** Pedestrian mortality rates in the United States are relatively constant across age decades until age 70, when deaths increase greatly. In the United States 40% of adult pedestrians killed have high blood alcohol levels. People who have been drinking should not walk near traffic. A sober person should accompany them to a safe place to recover. Always, walk on sidewalks or on the side of the road facing oncoming traffic. When walking at dusk or in darkness, always wear light colored reflective clothing. When bicycling, wear light-colored clothing and equip the bike with reflective tape or reflectors. In the rain wear bright yellow (not dark) raincoats.

*A prescription for anyone walking in or near traffic: Remain alert, no daydreaming, no distractions like headphones. Walk defensively. You are responsible for your own safety and survival.*

## THE ENGINEERING CHALLENGE

The greatest responsibility for containing—or "channeling—the threat of motor vehicles rests with the community. It is the community that builds, repairs (sometimes), and polices the roadways. Proper street and road engineering is the first step. This engineering has developed into an advanced science. Some of its newer techniques are low tech and inexpensive. It is better to build safely from the beginning, rather than to bequeath a blood-hungry infrastructure to future generations. When planning a new road, it is best to set aside a wide right-of-way, perhaps two to three times wider than the initial roadway. Most roads between busy cities need to be widened every 10 years because of increased traffic. This advance planning for space will save much money in the long run. Many expert consultative resources are available at little or no cost from ministries of transportation and international organizations such as WHO, PAHO, and the other Regional Offices.

Road features that limit speed are valuable—speed bumps, turns in the road, an unrepaired surface, all do quite well. Deep holes or ridges in the road surface are harmful, however, because they damage steering mechanisms and may cause cars to swerve and cycles to overturn. Another warning device called speed strips or rumble strips consists of strips or bands of rough or serrated pavement which create noise and vibration when crossed at too rapid a speed. This can be a warning that a stop sign is ahead or that the vehicle is going off the driving lanes, either to the left or right. Proper installation of warning signs and stop signs, painting lane lines on pavements, and creating turn lanes where traffic patterns require them cost little; their savings in human and property damage are comparatively greater. Head-on collisions—the impact of vehicles moving toward each other—are particularly lethal. Such crashes can be largely prevented by separating opposite traffic directions with barriers, fences, or wide spatial separation (e.g., dual-lane highways). In cities where speeds are less, similar benefits may result from one-way streets.

Other proven safety measures in roadway construction include:

- Make road curves of large radius, rather than small, and bank curves to reduce frequency of vehicles leaving the road.

- Make road shoulders hardened or paved.

- Use surfacing materials that provide good adhesion to vehicle tires to reduce skidding, especially in wet weather.

- Shield bridge abutments and immovable barriers with collapsible "bumpers" that reduce crash impact. A variety of bendable rails and plasticized barrels are produced for this purpose.

- Move poles for power and light well off the shoulders, and remove trees which might make an impact fatal.

A systematic life-saving program for towns and cities is to maintain records of locations of vehicular collisions causing deaths or disability. This includes injuries to people who are on foot or riding bicycles. Keeping track of minor collisions ("fender benders") may require much work, but they tend to correlate highly with places and times where major losses occur. One or two impacts or collisions might occur anywhere, but when a "spot map" shows larger clusters of incidents, helpful interventions can be made, often cheaply.

Vehicle engineering plays a major role in transport safety. The typical incident involves two crashes: first, the vehicle either hits an "outside" object (such as another vehicle, a post, barrier, wall, or a pedestrian) or it runs off the road; and second, the initial impact throws persons inside the vehicle against the dashboard, steering column, window glass, inner roof, or doors. Doors may swing open, and riders may be ejected outside onto unforgiving surfaces, depending on the speed of the vehicle on impact.

The exterior of the auto or truck can be designed and built to absorb as much shock as possible, thus reducing the crash acceleration of passengers inside. Similarly, the interior design can contribute to safety by cushioning the dashboard, steering wheel, and backs of front seats; constructing the steering column so that it slowly collapses on impact; installing crash-resistant door locks; and, most important of all, installing three-point safety seat belts that restrain both the shoulder and the waist. Such safety belts protect front-seat riders from crashing their heads on the windshield, and also prevent ejection out of the car, which too often has fatal consequences. Properly installed air-bags for riders in the front seats also add to safety, but only when the three-point seat belt is also worn at the same time. Seat belts are much cheaper than air-bags and far more effective as well.

In addition, new engineering changes are seeking to make vehicle exteriors less damaging to cyclists and walkers, by reducing protrusions on the front and sides of the vehicles and shaping the front to deflect the object struck to reduce frontal impact and move the object (or person) away from the wheels (Trinca et al., 1988).

## THE ENFORCEMENT CHALLENGE

Early in a nation's transition to motorization, it is essential for that country to develop, publicize, and teach its population a comprehensive, clearly defined system of laws relating to traffic behaviors of drivers, passengers, bicyclists, and pedestrians.

Enforcing such traffic regulations is an essential community function, which will have substantial effects in terms of lives saved. Consistent enforcement with locally appropriate penalties works on the principle of behavior modification by penalizing violations. Even though perhaps only a small percentage of such violations are initially punished, the effect on the total numbers of such behaviors will be substantial. Social learning principles will spread the effect to non-penalized persons, tending to change their behavior.

### Important Infractions from a Safety Viewpoint

- **Excessive speed for the section of roadway involved.** Higher speeds reduce the chance to avoid collision. They increase the distance it takes to stop. They make accurate steering more difficult. They increase the chance that an impact will be fatal both to those outside and inside the vehicle. Consider that two vehicles approaching one another, each at a speed of only 80 km/h (50 mph), collide with an impact equal to one car crashing into a concrete wall at 160 km/h (100 mph). Head-on collisions at such speed assure the destruction of both vehicles—and usually of the persons within.

- **Carelessness, risk taking, distraction, and attention lapses.** Stop and change drivers when the current driver feels inattentive, road weary, or emotionally upset. Where possible, it is wise to rotate drivers every few hours before fatigue sets in.

- **Impairment of drivers by alcohol or drugs.** This creates the highest risk of impact, crippling injury, and death. Severe penalties such as revocation of driving privileges or time spent in jail are appropriate. The legal definition of intoxication (and penalties) is a blood alcohol level of only 0.08% to 0.10% in most English-speaking nations. While other countries may have different standards, most places have definitions based on observable behavior, such as slurred speech, unsteady gait, odor of breath, slowed reflexes, or impaired thinking. Intoxicated driving is not that frequent in total populations, but because of its virulence, must be eliminated. Scandinavian nations have taken the lead in building zero-tolerance of impaired driving into their laws and culture (Evans, 1991, especially Chapters 7 and 8).

Social pressure and peer group helpfulness are far more effective than the law in keeping people who have been drinking alcohol from driving a vehicle. Media campaigns with the slogan "Friends don't let friends drive drunk" appear to be effective. Even persons not obviously intoxicated often have their senses, coordination, and judgment impaired just enough for a crash to happen. A group going to a party or event where alcohol will be served often appoints a "designated driver," who on that occasion will abstain from all alcohol and drive the group home safely. Using a taxicab or obtaining a ride from a fully sober person are other ways to avoid "drinking and driving" a motor vehicle. Even partly intoxicated persons walking along a roadway are at great danger because of their inattention and erratic walking pattern.

*Young drivers everywhere are involved in more crashes than older drivers. Delaying the eligible age for acquiring a driver's license will cut crash frequency.*

In places where traffic laws are new, largely ignored, or scoffed at, enforcement has a trauma-strewn road ahead of it. There are three specific antidotes to this problem:

- Establish the laws early in the area's movement into motorization and create a recognition of their practical value in the population.

- Teach schoolchildren and youth the rules of the road.

- Phase in enforcement by punishing the more serious infractions first, such as driving while under the influence of alcohol, reckless driving, speeding more than 30 km/h (or 20 mph) over the posted speed limit, and failure to stop at designated sign posts.

This kind of phase-in of enforcement has not been adequately evaluated in the field, but has the theoretic advantage of "making real" the fact of enforcement. First, it requires only a few arrests to spread the news widely. Second, it does not overwhelm traffic police and magistrates with large numbers of prosecutions. Third, a few arrests for obviously dangerous behaviors are less likely to create a community "backlash" of anger against authorities than many arrests suddenly.

After this level of enforcement becomes accepted as routine, traffic officials can begin enforcing less extreme violations, particularly if they result in a crash. Throughout each stage of the process, *consistency* of enforcement is essential. Later, officers also can begin issuing warning citations to persons with other infractions, such as making illegal turns and driving a vehicle lacking required safety equipment, such as burned out lights, ineffective brakes, or cracked windshields.

In some nations with a long history of motorization, new laws requiring seat belt use by everyone riding in the front seats of cars or trucks were phased in first by passing the law and providing public education, then by a month or two of "warning tickets" (citations), followed by comprehensive enforcement with monetary fines. For defective equipment violations, after the "learning period," enforcement consisted of issuing an arrest citation that the car owner could eliminate by coming to the police station within five days and showing a traffic officer that the equipment problem had been repaired.

## CROSS-CUTTING INITIATIVES

Other strategies for reducing vehicle injuries involve decreasing the number of individual vehicles on the road. Improving public transport systems in cities— bus or rail—and giving residents incentives for using them can be a valuable strategy. Bus and rail travel is not only safer per million passenger miles, it also reduces air pollution and traffic congestion in cities. Singapore, home to far more vehicles than city streets and boulevards could hold safely, pioneered restricting the use of private autos to alternate days, based on the last digit of the license number. Other cities provide remote parking and low cost commuter rail to the city. France has used a different tactic: taxing vehicles according to engine size. Since high speeds require large, high-powered engines, faster cars get taxed more. The result: fewer high-speed cars on the road.

Restrictions on drivers also have proven valuable. Young drivers everywhere are involved in more crashes than older drivers. If persons must be licensed before being allowed to drive (and violations are firmly penalized), delaying the eligible age for receiving a driver's license will cut crash frequency. Some states in the U.S.A. now have a stepped licensing program: 16-year-olds are eligible to receive a license after passing tests, but they can only drive an automobile if accompanied by an older licensed driver and can only drive during the day. Driving privileges are then incrementally expanded each six to twelve months. Other states only permit teenage drivers to carry one other teenager as passenger, because having several teenagers in one car has been found to create an especially high risk.

National, state, and provincial governments can help communities to reduce traffic deaths by introducing the vehicle equipment standards detailed below. After a run-in period sufficient for the early majority to obtain the recommended equipment, these standards can be required by law. **(Also see the section "Diffusion of Innovation" in Chapter 12.)**

- Motorcycles and their riders incur far more crashes per 100,000 km than do passengers in four-wheeled vehicles. Therefore, governments should encourage, and later require, drivers and passengers of any two-wheeled motor vehicle capable of going more than 50 km/h (30 mph) to wear safety helmets while riding. Helmets should be able to withstand impacts at the above speed without cracking open. The most frequent cause of death and most costly form of injury while riding motorcycles is head trauma with permanent brain damage. Helmets reduce the risk of fatality by about 28% in serious crashes. The most effective way to increase helmet use is to require wearing helmets by law, and enforcing it (Evans, 1991).

- Require all locally produced or imported cars or trucks to have safety belts installed, especially in front seats. In the United States, all but one state requires front-seat occupants to use seat belts. Three-point, harness type seat belts that restrain both shoulder and waist protect against the "second collision"—when the body hits the car interior after the car has hit an outside barrier or moving car. Shoulder belts protect the face and head. Restraints also keep the person inside the car. Ejections from the vehicle during severe impacts are very often fatal. Combined lap/shoulder belts reduce risk of fatalities to front-seat riders by about 40%, with half of this effect (based on United States national statistics) coming from preventing driver or passengers from being ejected from the vehicle (Evans, 1991, p. 247).

> *Traffic safety strategies that have worked in highly motorized nations may not be transplanted successfully without major modifications. Proven principles work, but not necessarily the details.*

- Smaller children require safety seats having their own restraints and being latched to seat belt anchors, preferably in rear seats. In the United States, all 50 states require that children be restrained in child safety seats or safety belts, depending on their size, or they must ride in the back seats. In a collision, an unrestrained child becomes a missile launched against vehicle windows, struts, and metal—often fatally. Areas mandating child safety measures quickly learn their value in lives saved.

- In developing areas many people ride in the backs of open trucks or cling to the sides of buses. Open trucks require protective railings, so standing passengers do not fall out at bumps or turns. Trucks and buses also should have sturdily mounted grab bars to assist people entering and leaving vehicles.

The problems associated with establishing and advancing traffic safety programs in developing nations are complex. Strategies that have worked in highly motorized nations may not be transplanted successfully without major modifications. It should be kept in mind that proven principles work, but not necessarily the details. More recently motorized areas need not reinvent the wheel, however. That would take unnecessary time and unnecessarily lose lives. The ideal is for the developing nation to face its problem early by constituting a panel of advisors combining international and national traffic safety experts, and work out cooperatively a year-by-year plan. The process is thoughtfully and critically described in the 1998 volume edited by the Global Traffic Safety Trust.

## CARBON MONOXIDE IN VEHICLES

Carbon monoxide (CO), an odorless, colorless gas, is the leading cause of fatal poisoning in the United States and is similarly serious elsewhere. Carbon monoxide occurs wherever fuels burn. CO poisoning of drivers, passengers, and auto repairmen is always a threat wherever motors are running in an enclosed space without sufficient free flow of outside air. Exhaust systems must be regularly checked for leaks, especially in buses or trucks where people ride in the rear. Of course, children are damaged by lower concentrations of CO than adults.

Early symptoms of carbon monoxide poisoning are drowsiness, dizziness, headache, or nausea. Anyone experiencing any of these common symptoms, should be questioned to eliminate CO exposure. Children arriving at school with these symptoms should have their buses checked. If repairs cannot be done the same day, bus windows should be kept open until the problem is fixed. Truck drivers with these symptoms should keep windows open.

## LOOKING AHEAD

Although the overall numbers of injuries may rise in a province or state as the numbers of vehicles increase, the future still looks more encouraging over time. The cultural changes of a motorizing society tend to reduce the burden of motor vehicle trauma in terms of hundreds of millions of vehicle miles driven. That means that nations become safer over time per unit of travel completed. In the United States between the 1920s and the 1990s, the motor vehicle death rate decreased from about 15 deaths per 100 million vehicle miles to about 2. This suggests that any nation committing itself to highway safety can achieve similar proportional reductions. This can be accomplished in fewer decades, now that research has identified which are the most successful initiatives.

## SUICIDE AND VIOLENCE

Worldwide, there were 786,000 deaths recorded as due to suicide and 563,000 due to violence (homicide) in 1990. According to the Global Burden of Disease Study, an additional 502,000 deaths were attributed to wars (see Table 11.1 for a breakdown of intentional and unintentional deaths). These worldwide figures mask the vast differences that exist in these rates across countries. Given such differences, each country must develop programs tailored to its own circumstances. (The sources consulted for this section were Bennets, 1993; and Murray and Lopez, 1996.)

Why anger emerges, how intense it is, and how it is expressed are tied to a person's cultural and ideological background. Interestingly, countries that have the highest suicide rates tend to have low homicide rates, and the reverse is true elsewhere. The same distinction between suicide-predominant versus homicide-predominant areas is observed among the 50 states of the United States. The social acceptability or degree of disdain toward suicide or homicide not only influences those persons who consider perpetrating the act, but also the validity of reporting. In most nations an unknown fraction of suicides and homicides are recorded as accidental deaths.

*Worldwide there were 786,000 deaths recorded as due to suicide and 563,000 due to violence in 1990, but these figures mask the vast differences that exist from country to country.*

The highest suicide rates among men occur in the former socialist economies, particularly among men aged 30–59 years old. Countries with the highest suicide rates in men are Hungary, Finland, China, and Japan. Established market economies, China, India, and other parts of Asia and the Pacific Islands follow. In most regions, the suicide rate increases with age, with China experiencing an annual rate of 104 per 100,000 for men over age 60.

The picture is very different for women, with suicide being infrequent, except for China, which has the highest rates, especially among young women 15–29 years old (44 per 100,000 in this age group). This compares to 23 per 100,000 in India, and 4 in the established market economies for women in the same ages. The highest suicide rate for women is 92 per 100,000 for women older than 60 years old in China. Suicide is extremely rare among women in Sub-Saharan Africa, Latin America, and the former socialist nations.

The cost of suicide goes far beyond years of life lost. While worldwide data are unavailable, many industrialized nations find that only about 5% to 15% of suicide attempts are fatal. The remaining 90% or so attempts incur many millions of dollars in medical expenses, and about 5% suffer permanent disabilities. Suicide rates have risen sharply the world over in the last 30 years, even affecting adolescents. However, suicide is still most frequent in the oldest ages. According to the GBD Study, suicide rates will continue to rise until at least 2020.

The ecology of homicide differs greatly from that of suicide. Highest worldwide risks are among men in Sub-Saharan Africa (176,000 deaths in 1990), where homicides outnumber suicides by 13 to 1. Latin American and Caribbean men have the second highest risk of violent death, at 89,000 such deaths in 1990 and a 5.6 to 1 ratio of homicide to suicide. In Africa, women die of assaultive violence 10 times as often as by suicide. These ratios are high because the number of suicides is extremely low. Men aged 15–44 years old are at highest risk for violent death worldwide, while women of all ages are relatively spared from homicide.

The challenge of reducing intentional deaths should consider primary and secondary prevention of aggressive conduct disorders. **(Also see discussion in Chapter 7.)** At the population level—the foundation on which cultural and health changes are built—the "culture of violence" must be systematically dismantled and replaced with tolerance.

> *It is at the population level—the foundation on which cultural and health changes are built—where the "culture of violence" must be systematically dismantled and replaced with tolerance.*

War is a health plague built on violence. In 1990 alone, wars were estimated to have caused 502,000 deaths (see footnote in Table 11.1). Although there were no world wars or major international conflagrations during that year, there were local conflicts in Africa and the Middle East. And yet, those 502,000 deaths in 1990 were more than deaths from site-specific cancers (except for lung and stomach), all the inflammatory heart diseases, or HIV/AIDS. Moreover, once permanent disabilities were added to the deaths, wars in 1990 accounted for 20 million lost years of health. And that continues year after year—a horrific epidemic, indeed.

War has been defined as, "Old men seeking power or revenge sending their young men out to kill, and be killed by, other young men." The GBD Study's accounting of war deaths belies this view. The 1990 tally was 211,000 men,

141,000 women, and 150,000 children under age 15 years. Clearly, women and children together die far more frequently than men by a ratio of 58% to 42%.

### Risk Factors

Data show that suicides outnumber other intentionally inflicted deaths by a 40% margin worldwide. Countries and areas within countries where suicide is a health and social problem, will find the discussion of depressive disorder useful, because that is the prime risk factor for self-inflicted injury. **(Also see the section "Neuropsychiatric Disability" in Chapter 7.)** Other factors that may precipitate suicide are (1) experiencing humiliation or defeat, (2) feeling trapped in a situation the person can neither overcome nor escape, and (3) believing that no close caring person is available who is able and willing to really help. **(Also see relevant text in "Major Problems at Ages 15–24" in Chapter 4.)**

The worldwide annual tally of suicides and homicides is huge—1.8 million in 1990. Nevertheless, small average cities of 100,000 residents might experience only about 15 suicides and 11 homicides in a given year. When incidents are so rare, it is difficult to predict them without labeling too many false positives—citizens who are categorized as "high risk," but who have no bad outcomes. With this caution held aloft, here are some of the "signs of risk" for suicide:

1. The strongest single predictor is a prior suicide attempt. Anyone who attempts suicide needs serious help, which should continue until the crisis is resolved.

2. Major depression confers an 18-fold lifetime risk over that of the population without any mental disorder.

3. Bipolar disorder confers 24-fold risk.

4. Chronic dysthymia—feeling sad and troubled for years—confers a 17-fold risk.

5. Persons who are currently depressed (suffering from any of the above three conditions), may have a 30-fold increased risk, according to one study (Guze and Robins, 1970).

6. Having overpowering feelings of being alone in the world, such as may occur after an acute life crisis.

7. A history of impulsive, damaging behavior.

8. A family history of suicide (gives patient a role-model).

9. A terminal illness or a disfigurement.

10. Belonging to a socially-alienated, stigmatized group.

11. Being hospitalized for alcoholism (70-fold risk), AIDS (36-fold risk), or renal dialysis (10- to 50-fold risk).

12. Availability of a lethal means of death: guns, poison, large quantities of a potentially lethal prescribed medication. Each culture has its own methods.

Family members, teachers, and health workers dealing with individuals or groups in which suicide risk factors are elevated should take into account the "natural life history" of this cause of death. The stages are as follows:

1. Thinking about death, dying, or reuniting with close persons who are dead.

2. Talking with others about hurting him- or herself and feelings of uselessness, failure, badness, abandonment, hopelessness, helplessness.

3. Making veiled or open threats of suicide.

4. Preparing for death: giving away favorite possessions, giving "final" advice, finishing up unfinished tasks (in the context of other signs). Using various indirect means of saying goodbye.

5. Making suicide plans: this is usually discovered only by asking, perhaps using several different approaches.

6. Attempting suicide; this is always a drastic step that needs treatment.

7. Completing the effort by another attempt.

Knowing the above sequence enables teachers, social workers, or health care providers to observe and inquire—and to help families look for and ask—for these signs and to intervene as early in the sequence as possible. Positive findings are a signal to obtain immediate help to halt and reverse the psycho-behavioral process. **(For further discussion, see the section "Major Health Problems at Ages 15–24" in Chapter 4, the section "Special Issues for Men" in Chapter 5, and Chapter 7.)**

# PART IV.
# INTERVENING MORE EFFECTIVELY

# 12. Principles and Methods of Behavior Change

## ETHICAL AND STRATEGIC PRINCIPLES

The main barriers to a community's health—no matter where it is in the world—are neither physical nor biological. Neither an unreliable water supply, living in crowded, substandard housing conditions, the presence of infectious agents or disease vectors, nor malnourishment are the most powerful hindrances to better health. Rather, the primary obstacles to improving a community's health are cultural, social, and interpersonal expectations and behaviors. Cultural expectations determine the priorities that social power structures allot to clean water supplies and raising housing standards. The values placed on average people—especially on children—shape how social groups and individuals interact with each other and what preventive health and educational services are made freely available to all.

Great scientific breakthroughs do not automatically "break through" to benefit the community. Many advances in environmental and health sciences have not yet been adequately put into practice. Witness the choking air pollution in many of the world's most rapidly growing cities, the famines due to food distribution failures rather than food scarcity, the continuing rapid spread of AIDS despite widespread knowledge about how to prevent the disease's transmission. In every one of these cases, science has at least a partial solution,

> *Because every individual or group behavior is learned, it has the potential to be modified or replaced with other, newly learned behaviors.*

but the will—or the skill—to change collective and personal behavior is missing. In short, every widespread human disease or health disorder owes it prevalence, at least to some degree, to social and behavioral processes. These processes may be involved in its causes, its transmission, or its treatment—and, hence, in its prevention.

Because every individual or group behavior is learned, it has the potential to be modified or replaced with other, newly learned behaviors. Learning principles also underline cultural changes. Every culture has changed faster in the 20th century than ever before. And the 21st century promises to bring even more rapid innovations, as satellites and the Internet instantly transmit ideas, images, and information across class, cultural, and political boundaries.

Persons, groups, and entire societies become exposed to alternative ways of doing things. If these new ways are seen as easier, less costly, or if they lead to more rewarding outcomes, persons and groups are likely to adopt the new approaches at the next opportunity. Each time people believe that a new behavior is less trouble and/or more rewarding than a former one, the new approach is strengthened—reinforced—until it becomes a habit.

**Culture** is defined as the total network of customs, beliefs, priorities and values, technology, social roles and behaviors, kinship, authority, and habits shared by people living together. Culture functions as an integrated system: if one part is changed, other parts alter themselves to fit that change. **Society** is the term for the content and structuring of interactions among the people involved.

When considering implementing a program designed to change behavior in individuals or groups, certain ethical questions come to the fore. For example, is it ethical and proper for health professionals to enter into an area with people of a different culture and try to change ways of living that the local group has practiced—and survived with—for many generations? Or, is it ethical—and justified—for local health workers to press individuals to change behaviors that are harmful to their own health but not harmful to anyone else? Shouldn't people still be free to do what they want?

In fact, it is the highest of ethics to set before groups and individuals the opportunity to make those choices that will better their health, their resources for happiness and productivity, and their futures. This might best be done by directly involving the various subcommunities in the area of the proposed intervention in the needs assessment, decision-making, program planning and implementation, as well as its evaluation and follow-up.

*The key to introducing ethical and effective changes depends on having health professionals work co-operatively with local groups and individuals.*

The key to introducing ethical and effective health changes depends on having health professionals, be they local or foreign, work cooperatively with local groups and individuals to provide informed choices. There are commercial, political, religious, and other groups locally active already trying to change residents' values and behaviors—sometimes for selfish reasons that may not advance the good of the community. In addition, various social, economic, or environmental trends also may be pushing their way through the community's thinking and lifestyle. Improving the entire community's health by working to change individuals, communities, or societies can be ethical and salutary, if the following five principles are kept in the forefront:

• involve the community,

• value people and their culture,

- offer choices,

- develop informed consent, and

- keep the purpose, actions, and planned outcomes open to everyone that will be affected, including local citizens, their opinion leaders, health officials, and professionals.

The world seems to have shrunk to become a global village. A cholera outbreak in one community can spread to many nations, and winds can carry nuclear fallout to every corner of the world. The deadly Ebola virus and novel strains of influenza now jet from country to country, rapidly spreading disease across international boundaries. And, irresponsible, unprotected sex spreads HIV, breaking up families, leaving orphans, and taking a tremendous toll on communities. Traditional local solutions—or non-solutions—to health crises may prove inadequate for coping with these global problems. They may need to be replaced by newer scientific solutions, solutions that depend on changing societal and personal behaviors.

## MOBILIZING THE COMMUNITY

As health research continues to discover more pathways to disease prevention and health promotion, it becomes clearer that health workers alone cannot accomplish all the work ahead (Rojas Aleta, 1984, p. 3). In addition, worldwide population growth and spreading poverty make the task formidable.

The world's population continues to expand, migrations and wars cause increasing family dislocation, shantytowns in and around cities multiply and are reservoirs of disease and social pathology, and a million communities need pure water and waste disposal. Hundreds of millions of people have mental health problems; three or four billion need to change to healthier lifestyles. In short, throughout the world profound changes in societies, cultures, and ways of living are imperative if we truly are to achieve "health for all."

The World Health Organization and the United Nations Children's Fund jointly organized and sponsored the 1978 landmark International Conference on Primary Health Care, held in Alma Ata in the then USSR. Delegations from 134 governments and representatives of 67 United Nations organizations, specialized agencies, and nongovernmental organizations gathered there to affirm the key role of primary health care in reaching the goal of "health for all." They urged the health sector to cooperate with other public sectors (agriculture and industrial development, education, economics, transport, communication, and labor) to accomplish shared health goals. The vital thrust of the report was that generating the community's participation was critical to successfully having the entire community adopt healthier ways and sustain them even after outside project workers had gone home.

To make this happen, agencies from outside the district or nation must channel their energies on training local persons in community participation and group organizing (in addition to health service skills), so that both technical knowledge and community momentum can be sustained. This process already has proven successful in the Caribbean for training national health educators to spread their outreach and generate budget support for program continuity.

Community participation was seen in the 1970s as the magic vehicle that would carry the developing world toward the goals of "health for all." Efforts to put this approach into practice have been carried out in many localities and by many cultural and political systems. With each effort, the meaning and implications of "community participation," "community involvement," "health consumerism," and "primary health care movement," have broadened, as have the other labels given to this general philosophical approach. The result is a complex concept, not usually clearly defined and hence difficult to evaluate in terms of its inputs, processes, and outputs (Morgan, 1993).

After 25 years, the concept of achieving health for all through community participation and intersectoral cooperation remains almost universally accepted ideologically, although its application has been more debated and has generated more conflict (Morgan, 1993; Stebbins, 1997). There has even been debate about whether community participation generates better health outcomes than does standard health services delivered by the government. In 1985, Professor A. Ugalde wrote that, promotional efforts by international agencies notwithstanding, at that time there were no success stories proving that community participation had incrementally improved outcomes in Latin American health programs (Ugalde, 1985).

Either way, those committed to the concept argue, largely on philosophical and political grounds, that community involvement is valuable in its own right, irrespective of health outcomes. They add that the process of sharing mutual concerns and developing internal leadership will assist in later community development efforts.

A 1998 literature search conducted for this Handbook identified many hundreds of publications referring to community or consumer participation. The latest reviews of this literature in scientific journals and books dwell on the problems of conceptualizing and implementing research and evaluation, rather than on the health results of controlled studies. Ideological consensus does not prove that community participation delivers measurably better health outcomes, however (see also Morgan, 1993; Ugalde, 1985; Rifkin, 1990). Nor does

BUILDING BETTER HEALTH

a lack of rigorous data prove that the community involvement approach has no incremental values beyond the traditional provision of health services. Instead, the fundamental questions—as yet unanswered—are more along the order of the following: In what social environments and among what cultural and educational groups do specific community involvement programs result in changes in pre-defined group health conditions?

Full discussion of the theory and practice of "community participation" is beyond the scope of this Handbook. The consensus inferred from the 1998 literature review, however, is that the planning of any specific local program must take, as a minimum, all of the following factors into consideration:

- the current level of community development,

- the community's educational levels,

- cultural practices,

- openness to new ideas,

- the economic situation,

- the past history of political or decision-making involvement by all the community's subpopulations.

The array of published materials reviewed about community involvement came from left, center, and right of the political spectrum, and from a variety of academic disciplines and field workers. Nevertheless, there seemed to be broad agreement on some principles and concerns. We list below a series of brief statements that reflect recurrent themes in the literature, which are supported by psychological and sociological research on related issues.

- It is more effective to do things *with* people rather than for people.

- Where at all possible, the public should participate actively at all four stages of a health project: situation diagnosis and problem identification, decision making and program formulation, implementation, and monitoring and evaluation.

- Community participation is not a "one-size-fits-all" approach.

- Health cannot be imposed on anyone.

- Health is not only a right, it is a responsibility to be shared by every segment in the community.

- To be balanced and successful, community projects should integrate three kinds of talent around a common goal—"Head, Hands, and Heart"—or as academics might word it, theory, practice, and commitment.

- Communities without previous experience of having all social levels working together will be more likely to support activities addressing their needs than to initiate them.

- Start with a small program that can show visible results rather quickly. A small success builds a sense of self-efficacy (group competency), cooperative skills, and leadership experience that equip the group for sustained longer-term projects and larger successes. Visible success helps a group survive.

Agricultural extension agents in rural North America started this kind of work in the 1930s. They found their first tasks involved bringing people together to show them how to interact and do projects cooperatively, as well as how to make step-by-step plans. This was not didactic teaching, but a "let us do it together" approach. The first project may have been to get rural women to share their skills in helping each participant to plant a small vegetable garden (see section on cancer prevention). Later they were taught how to preserve foods by boiling them in jars. The content of each project was determined by the group's perceived needs. The most valuable products always were the organizational and leadership skills the participants learned.

*In many places, women are more ready to participate, work, and learn together than are men—in those localities, agencies should start working with the community's women.*

In many localities, women are more ready to participate, work, and learn together than are men. In such situations, agencies start with the best motivated people. After a year or so, other sorts of people will want help to get themselves active, too. The outside trainer who fits in best is usually a person of the same culture and gender as the participants.

- Sustaining community participation depends on attitude and behavior changes, building organizational skills, and the patience to keep working for longer-range outcomes. All these take time to happen.

- Existing social groups, organizations, and agencies should be sought out to help promote the health programs before trying to bring together a totally new action group.

- Community participation in identifying a need and planning to remedy it takes more time and effort than bringing in a ready-made program from the central government. However, community participation at the formative states gives the community a sense of ownership of the effort, self-esteem, and power that pays off in better popular response to the program, and much longer continuation of the program activity.

- When encouraged to participate in health programs, especially prevention efforts, people will be educated by means of their participation.

- All behavior—including project participation—requires rewards in order to be sustained. The following list offers some clear rewards for groups and individuals to keep them putting in their efforts: (1) they make new social contacts and friends; (2) they build self-esteem and self-efficacy; (3) they enhance their personal image in the community; (4) they satisfy the desire to do something new, to be pioneers, leaders; (5) they help solve a common problem or leave a lasting improvement in their community; and (6) they share in the energy generated by group activity (this list of benefits has been adapted from I. Rojas Aleta (1984).

Persons interested in learning more about employing community participation as part of changing infrastructure, lifestyle, health behavior, and overall well-being may consult the numerous monographs and scientific articles published each year. Focus on the ones that include practical guidelines and/or data showing efficacy. One of the best practical guides is Anne V. Whyte's "Guidelines for planning community participation activities in water supply and sanitation projects" (Whyte, 1986). Although this 53-page monograph is addressed directly to environmental projects, the flow charts, data collection instruments, and twelve stages of activity can be readily modified for other health goals. If a new program could supply only one pre-1996 resource to its workers, this would be the most helpful operationally.

Up to now this chapter has reviewed ethical and strategic principles of health programs and some strategies for becoming partners with the community. The following sections will flesh out these principles with strategies for conceptualizing and achieving the changes in perception and behavior that build better health.

## OVERLAPPING THEORIES OF BEHAVIOR CHANGE

Over the centuries, teachers have developed ideas about how children learn. Philosophers and psychologists organized these ideas and practices into theories and teaching guides. But it was not until the 20th century that a garden of learning and behavioral theories came into full bloom.

As is true for many fields having competing theories, different learning and behavior theories are more or less applicable depending on what is to be learned, the kinds of people involved, and the circumstances present. Therefore, this chapter will treat the host of available models and theories about health-related behavior like a workshop, displaying many tools shown useful in clinical and community settings, without regard to philosophical consistency or comprehensiveness. These tools can be used in various combinations to construct local programs. Readers interested in systematic presentation of theories of health behavior may consult books devoted to this topic, such as *Health Behavior and Health Education* (Glanz, Lewis, and Rimer, 1997).

## OVERALL ORIENTATION

Enlisting the cooperation of communities, families, and individuals in changing behaviors to improve health is more complex than it seemed 70 years ago. At that time, providing information about a disease and the necessary actions to prevent it appeared to be enough to bring about substantial public acceptance. Thus, the simpler epidemic diseases came under control. As multicausal diseases and injuries began to be targeted and public and personal agendas became more complex (including conflicts between corporate profits and public health), group and individual health-related behaviors also became more difficult to change.

Figure 12.1 diagrams key areas to address when seeking to change health-related behavior. By filling in specific content the table can be used as a guideline to planning programs ranging from immunization to smoking cessation.

As many field trials have demonstrated in recent decades, merely providing information is not enough to improve health behaviors. There is an essential next step to changing any behavior—motivation. The health promoter analyzes community and individual priorities and either tries to make pro-health motives stronger than existing priorities, or harnesses existing priorities and needs to push forward the health promotion program. The existing motivations need not be health related in order to be used successfully. They can be based on a desire to be a good parent, a good athlete, or a good teacher; or they can be tied to community pride, wanting a healthier work force, or raising productivity. Once a health promotion activity has been carefully evaluated for its chances of success, risks of failure, and possibilities of unexpected side effects—and the balance is found to be clearly positive—then health workers should be open to carefully select all those motivations, perceived needs, and priorities that will advance the community toward successful health improvement. The following example illustrates these points.

In a WHO Region in the 1970s, an international consultant sought to expand staffing for local health promotion efforts. He used the standard approach and conducted workshops and training sessions for staff at the ministries of health and related government agencies in 19 emerging states and territories. Despite almost universal enthusiasm for increasing health promotion, only two of the 19

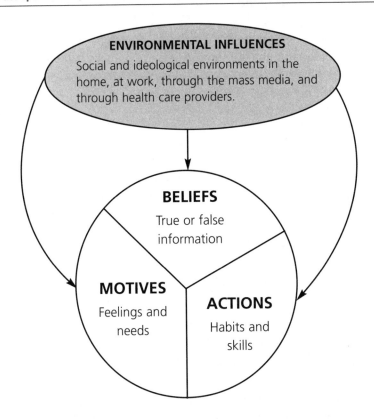

jurisdictions started any new program. To pursue the goal at a regional conference of health ministers, an international staff spent months and much money preparing an elaborate presentation about all the valuable things health education/health promotion teams can do to prevent disease. The effort was greeted with polite approval and thanks. In contrast, at the same meeting, a Minister of Health from one of the smallest and poorer states gave a simple "show and tell," praising the contributions made by his few health educators to the outreach of his entire health program. His simple report drew standing applause, and he— not the international experts—became the magnet for informal discussion during the recesses. And yes, several other countries soon had programs running. Ministers of health from nearby countries and territories said, "If that little place can have such a program, our proud state must have it, too."

The moral—the bottom line—of this true story? Please draw your own conclusions . . . then consider the following:

- Group insiders have more motivating power than outsiders. This is because they are well known within the community and their enthusiasm is experienced within the context of the group's shared experience and culture.

- Logic and facts can be slow motivators. Personal experience, anecdotes, and enthusiasm work more quickly.

- Workers and administrators expect experts and resource persons to present always new (always additional workload) programs in an elaborate and urgent way. That is what they are paid to do, and they never disappoint. But when respected individuals step outside their expected roles and scripts to report something that touches a shared need, that is when ears and minds open.

- Competition, and maybe a touch of envy, can motivate more strongly than logic. First, weigh the ethics and the long-term implications; then utilize each true and fair motivator that advances personal and public well being (and disadvantages no one) to get movement to resolve health problems.

## MAKING PROGRAMS HAPPEN AND FLOURISH

The final stage for health promotion is to teach the actions, habits, and skills required to keep communities, families, and persons acting permanently in healthful ways. Many communities and individuals already know what they need to do to reduce health risks, and they clearly want to achieve that goal. They just don't quite know how to make it happen. For individuals, this means learning and practicing some of the techniques for changing behavior. For communities, it may mean learning how to stimulate and organize community participation which, in turn, generates the structure and plan to carry out the program of health enhancement.

*Many communities and individuals already know what they need to do to reduce health risks, and they clearly want to achieve that goal—they just don't quite know how to make it happen.*

Figure 12.1 reminds us that all goal-directed efforts designed to transmit knowledge, motivation, skills, and habits take place in environments that simultaneously have interpersonal, community, social, cultural-ideological, and physical (infrastructural) properties. Health messages are spread through interactions taking place in these environments.

All training of actions, habits, and skills ultimately occurs at the individual level—one brain at a time. Depending on the roles of the trainees involved, however, the skilled performance of these actions may have an impact on the entire community, on various families, or just on the individual trainees. The following paragraphs explore each scenario.

At the community level, city workers can be taught to repair water pumps and pipes, and safely and regularly treat water with chlorination and, if needed, fluoridation. Such an effort also might involve teaching clinic managers how to keep vaccines at the proper temperature, prevent loss and waste of clinic supplies, or keep clinics staffed and open on schedule. Perhaps most critical for the long term is providing information, motivation (i.e., a sense of mission), and skills-training to schoolteachers and community leaders to prioritize health, model healthful ways, and finally spread them, especially to children and youth.

At the family level, some of the habits and skills that need teaching include how family decision makers can plant gardens and provide the most needed foods for the family, such as legumes to provide proteins and fruits and vegetables that can prevent many chronic diseases later in life. Mothers also can be trained to prepare and use oral rehydration fluids. Skills that preserve health within the family include ensuring the home's safety by removing hazards that might allow falls, cuts, burns, poisonings, insect bites, and exposure to human wastes. The benefits of such trauma prevention are crucial for children, yet also extend to all ages.

Finally, individuals must be motivated, informed, and trained on how to take care of their own health. They must be encouraged to ask themselves, "If I don't take care of my own life, how can I expect anyone else to do so?" General health improvement for the more than six billion voyagers now on our planet demands a tremendous increase in effective health self-care. The responsibility of health professionals goes far beyond delivering health care themselves. Perhaps more importantly, they must enable and stimulate communities and individuals themselves to deliver preventive and primary self-care. Self-directed behavior change has been proven to work. It should be more widely taught and used throughout the world.

## COLLECTING INFORMATION FOR PLANNING AN INTERVENTION

Based upon the overall orientation presented in Figure 12.1, what needs to be known about the target population to be used to shape an outreach program? A comprehensive understanding of the group to be reached, the helpful or hindering aspects of their environment, the group's beliefs about the threat posed to them by a health problem and its causes, and the attributes of the desired health action in behavioral and social terms, all need to be entered into effective outreach programs. Figure 12.2 shows the three areas of information needed, their interactions, and their impacts on developing outreach programs. This background information will identify what kinds of messages and persuasions need to be delivered to change knowledge and beliefs and to teach motivations, skills, and finally to trigger behavior. The categories, detailed content, and the interactions suggested in the figure have been assembled from the health-belief model, social learning theory, and the theory of planned behavior and social marketing. The following text expands on the figure.

FIGURE 12.2. Model for encouraging community changes toward healthful behaviors.

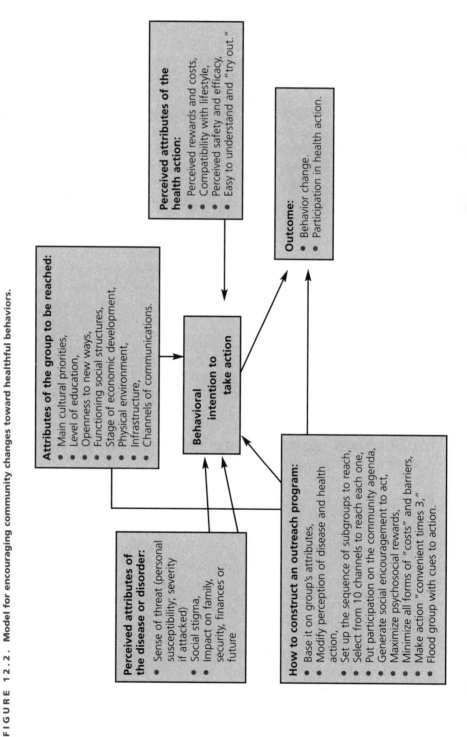

**Attributes of the group to be reached:**
- Main cultural priorities,
- Level of education,
- Openness to new ways,
- Functioning social structures,
- Stage of economic development,
- Physical environment,
- Infrastructure,
- Channels of communications.

**Perceived attributes of the health action:**
- Perceived rewards and costs,
- Compatibility with lifestyle,
- Perceived safety and efficacy,
- Easy to understand and "try out."

**Perceived attributes of the disease or disorder:**
- Sense of threat (personal susceptibility; severity if attacked)
- Social stigma,
- Impact on family, security, finances or future

**Behavioral intention to take action**

**Outcome:**
- Behavior change.
- Participation in health action.

**How to construct an outreach program:**
- Base it on group's attributes,
- Modify perception of disease and health action,
- Set up the sequence of subgroups to reach,
- Select from 10 channels to reach each one,
- Put participation on the community agenda,
- Generate social encouragement to act,
- Maximize psychosocial rewards,
- Minimize all forms of "costs" and barriers,
- Make action "convenient times 3,"
- Flood group with cues to action.

The stage of the program and the nature of the health action required define the group to be reached. Early in program planning the groups and persons whose support and participation will be needed first must be reached. Doing this will help later forms of outreach to proceed successfully. Initial groups include the community's formal and informal power structures, health professionals, and opinion leaders. At some point between planning the intervention and delivering it, the essential person or group to be reached convincingly is the one who controls the required resources—power, money, or personnel. This person or group may be outside the organizational chart of the health and medical systems. It might be a chief executive, a village chief, the wealthiest family in the community, or a political party. The program must offer a win-win-win situation for those with power, for the public, and perhaps even for the health proponents.

The subpopulation at risk of the health problem may be addressed later. Health efforts such as financing maternal and child health clinics, setting up school immunization services, or building sewage treatment plants, usually must win over community and fiscal decision-makers before an appeal can be made to the general public. For child health programs, parents and community leaders are involved first and the young children, later.

The population's educational level and the communication channels that most effectively reach community members influence both the sophistication of the messages and how they should be formatted. For example, some subpopulations may be better reached by posters than by television, or by radio rather than through the print media. Sometimes, the media can best set the agenda for public discussion. Word-of-mouth through social networks can spread the desired motivations and readiness for action. The group's sense of self-efficacy—the power to accomplish tasks—will shape the messages (and the programs), such that each subgroup will feel that what it is called upon to do is both feasible and valuable.

The existing infrastructure in a location where a program is being launched is an important environmental determinant. Are roads and public transportation sufficient to provide the public easy access to program sites? Should the program be run from mobile clinics? Can vaccines or drugs be kept under refrigeration? Can local personnel be hired or must all staff be brought in? Are telephone facilities adequate for program coordination?

Each leadership echelon and each segment of the community has its own priorities. For elected officials this might mean pleasing the community, their political party, the central government, or a few financial supporters. For health professionals it might mean pleasing local opinion leaders, gaining professional prestige, or reducing the frequency of a widespread disease. Schoolteachers, factory owners, and community agencies all have good reasons for helping to improve the health of those with whom they work. Calling upon enlightened self-interest usually makes people more willing to become involved, than does simply asking people to do what is good, right, or charitable.

Proposed health interventions should be promoted not only for the health benefits to the "treated" subpopulation, but also as steps toward meeting the self-defined goals of each assisting, contributing group. Thus, while anti-diarrheal programs for infants or anti-HIV programs for teenagers each have similar plans of action wherever on earth they are conducted, the promotion of the interventions and the reasons given for enlisting different parts of the community will work best if tailored to the local setting.

## ATTRIBUTES OF THE DISEASE OR DISORDER

Some health interventions, such as immunizations, target specific diseases. Others, such as smoking cessation campaigns, target many diseases with a single program. Still others, such as nutrition and exercise programs, aim more at immediate health improvement, although they are also well proven long-term preventers of chronic disease conditions.

The "health belief model" (Becker and Maiman, 1980) emphasizes the program recipient's perceptions, beliefs, and feelings about diseases—specifically, what are the chances of getting the disease (susceptibility) and how damaging would it be (severity). Diseases to which people are highly susceptible, but whose severity is almost nil—such as the common cold—don't move people to preventive action. Neither do severe or fatal diseases that are extremely rare—such as rare cancers. Diseases or conditions that combine moderate susceptibility and moderate severity seem to generate a perceived threat that moves people toward acting in preventive ways (depending on other simultaneous factors, such as those listed in Figure 12.2).

Something about the community's beliefs and feelings about the targeted disease or condition can be learned by bringing together focus (discussion) groups, each one representing a sub-community defined by neighborhood or social status. This is a good way to learn local names for the condition, its presumed causes, the qualities (often negative) of the people at highest risk, and any "inside rumors" regarding proposed prevention or cure. The most important information for designing program communication and plans is usually internal to the targeted group, is rarely volunteered to health professionals, and often is expressed in simple slang terms.

A human group is never an "empty pitcher" waiting for health professionals to pour information about an illness. Every group is already full of beliefs and feelings about every health problem their group has experienced. The current folk

BUILDING BETTER HEALTH

wisdom may need to be replaced, at least in part, with more effective preventive beliefs and behavior.

## ATTRIBUTES OF THE HEALTH ACTION

Beliefs and feelings about recommended health actions also enter into this model's equation. Ideally, the targeted population must perceive the health action as effective. The action also must be safe and socially acceptable. For example, parents won't boil water if they don't believe that doing so will help prevent diarrhea in their children. Nor will they get immunizations for their children if they think this might have bad side effects. Some preventive behaviors may violate local norms unless performed according to culturally required restrictions, such as having female caregivers administer Pap smears.

A health program may seek to introduce a new provision or behavior (say, a new vaccine, a new food to be eaten more often, or additional sanitary standards) or to eliminate a current habit or condition (such as tobacco use, withholding food from infants with diarrhea, sedentary lifestyle, or obesity). Another consideration is whether what is being introduced or eliminated is a daily behavior or an occasional one, like a mammogram every two years or checking the safety of a heat stove at the beginning of winter. Tactics and reminder cues need to be different for daily than for occasional health behaviors.

Adding a health behavior requires positive cues and rewards to remind people to perform them, either on a daily basis or at proper intervals. Removing unhealthy behavior requires different strategies, including withdrawing cues and rewards for the existing habit, replacing the old habit with a healthier one (such as eating fruit instead of fatty snacks), and providing cues and rewards for the healthier substitute. Conditioning and behavior change studies have consistently shown that rewarding a substitute, healthier behavior brings about a quicker, more enduring change than punishing the old behavior or making it more difficult or costly.

A general principle in a person's decision to perform a given action or change a behavior is that person's reckoning whether the benefits to be derived from the action are greater than the effort and "cost" involved for him or her and for those for whom the decision is made. Thus, a parent will tally (often unconsciously) the total time, effort, and cost of taking a child for a regular health check-up and compare that to the total anticipated benefit to the child's health and growth and the reduced risk of future burden upon the parent of having a sick child. Similarly, when weighing how to spend their budget,

> *Studies have consistently shown that rewarding a substitute, healthier behavior brings about a quicker, more enduring change than punishing the old behavior or making it more difficult or costly.*

**FIGURE 12.3.** Use of rewards and costs to change the balance between healthy and harmful behaviors.

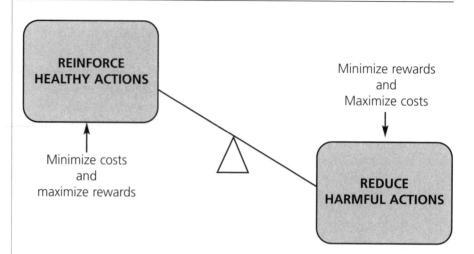

district officials may consider the benefits-to-costs ratio of a spraying program to control mosquito-borne diseases versus building a new road. Health advocates need to document benefits and costs of health interventions and the number of citizens who would benefit from them as effectively as other interests do when trying to persuade regional, community, corporate, or sectoral decision-makers. Economists at local universities (or the students they supervise) can help immensely with this process as part of their public service.

People and groups may move toward improving their health or that of the community for health-related reasons or for reasons that don't really have to do with health. Teenagers, for example, may brush their teeth more to have an attractive smile than for dental health. A man may reduce his risk factors for chronic disease, even though he doesn't enjoy it, because he believes his children need him healthy and working for two more decades. In an early oral polio vaccine program, many adults felt they might not need the vaccine, but took it "because that's what everybody is doing." A politician may support building a new water purification plant in part because he wants his name engraved over the entrance.

Figure 12.3 illustrates how "rewards" and "costs" (broadly defined) affect the performance of healthful and harmful behaviors. To increase healthful behaviors maximize the rewards and minimize the costs (e.g., time, effort). To reduce harmful behaviors maximize costs and reduce their rewards—for example, taxes on cigarettes and alcohol can be raised and severe penalties against reckless or drunken driving can be consistently applied.

Taken together, the characteristics of the group to be reached, its environment, and the perceived attributes of the disease and the health action required interact to generate a disposition to act or not to act (Figure 12.2). The "Theory of

Reasoned Action" refers to this as a "behavioral intention" (Glanz, Lewis, and Rimer, 1997). All these attributes and perceptions can either be modified or taken into account as the behavior change program is shaped. The following section discusses how to use this information in making a diagnosis of the health behavior problem.

## MAKING A BEHAVIORAL DIAGNOSIS

Physicians are most successful in treating disease when they first work to make the correct diagnosis. The same is true for health professionals trying to change illness- or trauma-promoting behavior. Before laying out an intervention or program, a health worker must do what is necessary to understand the determinants of the current behavior (or lack of behavior) and then work to introduce and consolidate the new healthier actions.

Figure 12.1 presents a framework listing possible ingredients of the problem of unhealthful behavior. To make a behavioral diagnosis, program planners identify the barriers to health-promoting changes that are present in terms of beliefs, motives, skills, and physical, social, and cultural environmental influences. The shortcomings of previous interventions often point out these barriers. The diagnostic process has the following steps, whether they target individuals or groups. (The following scheme for diagnosing health-behavior problems and shaping intervention is described more fully in Last, 1986, Chapter 30.)

- **Fully describe the problems of health-related behavior in operational steps.** This is the equivalent of clarifying the "presenting complaint" a patient brings to a doctor. In the control of schistosomiasis, for example, this calls for conducting studies of local habits of urine and feces disposal, as well as understanding individual and community contact with rivers and lakes, which are the reservoirs for the agent. In control of obesity, operational issues include the amount and quality of calories eaten, their "vectors" (foods), and the circumstances encouraging and discouraging their consumption.

- **Obtain a history of the problem.** How long has it gone on? Is it consistent? Is it intermittent? Is the entire community affected? Does it only affect a subgroup? Did some event precede or coincide with the onset of the problem?

- **Determine the behavioral dynamics.** What encourages change versus a continuation of the problem? What are the rewards and costs that maintain the old way? What subgroups want change? Which subgroups obstruct change?

- **Arrive at a behavioral diagnosis.** What needs to be changed? Who can best make this happen? Where are the barriers? More educated subgroups may need only skills learning, while others may lack strong enough motivation.

Too often health professionals want to change the patients or the target group, when what needs to be changed first is the health worker, aspects of program delivery, or other concurrent community problems.

- **Make a "treatment plan"—i.e., design an intervention—in cooperation with the program's recipients.** Involve patients, families, and the community as active participants, so that everyone owns part of the success of the health improvement. The program should consist of specific small steps, thus providing many occasions for success and rewards, and giving all concerned a sense of moving forward with a greater sense of self-efficacy and empowerment. (Also see section "Conveying Learning and Values to Overcome Health Vulnerabilities" in Chapter 4.)

- **Always pilot test the program on a small group.** "Patch the holes" in the plan before launching out into the deeper waters of the whole community.

- **Deliver the program and evaluate its effectiveness.** Adjust or repeat the effort as needed, then move forward to the next milestone.

## PRESENTING PROGRAMS SUCCESSFULLY

Program planning covers two components—the program's presentation or marketing to the group to be reached, and the program's organization and delivery.

Prior to actually delivering services, program promoters should make a "community diagnosis," both as discussed in the previous section and as displayed in Figure 12.2. This will not be an umbrella diagnosis covering the entire community, but rather a specific diagnosis targeting different subgroups. At this stage, one inputs the following information, as collected in the section on "Collecting Information for Planning an Intervention":

- the characteristics of the groups to be reached and in what sequence they will be targeted;

- the groups' perceptions and feelings about the health problems being addressed;

- the health cooperation and social and behavior changes being sought; and

- the groups' feelings of liking or disliking, trusting or doubting, the people and the agency bringing the proposed program.

People act on the basis of what they believe and feel, even if it is not accurate. The task of the intervention's pre-delivery stage is to motivate and educate the selected subpopulation by getting it:

- to learn about and relate positively with the health-promoters;

- to hear, read, and discuss together the agenda of the program;

- to replace erroneous ideas with accurate beliefs; and

- to replace apathy and fearful avoidance with positive motivation to do what is needed to prevent disease and promote health.

People at all educational levels are full of ideas about their health, their illnesses, and their world. From a health professional's perspective some of their ideas may seem wrong; that is, less likely than other ideas to lead to behaviors that reduce health problems. For both the group being helped and the group seeking to be helpful, lacking accurate information is less of a barrier than is clinging to misleading ideas.

*Sharing the need to have a program with opinion leaders from the selected subpopulation and enlisting their support will open the door to quicker public cooperation.*

Sharing the need to have a given program and that program's goals with opinion leaders from the selected subpopulation and enlisting their approval will open the door to quicker public cooperation. Asking those same local leaders for advice on how to promote and deliver the program—and using some of that advice—will help avoid cultural and local political blunders. Another bonus: program planners also will be held in much higher esteem by the public. After all, people always respect the wisdom of those who ask their advice.

The strategy for intervention will differ by the stage of disease—primary, secondary, or tertiary—at which intervention is aimed. It also will differ depending on whether the health behavior change involves doing something new or differently, or whether it consists of stopping an established, unhealthy practice. Finally, it will differ depending on whether the targets for change are political and community leaders, health professionals, parents of children, or individuals in the at risk group.

Three program traps to avoid:

- Never start a screening program unless there are ready-to-function facilities for following persons who screen positive.

- Never raise public demand for a health service unless its personnel and facilities are ready for the influx of users.

- Never raise fears of a disease or epidemic unless the services needed to reduce such fears and risks are readily available.

Errors such as these not only cause an immediate backlash by persons and their families stirred to action and then not helped. They also plant a distrust for future programs proposed by the agency.

## COMMUNICATING HEALTH MESSAGES

There are at least twelve channels for getting messages to populations or subgroups (Jenkins and Hewitt, 1992). Some communities may lack some of these, but may have other, locally unique ones to add.

### Twelve Channels for Communication

1. Regional and national government.

2. Nongovernmental organizations.

3. The mass media.

4. Community leaders.

5. Businesses and labor groups.

6. Schools and teachers.

7. Those who set health care standards (e.g., insurers or managed care and accreditation agencies).

8. Health professionals—medically trained, alternative, or traditional healers.

9. Local informal or formal social groups, including clubs and local religious congregations and their leaders.

10. "Gatekeepers" to seeking help, such as clergy, counselors, pharmacists, schoolteachers, nurses, athletic coaches, beauticians, barbers, bartenders.

11. Families, friends, coworkers.

12. Individuals.

Health program planners should select only those channels that seem appropriate at each stage of their specific program. Adding channels usually costs additional resources, but that investment may be warranted if the program receives only half-hearted support after using the channels first selected. In a multicultural area, make sure that the messages are delivered in all dialects and cultural styles present in the population, using terms that even those groups with the lowest educational levels can understand.

## TAILORING PROGRAMS TO THE TARGETED GROUP

Disease and disability do not rain down randomly across the community. Often, an identifiable subgroup representing some 20% to 30% of the population will experience 70% to 80% of certain conditions, for example, infant mortality and deaths due to certain infections (e.g., tuberculosis, AIDS), fires, homicides, certain cancers, and industrial toxicities (Jenkins, Tuthill, and Tannenbaum, 1977). The high-risk subgroup might be identified by geographic area or demographic characteristics. Special programs, community involvement, effective outreach, and continuing follow-up are required to reach these subgroups and change their behaviors. Involving the targeted subgroup in the design and operation of its program will speed adoption through the social network, as will the sense of ownership conferred by involvement of local opinion leaders.

Presenting and delivering health programs requires the same flexibility as tailoring a suit of clothes. Different customers prefer different colors and textures of fabrics. In marketing health programs, the customers help determine the style and content of the messages and the channels through which they are delivered. Health interventions also can be tailored for size and shape. When, where, how, and by whom the intervention will be delivered should be "fitted" to the medical history, presenting complaints, beliefs, feelings, motivations, and convenience of the publics to be reached. This results in greater program effectiveness (Campbell, 1994).

> *Presenting and delivering health programs requires the same flexibility as tailoring a suit of clothes. In marketing health programs, the customers help determine the style and content of the messages and the channels through which they are delivered.*

Those who work in the real estate business often say that the three most important things to consider when buying property are location, location, and, once again, location. Health service planners trying to obtain maximum participation likewise have three most important things to achieve—convenience, convenience, and convenience. Consider the following:

- Convenience in location. Places should be easily accessible by walking, public transportation, and other means.

- Convenience in times when the service is provided. Schedule services during evening hours for daytime workers, weekends so rural residents can get into town, and at schools and during school time for the benefit of school-children.

- Convenience and comfort in participating in the program. Conveniently sited and scheduled services also should be delivered without bureaucratic complexity or long waits, and should be offered in a friendly, locally appropriate style that makes clients comfortable, pleased with the service, and inclined to return for this or other programs—these aspects of convenience and comfort may be described as "user friendly."

Educational and motivational efforts at the beginning of programming should establish the public's expectancy that participating will be rewarding, safe, and convenient. The delivery of the health service should be designed to make those promises come true. The design and delivery should minimize effort, inconvenience, and cost, and maximize the perceived rewards and aptness of the health action, as well as the helpfulness of the health workers involved.

The importance of "convenience, convenience, convenience" in promoting the actual behavior desired from the target group by no means should be the last consideration among those listed in this section. Leaving convenience to last would be easy to do, because most health behavior theories, including the intrapersonal and interpersonal theories reviewed in the volume edited by Glanz, Lewis, and Rimer (1997), are heavily weighted by cognitions, decisions, and intentions. Field workers with broad experience in health programs may conclude that the more complex of these theories apply only to persons who think with the same complexity as the psychologists who contrived the theories. This belief has not as yet been disproved by field studies. People participate in health actions for many reasons, including some not related to health. With a well-marketed program that is conveniently available, many participants will make their decision on the spur of the moment.

Field studies such as that by Montano and Taplin (1991), dealing with use of mammography, have found that "facilitating conditions" (convenience) were the strongest of the many predictors in their relation to actual behavior. In fact, the simple use of reminder postcards nearly doubled the probability of having a mammogram in this study.

A very successful immunization program in Florida (USA), carried out when oral polio vaccine was first introduced in the 1960s, was based on the principle, "Make it easier to take the vaccine than to avoid it." This was followed by a second principle, "Teach the people only what they need to know to make an informed decision to take the vaccine." By focusing on these two principles, health educators could avoid detailing polio's pathogenesis or the biology of vaccine preparation, and instead focus on the simple message: "A virus causes polio.

This vaccine contains a weakened kind of virus that will safely and effectively prevent polio and its damage. And many people will be taking the oral vaccine." This anecdote underlines the fact that the focus of health education/promotion efforts must be on changing behavior, not on teaching medical science. The Florida program concentrated on setting up hundreds of distribution sites that were open both days and evenings. The effort was supported by mass media coverage and the involvement of community groups in every definable socio-cultural niche (Johnson et al., 1962). To extrapolate from this example, if a program were initiated to convert a village to use a pure water supply, it is important to place pipes and water taps so that no matter where a family lives, the pure water source is more convenient than the old sources of polluted water.

And going back to the polio vaccine example, one of the strongest predictors for adults taking the polio vaccine was their reporting having friends who also were taking it. In fact, 90% of adults who reported that "all or almost all" of their friends and acquaintances had taken the vaccine, did so themselves; whereas only 11% of respondents saying that none of their friends and acquaintances were taking the vaccine had taken the vaccine themselves. Participating in informal networks and belonging to organizations served to connect people to what was happening in their community, thus raising the probability that they would take the vaccine. These observations support the idea of enlisting groups organized for other purposes to spread positive, encouraging information about the health program on a temporary basis. Civic clubs, labor groups, local religious congregations—in fact, most of the 12 channels of communication detailed in the section "Communicating Health Messages" earlier in this chapter—are willing to promote health interventions for a limited period of time. This approach also makes individuals feel that people like them will participate in the program (Northcutt et al., 1964). These strategies diffuse new ideas and actions throughout the population (Glanz, Lewis, and Rimer, 1997, Part 4).

## A SAMPLING OF SELF-DIRECTED BEHAVIOR CHANGE TACTICS

Most cigarette smokers in most nations (perhaps 90%) already know that smoking harms them in many ways. Most also claim that they want to quit, and many add that they have tried, but lack the willpower to stay quit. The teaching of habits and skills to remain tobacco-free will be of greatest benefit to these people.

There are a host of such simple habits, counterarguments, and counteractions that have been found helpful in many successful, effective smoking cessation programs. These will be discussed more comprehensively in Chapter 13. The following section outlines a few examples of simple action steps that could contribute to smoking cessation. They can easily be extrapolated for changing other unhealthful behaviors, such as careless driving, eating junk food, indulging in unsafe sexual activity, or forgetting to take essential medications. The psychological purposes of each action will be listed first followed by the content each might assume in a smoking cessation program.

- Raise awareness of the extent of the problem—i.e., have trainee record on a paper every time he/she takes a cigarette.

- Build commitment (motivation) to change to better health—i.e., have trainee list all the benefits of stopping smoking, especially immediate ones such as saving money, having cleaner breath and teeth, recovering a taste for food, setting a good example for children, avoiding burns on clothes and furniture, and increasing one's sense of effectiveness and power. These benefits should be raised to a high priority in the trainee's life.

- Encourage trainee to make a public statement to family and friends of his/her new healthier behavior. Public commitment intensifies personal compliance. In some communities the graduating class of each smoking cessation course is congratulated, individually named, and interviewed by the local newspaper. This praises graduates and enlists the support of their friends for the new health plan.

- Dissuade automatic, reflex repetition of habit; rather, teach trainee to make a conscious choice to smoke. For example, have trainee wrap pack of cigarettes in two layers of paper held by elastic bands, to give trainee a few seconds to think about the decision to smoke. Trainee can smoke anytime he/she wishes, but the pack must be rewrapped after each use.

- Replace any motor behaviors associated with the habit—e.g., chew gum, suck toothpicks, keep hands occupied, rather than smoking.

- Counter physiologic smoking withdrawal cues—e.g., drink water frequently to eliminate dry mouth, sip on a flavored sugar-free drink to give a pleasant taste and take the edge off hunger, and get busy with something as a distraction from boredom.

- Enlist social support for changing into new behaviors. For example, have trainee find a family member, coworker, or friend to give emotional and practical support. Two persons sharing the same problem and wanting to change together can really help each other—witness weight-loss clubs or the twelve-step programs to stop alcohol and drug use.

- Help trainee develop a specific "quit plan," using the steps above, and have him or her set a schedule on paper, including a final "quit date" when all tobacco use will stop.

- Modify the immediate environment to support the changed behavior—e.g., encourage trainees to remove ashtrays from home and workplace, give away lighters, ask other smokers not to smoke near them or give them a cigarette.

- Set up a series of self-rewards for achieving each milestone in the plan. This could include going to an enjoyable event, or buying a piece of clothing or small gift.

## SPREADING NEW HEALTH BEHAVIORS THROUGH THE COMMUNITY

Many health promotion programs are not brief, nor intensive, nor time-limited efforts, as are immunization campaigns. Rather, they may involve continuing change, as does smoking cessation; or ongoing community change enlisting successive waves of individuals, as in obtaining prenatal care or following safer sexual practices. For such efforts to change and maintain healthier community norms, the studies of diffusion of innovation are instructive.

Studies of the adoption and spread of new ways of doing things were first conducted in rural areas, as farmers adopted new agricultural practices. The ideas and techniques learned there have been used in health programs for about 40 years. These rural origins make promoting "innovation and diffusion" well fitted for rural as well as urban health interventions.

Because the mass media now has almost universal penetration, it is useful to enlist persons well known locally or nationally to appear on TV, radio, the print media (including billboards), and public gatherings to explain and display the new health behavior, to "model" participation in health programs, and to live in healthy ways themselves. Persons selected to present the messages for health programs should be: widely known, respected and trusted, honestly reflecting their own health behaviors, and willing to spread their messages through at least some of the channels of communication. (See the section on "Communicating Health Messages," earlier in this chapter.)

Studies on how new beliefs and behaviors are spread have shown that there is an established sequence through which groups become "converted." In most diffusion studies already published the rate of adopting the "new way" over time forms something like a bell-shaped normal curve, but often with a longer, slower rate of adoption at the beginning. The rate of new adoption slows after the peak of the curve, when the majority of the population are already practicing the new way. See Figure 12.4 for a schematic timeline of the diffusion of a behavior innovation in a community.

Everett Rogers, the pioneer researcher in this field, in his book *Diffusion of Innovations* (1995), sets out five successive theoretical community groups in terms

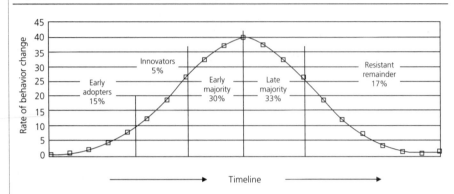

of their sequence of adopting new ways, some of their typical attributes, and approximate size in past studies. The following sections review these categories. This knowledge can help health leaders to design the sequential outreach efforts of health improvement programs. The basic work on the Rogers diffusion model was performed mainly in industrialized nations. Some modifications may be needed for different cultures and stages of development.

## INNOVATORS

These are venturesome people who have more than the average number of contacts outside their community. They have access to outside news and discuss it with friends who are often also seeking to learn more about the outside world, new developments, and a better life. The majority often views them as having "only one foot inside the local culture."

*Persons selected to present the messages for health programs should be widely known, respected, and trusted, and willing to spread their messages through at least some of the channels of communication.*

Innovators (compared to the rest of their community) tend to have more education, more access to the mass media, and larger homes or farms. They also tend to feel and act more independently, feel secure for reasons other than social conformity, and are willing to live with some uncertainty. Innovators are a very small group, usually less than 5% of a community.

Along with "change agents" (who often are outsiders) and local sponsors of health programs, innovators are those who first demonstrate the new way to the community. They are the persons from whom the next category of persons—the early adopters—take their cues.

## EARLY ADOPTERS

These individuals are opinion leaders who have more comprehensive contact networks in the community than the innovators. They tend to have higher educational levels, control more resources, and receive greater respect than most other citizens. The majority regards early adopters as good sources of information and guidance, and as more dependable and prudent than innovators. Early adopters represent between 10%–15% of the population.

Early adopters have a greater sense of self-efficacy—a sense that they have more power to control their circumstances—than do later adopters and the reluctant remnant (the laggards), who may be the last to make the change. Early adopters are less tied to the past, think abstractly as well as concretely, and place more trust in science. They travel more and participate in more social activities than those who delay acceptance of the new way.

Health program change agents sent into the community can speed up acceptance of a new health intervention or behavior by aiming the early stage of the program at innovators and early adopters, who share many characteristics. In cities, this early targeting can be done by making presentations to organizations holding meetings, and asking at each place, "What other groups or persons should have a chance to discuss this program with us?" In rural areas, informal inquiries can be done to determine who were the first persons to accept prior new innovations and

> *Be prepared to modify program strategies to later reach the skeptical late majority and the resistant remainder.*

whom would people ask about the advantages and disadvantages of a new program. The persons most frequently mentioned favorably are the early adopters. Program planners should meet with them to learn how the "new way" should be positioned and presented so as to best reach the entire community. Moreover, potential early adopters should be involved early on in program development. Typically, early adopters seek out information about innovations, while early and late majorities tend to wait for results of early adopters' experience before trying new ways themselves.

Keep in mind that people may adopt a new health behavior at any stage in this process for reasons that are not health related. For example, they may want to be seen as leaders, may want to please the change agent, may want to be part of a stimulating social activity, or may want to do something important for their children. Be prepared to modify program strategies to later reach the skeptical late majority and the resistant remainder.

## EARLY MAJORITY

Rogers (1995) characterizes the early majority as a group more deliberate and hesitant than those described above, but one that does not fear new things and is not blindly committed to old traditions. The early majority comprises about one-third of the population. Once won over, half of the target group will have at least tried out the new way.

The early majority are "average folks." They prefer to observe an innovation until they know it works well, rather than accept it because science or local experts say it will work well. The early majority has fewer connections with the outside world and is less willing to take a leadership role. Nevertheless, they have adequate education to accept the logic of the new way, once it has been shown safe and practical. Social communication networks between early adopters and the early majority will contribute greatly to the formal program, urging acceptance of the new approach.

## LATE MAJORITY

This group tends to have lower social standing, less education, and a more local outlook. The late majority thinks concretely and skeptically, and has a less active social communication network. They may have been misled in the past and so may harbor some resentment of higher social groups; hence, they are skeptical. This group comprises roughly one-third of the community. By this stage, the innovation program should have gathered enough momentum to continue spreading through the social channels of the first three change groups. At this point, the time has come for program managers gradually to change the emphasis of the public education and motivation campaigns. Less attention should be given to abstract or scientific arguments and more to observable results. Testimonials about local people experiencing the high rewards, low cost, low complexity, trustworthiness, and flexibility of the new approach or behavior should be highlighted. Locally popular figures and average citizens should deliver these messages. Respected teachers, coaches, skilled athletes, and admired community opinion leaders have more impact than do political officials or health professionals at this stage.

The idea that about half the community is already doing the new thing and liking it, and that more people are starting every day, adds to the effort's social momentum, convincing the followers, the postponers, and the skeptics that it is safe to try the new way. After all, the sense of uncertainty about this new thing has been dispelled. This is the time for health programming to change its message, but not to slow down. The late majority may have more health problems (higher prevalence or incidence) and so may be more helped by the innovation than previous acceptors. The redirected program must help them to try the new way and to stay with it long enough so that they begin to see its benefits and feel comfortable with it as part of their way of life.

This 10% to 20% of the program's total target population is usually not actively opposed to the innovation, but they may not have been reached by the program; if reached, they may not yet be convinced. Many in this group are socially isolated, uninvolved in the rise and fall of community agendas. Moreover, they may not even bother with mass media. They may be struggling just to keep their family going and may not have the money or the time to come to a health center, buy different food, or have plumbing installed in their homes. In the previously described programs to distribute free polio vaccine in Florida in the 1960s, young adults aged 20–40 years old who did not obtain the vaccine were most frequent among persons with few or no friends and who were not members of organized groups, persons with low education or relatively unreached by local media, persons who had a greater degree of skepticism and fear of exploitation, and persons who said that none of their friends or family had participated in the program (Johnson et al., 1962; Northcutt et al., 1964). These categories have been found predictive of non-response to health programs in most research reports in the last 40 years.

What can be done about this "hard-to-reach" minority? Control of some infectious diseases in a community can be achieved with only 70% to 80% coverage. This is due to a phenomenon known as "herd immunity." But for other conditions, such as noncommunicable causes of sickness and death concentrated in poverty-stricken sections of inner cities, it is necessary to redefine the community as those persons living or working in the high-risk area. Among them community-oriented programs can identify innovators and early adopters with whom to develop culture-specific programs to reach the resistant group.

Medical anthropologists are an important resource for any cross-cultural work. They can identify which key elements of beliefs, motives, and skills may need changing, and by what social processes this can most easily be accomplished. They also can train local health workers. Many large universities have medical anthropologists on faculty, and they can consult directly or provide the names of past graduates. In developing countries, health leaders can request such a consultation from their ministry of health or request international agencies to help find a specialist.

In summary, a group's willingness to accept and practice a new way of doing things—for health or other goals—and the speed with which the change spreads to all parts of the community depends in part on the properties of the innovation and the way it is presented or marketed. An innovation's diffusion can be accelerated if the target group perceives it has the following attributes, when compared to the existing way of dealing with the problem:

- **The new way is more rewarding.** Show that the innovation gives better results than the old way. Make it easy to understand. Help people to see the benefits of the new health behavior. If benefits are not perceived at the individual level, publicize reductions in the community's illness rates as they happen. Use testimonials of local people.

- **The new way should be less trouble and less costly.** Does the new health behavior (by agencies or individuals) require less equipment, drugs, and services, than the old way? Will it require less time and effort; is it easier to do? Show how the new way is less expensive than the old way, and how it can be tried with minimal risk, uncertainty, and anxiety. Emphasize whatever points of improved convenience are valid.

- **The new way "fits in" with current local culture and social structures.** Shape the innovation so it "feels like it's OK" with the group to be reached. Can the new way be carried out without creating social conflicts locally. Modify the new way if necessary, and present it so as to fit in with local values, beliefs, and ways of doing things, then it will be promoted by the culture rather than resisted by it.

- **The new way is flexible.** It is not irreversible. The new behavior or system can be tried out, modified, or even discontinued without damage to the health system or community if it is not successful. It also can be updated over time. The front-end costs of trying out the change in terms of money, institutional commitment, and changed role functions are not overwhelming (these attributes are adapted from Oldenburg, Hardcastle, and Kok, 1997).

## STAGES IN HEALTH BEHAVIOR CHANGE

Just as it is useful to know the stages that a community goes through in adopting more healthful behaviors, programs can benefit from understanding the five stages that an individual passes through in incorporating new healthful habits. This model, which was developed and tested by Prochaska and DiClemente,[1] applies primarily to long-term lifestyle changes, rather than to sporadic actions such as cancer screening. The model's five stages are as follows:

- **Pre-contemplation.** This is the stage at which individuals are not even considering the idea of a change. Unfortunately, some persons remain always at this stage.

- **Contemplation.** At this stage, people begin to think actively both about the health risk and the actions required to reduce that risk. The issue is now on their agenda, but no action is planned.

---

[1] Their publications can be seen in *The American Psychologist, Health Psychology,* and other sources from 1992 to the present.

- **Preparation.** At this point, contemplation moves into early action, such as developing a plan, joining a class or group, and getting materials (new foods, nicotine gum, or self-help booklets). Action is planned for the coming month.

- **Action.** This stage is marked by observable changes in the health-related behavior itself. The battle is under way. There may be relapses, but these should be dealt with as part of the change process and not as an excuse to slide back into contemplation. The action stage may go on for about six months. If successful, the person, or group, moves on to the less intense maintenance stage.

- **Maintenance.** At this stage the new health action needs to be firmly consolidated as a permanent lifestyle. Prevention of relapse to the less healthy behavior is essential. A return to smoking, alcohol abuse, or sedentary habits, or failing to complete a series of immunizations, may erase all the progress from earlier stages. Confidence and self-efficacy increase. Temptations to relapse are dealt with more routinely.

The strategy of the health promotion program or the health counselor is to move groups and individuals forward one step at a time through the stages of change. Success will be unlikely if the health counselor tries to move a person from pre-contemplation to action in a single leap. The health planner or counselor should establish where the individual stands in his thinking about the health changes and then provide knowledge, motivation, and skills to move on to the next stage. In terms of smoking cessation, for example, repeating the list of all the diseases and disorders cigarette smoking can cause will not help a smoker who needs help at the action stage. Nor will maintenance skills help a smoker who is not interested in stopping. Ask questions of individuals or groups, or survey a community to determine at which stage of change (see 1 to 5 above) the majority place themselves. Determine the barriers that keep them from the next step. Then work with them to overcome those barriers.

> *The strategy of the health promotion program or the health counselor is to move groups and individuals forward one step at a time through the stages of change.*

This model of the stages of change fits into the model of diffusion of innovation in the community. At any point during a community health promotion program, different people find themselves at different stages in the process of changing their behavior. At the beginning, most may be in pre-contemplation. As the program continues, however, more and more persons contemplate change and others are ready for action. Early adopters, for example, may have already adopted the change, while those in the late majority may not even be considering change. A family's position in the diffusion continuum is roughly correlated with its advancement along Prochaska's stages of change.

This understanding has important implications for health promotion programming. The public communication and service delivery activities must move forward one stage ahead of the growth of the advancing innovation/diffusion categories. As soon as 20%–30% of a population (which may be as small as one neighborhood or one factory) is thinking about (contemplating) a new health behavior, the program should be teaching this group preparation for action and the steps involved in making the change. At the same time, the program should continue to stimulate the remaining 70% to start considering action. However, that task should become much easier and less expensive because the natural flow of social interaction will spread the message from people already making the change to the late majority.

The messages communicated by the program should be separately conceived and delivered—some to reach uninterested people; some to move contemplators to action; and, later, some to deepen the commitment of people who have already changed to maintain their new attitudes and behaviors. The fact that in the early 1990s in the United States, 90% of active smokers knew smoking was harmful, but had not decided to quit, reflects the failure of the country's program to move from merely informing to motivating and teaching the skills to quit. The models for stages of change and community diffusion of innovation tell us that one kind of message does not fit everybody. People whose thinking is at a given stage of the change process require a message specifically tailored to move them to their next stage. Education, after all, is but one leg of a three-legged stool. Without adding the other two legs—motivation and skills training—a program's efforts are precarious, indeed.

No matter what the characteristics of intended participants, the issues of perceived threat of the disease, perceived benefits and costs of the new health action, reduction of uncertainty, and increase in perceived self-efficacy and empowerment must be taken into account (as explained earlier in this chapter). The treatment of each issue must be tailored to the belief and action system of the desired participants.

In technologically advanced areas, many physicians have adopted the roles of scientist and decision-maker, and moved away from the traditional role of personal healer. When it comes to changing health behaviors of individuals or communities, science provides theories and guidelines, but only a sensitive, enthusiastic, personally involved guide can actually make behavior change happen and ensure that healthy changes are maintained. Since in our present world, changing human behavior is the superhighway to Health for All, perhaps a new discipline of interpersonally talented, behaviorally-trained health counselors should be created to serve this essential function. Community development field workers, health aids, nurses, psychologists, and physician's assistants may provide the major pool from which this new profession can be selected and trained. The gross anatomy of behavior change presented in this chapter will be fleshed-out with specific examples for an array of different health promotion interventions in Chapter 13

# 13. Getting Specific: Actions to Reverse the Most Destructive Risk Forces

This Handbook focused on the stages of the life cycle in Part II and on specific major disease outcomes in Part III. Throughout, it has offered lists of risk factors and recommendations such as how to get people to stop smoking tobacco or how to improve children's nutrition. Chapter 12 explained the principles and methods of behavior change. This chapter puts together the easy-to-say, but hard-to-implement, recommendations (such as how to cut down the prevalence of alcohol use in a community) and the principles of behavior change, and organizes them around mega risk factors—risk factors that operate around the world and each of which produces multiple disease outcomes.

Table 13.1 shows the burden of death and disability attributed to ten major risk factors according to the GBD Study (Murray and Lopez, 1996). The forces that damage health are extremely different in the developing world than in the industrialized world. For developing nations, most of them impoverished, undernutrition and lack of safe drinking water and waste disposal services are the leading killers. Along with sexually transmitted infections, they are the top three causes of years of healthy life lost (Disability Adjusted Life Years, or DALYs). On the other hand, in industrialized nations—those that the Global Burden of Disease Study defines as "established market economies" and "former socialist economies"—the leading mega causes of death are tobacco use and hypertension. Tobacco use and alcohol use are the leading disablers there.

It should be kept in mind, however, that attributing death to various causes is somewhat arbitrary, especially when two or more pathologies are active simultaneously. For example, there are fewer than 1,000 deaths attributed to undernutrition in established market economies and former socialist economies. And yet these deaths do occur, and by the thousands, among the poorest people in these regions. DALYs estimates also are very loose. And yet, even though the numbers may be only shadows of the reality, even a glimpse at shadows can reveal whether a problem exists and something about its profile.

## MALNUTRITION

Of all the destructive deprivations in human experience, starvation for food ranks second only to starvation for love. Food malnutrition can show itself in several forms.

**TABLE 13.1.** Burdens of death and Disability Adjusted Life Years (DALYs)[1] attributed to ten major risk factors, worldwide (estimated counts, not rates).

| | Deaths (in 1,000s) | | DALYs (in 1,000s) | |
|---|---|---|---|---|
| Causes | Industrialized nations | Developing countries | Industrialized countries | Developing countries |
| Malnutrition | ... | 5,881 | ... | 219,575 |
| Poor water supply, sanitation, and hygiene | 4 | 2,665 | 229 | 96,169 |
| Tobacco use | 1,577 | 1,460 | 19,410 | 16,772 |
| Unsafe sex | 87 | 1,008 | 3,326 | 45,376 |
| Alcohol use | 137 | 637 | 15,398 | 32,289 |
| Hypertension | 1,406 | 1,512 | 7,577 | 11,499 |
| Occupational injuries and illnesses | 230 | 899 | 7,330 | 30,557 |
| Physical inactivity | 1,099 | 892 | 6,453 | 7,200 |
| Air pollution | 275 | 293 | 2,426 | 4,828 |
| Illicit drug use | 38 | 62 | 3,108 | 5,359 |

**Source:** Murray and Lopez, 1996, Chapter 6, pp. 295–324.

[1] Disability Adjusted Life Years is a measure that combines years of healthy living lost due to premature death and years of disability (graded from 0.10 to 1.00, based on severity).

1. **Protein-energy Malnutrition.** In this condition, there is not enough food of any kind for groups of people to maintain weight for extended periods. Protein-energy malnutrition is an academic label for starvation.

2. **Specific Nutrient Deficiencies.** This category includes such conditions as pellagra, beri-beri, iron deficiency, or iodine deficiency. In these cases, there are enough available calories, but specific essential vitamins, minerals, or amino acids (from proteins) are missing.

3. **Malabsorption Syndromes.** These are associated with diarrheas, parasitic infestations, or other conditions that prevent the absorption of consumed foods.

4. **Overnutrition.** This condition is due to an overconsumption of foods (especially calories) far beyond what the body needs for growth and activity. It is primarily a problem of post-industrialized areas, which are experiencing obesity epidemics, but it also can be found elsewhere in the world.

By far the greatest contribution to premature death and continuing disability comes from the first three forms described above, and the three are intertwined. Where there is marginal starvation, there also are specific nutritional diseases.

Where people are undernourished, resistance against infections and parasitic diseases is lowered. Infections and parasitic diseases, in turn, cause malabsorption syndromes. Even if previously adequate levels of food are made available at this point, the bodies remain undernourished.

Table 13.1 shows the burden of malnutrition on world health. The figures are calculated only from information on children undergoing degrees of starvation. The impact of undernutrition on adolescents and adults is admittedly both damaging and widespread, but quantifying it is difficult (Murray and Lopez, 1996, p. 305). Despite this narrowed scope of data, malnutrition is rated as the leading cause of death (nearly 6 million per year) and of disability. Poor nutrition in infancy causes retarded physical growth (stunting) and impaired neural development. It opens the door wider to many childhood diseases, which leave organic and functional scars that remain detectable throughout life. Hunger contributes to deaths coded as infectious and parasitic diseases, respiratory infections, perinatal conditions, and congenital anomalies, in addition to those directly coded as nutritional deficiencies. Hunger is the most active co-conspirator in millions of childhood tragedies each year.

> *Hunger is the most active co-conspirator in millions of childhood tragedies each year.*

According to the Hunger Project's data (Hunger Project, 1985):

- there is enough food produced in the world each year to feed every living human and

- there is enough potential farmland as yet unused or inadequately used to increase production enough to feed all people even if moderate population growth continues.

Why, then, is it not getting to people—predominantly children—who are hungry? Economics and distribution problems are the main barriers. Corporations that produce foodstuffs require payment, as do those who transport and distribute them. Actually, world hunger should not be blamed on famines, because these are usually localized to part of a nation and limited to a year or two. Importation of stored foods from other regions could save famine victims, were it not for those two barriers—and the decisions not to use money to overcome them.

World hunger has been a scourge for millennia, at least going back to Ancient Egypt. In this century, world hunger has been variously blamed—sometimes conflictingly so—on the world's capitalist economic system, or on a lack of a capitalist economic system in a given region, or on excess population growth due to high birth rates, or on a lack of foreign food aid, or the presence of foreign food aid that has fostered dependency. To try and deal with hunger, we have seen decades of international conferences, expert committees, books, United Nations resolutions, and draft programs. But after all is said and done, much more has been said than done.

Although world hunger has pandemic health consequences, it is primarily a political and economic issue. This is true among countries, as well as within countries, inasmuch as most nations have within them a comfortable fraction of overly fed people and a larger fraction of chronically hungry persons. And yet, nations have it within their power to solve this global scourge. The technology for producing and distributing enough food for everyone on the planet has been available for decades, in fact. The only thing lacking is the popular and political will of the people who have the power in their hands.

## DIAGNOSING AND TREATING HUNGER EPIDEMICS

The following approach may help identify partial solutions for hunger at the provincial, state, or metropolitan levels. Of course, the suggestions must be part of a comprehensive plan.

1. Treat hunger epidemiologically, as befits the disease that it is. Identify the host, agent, and the environment. Answer the Who? What? When? Where? Why? and How? of the situation. Identify the risk and protective factors that separate the hungry from the well fed—and that separate the hungry poor people from the non-hungry poor people elsewhere in the country.

2. Trace the flow of food from its place of origin (local or distant) to the target subpopulation that is malnourished. Are there adequate supplies elsewhere in the country? In the province? In the city and its surroundings? Locate the distribution barriers; the cost-barriers. How might each be overcome? You may need to consider an entirely different framework of possibilities than people have previously used. Past ways of thinking did not solve the problem then; they are unlikely to solve it now or in the future.

3. Consider how foods are being lost after harvesting through spoilage, exposure to insects and rodents, or due to theft and diversion. Encourage the community to consider drying grains by using ventilating equipment or natural means to prevent most spoilage, including aflatoxin which causes fatal liver diseases. Or suggest storing foods in screened areas or off the ground to help keep raw foods dry and safe from larger insects and animals. Storing crops locally in small bins also may reduce both shipping and storage problems. Remember that local farmers will keep closer watch to prevent spoilage than managers of a centralized facility. Having checks and balances in accounting, storing, and shipping of foods should reduce diversions. Providing

rewards for reporting instances of theft should reduce its frequency or make bribery too complex and expensive to be economically sensible.

4. Determine what crops can be grown under local conditions and support their production in family gardens. Once the techniques and skills for those foods are developed, larger scale production can be encouraged. The impact on local hunger will be substantial, because many people have been trained how to raise a food they have already learned to eat at home. Agricultural extension workers will be needed to teach the new methods. They can be selected and trained from among the more enthusiastic local farmers. **(Also see the section "Spreading of New Health Behaviors through the Community" in Chapter 12.)**

5. Look for available fruits, vegetables, and grains that local people are not accustomed to eating. In rural Puerto Rico a few years ago, farmers had grapefruit trees, but allowed the cattle to eat the fruit. They called grapefruit "animal food," and steered away from eating them, thus losing their nutritional benefit. Even now, many people in Western Europe consider corn (maize) as animal food. They continue to miss out on the joys and values of this delicious food. For centuries, tomatoes were thought to be dangerous to eat.

*Although world hunger has pandemic health consequences, it is primarily a political and economic issue.*

Could there be some partial solutions to local hunger being trodden underfoot? Again, new learning is required. Very successful "new food" programs have used cooking classes and tasting parties to introduce foods. The social context gives people the courage to try something new, and peer reaction encourages a shared positive evaluation. New recipes for use of the new food often allow it to be prepared in a style similar to currently favorite foods and with similar spices and sauces to make it look and taste more familiar and traditional.

6. Can current practices for growing food be made more productive? Are there fertilizers available, such as animal dung, compost heaps of decaying grasses and leaves, wood ashes, crushed limestone, which could increase yields? Can better quality seed be provided? Would crop rotation restore worn-out fields? Would terracing, contour plowing, or erosion control keep cropland from losing its fertile surface? Are modern dry farming techniques being used in arid climates? Can limited seasonal rainfall be conserved behind earthen dams or in local ponds?

Trained agriculturists will be able to answer these questions, as well as questions that are even more relevant for each local setting. There is an opportunity for intersectoral cooperation among agricultural specialists, community development agencies, and the health system.

The above approaches cannot totally solve world hunger, but thinking and acting locally is a good start. The number 6,000,000 means little to most of us, even when each one is a death from hunger that occurs each year. If we could see our own children's faces in each of those 6,000,000 deaths, however, how different the impact would be. Communities that can see the faces of their own children among hunger's potential victims may be the first to have the willpower to overcome hunger, working locally. **(Also see the section "Mobilizing the Community" in Chapter 12.)** Perhaps some of the ideas given above will help in that effort—at least until the cold, calculating iceberg of human unconcern melts.

## INADEQUATE WATER SUPPLY, SANITATION SERVICES, AND PERSONAL AND DOMESTIC HYGIENE

Industrialized nations have these environmental and behavioral risk factors well under control, except in their areas of poverty. Frequently, rural areas in industrialized countries are not well served with drinking water and waste disposal services either, but their low population density lowers the risk of disease outbreaks spreading there.

In less developed nations and areas, however, these conditions rank as the second leading causes of death and of disability. The overall estimated burden of healthy years lost through death and disability (DALYs)—96 million person years—is particularly disturbing.

### CLEAN WATER SUPPLY

Reasonably clean water is needed for washing, bathing, and cooking. Pure, boiled, or disinfected water is required for drinking. A. V. Whyte's guidelines (1986) are a particularly useful reference in regard to the community's participation to facilitate the installation and operation of public works necessary for a safe water supply. **(Also see the section "Mobilizing the Community" in Chapter 12.)**

Providing safe water does not always mean building purification and piped systems. In some places, it may be enough to use currently available clean water sources and shut down those sources that cannot be cleansed.

The low technology, highly logical processes used by the giant of epidemiology, Dr. John Snow, in London in the 1850s can be applied to many situations now. Every nation has its cadre of powerful logical thinkers whose help can be enlisted. The formula is to locate people who are getting sick, most of whom will be children (a spot map of the cases in the area helps greatly). Then, determine the source(s) of the noxious agent. In infections and parasitisms following the fecal-oral route, keeping those agents out of the fresh water supply will help solve the problem. **(Also see Table 2.1.)**

> *Providing safe water does not always mean building purification and piped systems. In some places, it may be enough to use currently available clean water sources and shut down those sources that cannot be cleansed.*

The job is not finished when safe water becomes available. Many programs declare success, but then the local people don't use the safe water exclusively. They may continue to use the former source because it is more convenient; because it tastes more familiar; because they say, "I drank it all my life and I'm alive and well"; or for other reasons. This is where health educators can help diagnose the behavioral resistance and teach and reinforce the healthier ways. **(Also see Chapter 12.)**

---

**SAFE WATER MEASURES THAT A COMMUNITY MIGHT CONSIDER**
- Provide pit latrines in safe locations convenient to currently used places for defecation.
- If a community uses a river as its water source, work to get all upstream dwellers to dump human, animal, and industrial waste in places that do not drain into the river.
- Dig new wells in safer places.
- Boil water that is to be drunk or used to prepare food.
- Use chemical additives such as chlorine to purify drinking water.
- Consult a sanitary expert for additional local solutions.

---

**SANITATION**

The goal is to keep land, water, and air free of waste harmful to health. Major concerns are human, animal, industrial, and sometimes radioactive wastes.

- Social and behavioral change are the key to improving human waste disposal. As a rule, the sequence of development is as follows: (1) building privies; (2) using "night jars" to collect children's and adults' night-time wastes, later to be dumped in the privies; (3) introducing septic tank systems (low-tech, no moving parts); and, finally, (4) installing community underground sewage collection and treatment systems. Many cities in developed nations make money from their sewage treatment facilities by selling fully dried sewage sludge as farm and garden fertilizer.

- Animal wastes can pose a problem on family farms if they are allowed to drain into the water supply. Large commercial farms raising livestock must be monitored to prevent them from dumping large amounts of waste, thus polluting small streams and the rivers into which they flow. Relocation of waste lagoons, provision for longer filtration times, and relocation of water supplies all can help solve pollution problems.

- Industries and communities that generate waste must be responsible for controlling it safely. Many companies opt for maximizing immediate rather than longer-term profits, and fail to act in responsible partnership with the communities and the people around them. Hence, governmental regulations and their enforcement are required, if not for the current corporate residents, then for future ones that may not be such good neighbors. Sanitary and environmental engineers and public health experts can provide detailed guidance.

All these steps to maintain a healthy environment help ensure safe water, thus preventing infectious, parasitic, and toxic disorders. They also assist in providing clean air, thus preventing both pulmonary and cardiopulmonary diseases.

## PERSONAL AND DOMESTIC HYGIENE

Hygiene leaves much room for improvement in every nation, no matter the level of development. Even in industrialized nations, some locations may be overlooked—nurseries and child care centers, which are at risk for the spread of fecal-oral diseases; schools, where diseases can spread among non-immunized children; hospitals, where iatrogenic infections are carried by workers' hands, bedding, ventilation systems, improper handling and disposal of medical wastes; nursing homes, especially around incontinent patients; and public eating places. But it is in the home—where most of the people spend most of their time—where most of the exposure to unsanitary conditions usually takes place.

### Handwashing

The call of Ignasz Semmelweiss echoes across two centuries—"Wash your hands: more often and more thoroughly"—and still resonates with us today. A quick soap rub and a flush of water was not enough to prevent childbed fever from spreading through obstetrics wards, Semmelweiss found. He added chlorinated

---

### THE MESSAGE TODAY

- Wash adequately with anti-bacterial soap.
- Wash thoroughly.
- Wash after caring for each child or patient.
- Wash before handling food, beverages, or objects that must stay clean (such as eating utensils, toothbrushes, cloths for washing irritated, abrased, or wounded skin, any items children might put in their mouths).

Health care workers who have sensitive skin may need to wear latex gloves and change them or wash them thoroughly after each use.

lime water to the washing process in the 1850s in Austria-Hungary, and required thorough handwashing more often. His methods stopped outbreaks of childbed (puerperal) fever in his day and still do wherever they are used.

### Food Handling

Store foods in insect-proof, animal-proof, waterproof containers. Maintain food cleanliness when dispensing portions for immediate use. Keep clean surfaces on which food is cut up, mixed, or prepared; pots and pans in which it is cooked; and dishes and utensils with which it is eaten. Avoid unclean or spoiled foods.

### Household Cleanliness

Keep the living space of the home cleaned of any materials that would attract insects, mice, rats, etc. Keep domestic animals outside the house, unless they are trained not to defecate or urinate inside. Be careful that household animals not be carriers of fleas, ticks, triatomids, or other insects that can infect humans. If using insecticides, be careful not to spray them where food is to be exposed or children might handle sprayed objects. **(Also see relevant text in the section "From Birth through Age 4 Years" in Chapter 3.)**

All these measures require changes in thinking, in appraising (evaluating) circumstances, and in behaving. To mass audiences these changes are best spread by changing social expectations and cultural patterns. Local mini-cultures exist in each hospital, school, day-care center, or family. Once incorporated into a local group's cultural web of behaviors, hygiene practices will become second nature to the people involved. Again, incremental changes are the order of the day—cultures are changed one mini-culture, one outpost, one family at a time. **(Also see Chapter 12.)**

> *It is in the home—where most people spend most of their time—where the greatest exposure to unsanitary conditions usually takes place.*

## TOBACCO USE

Tobacco-related diseases were responsible for about three million deaths worldwide in 1990, half of them occurring in industrialized nations, more than 800,000 in China, and many more of the remainder in other parts of Asia. In the Americas, almost 15% of men's deaths and 7% of women's were attributed to tobacco (PAHO, 1992). By 1990, worldwide one person died every 10 seconds due to tobacco.

Using the statistical projections of Peto and Lopez (cited in Murray and Lopez, 1996), tobacco mortality will rise rapidly, reaching about 8,400,000 deaths per year by 2020. This means that the world is steadily moving towards being able to count one tobacco-related death every 3.6 seconds. More alarming, this figure does not include the many additional years of disability due to smoking and chewing tobacco, estimated at slightly less than 10,000,000 person/years (Years of Life Disabled, or YLD) in 1990. Thus far, 43 carcinogens have been identified in tobacco smoke.

## EFFECTS ON USERS

As discussed in chapters 7 through 10, tobacco enters into the causal picture of many diseases—ischemic heart disease, stroke, pulmonary heart disease, peripheral vascular disease, cancers of the trachea, bronchus, and lung, head and neck, cancer of the bladder, cancer of the uterine cervix, peptic ulcer disease, chronic obstructive pulmonary disease, and emphysema. It also increases susceptibility to respiratory infections, aggravates asthma, contributes to low birthweight and developmental problems in babies whose mothers smoke during pregnancy, and can lead to higher risk of infant respiratory disorders from second-hand smoke in the home. And the list goes on.

Smoking raises the risk of fires in the home. Vehicle drivers who smoke are more likely to have crashes. In areas where birth control pills are commonly used, even stronger arguments can be made for women to stop smoking—the combined biochemical effect of birth control medications and tobacco smoking multiplies the risks of cerebrovascular strokes and myocardial infarctions in younger women. Additionally, those who chew tobacco or use snuff put themselves at high risk of cancers of the oral cavity. This practice is responsible for the very high rate of head and neck cancers in India and other parts of Asia.

## EFFECTS ON NONUSERS

Some smokers claim that their habit harms only themselves and that they should be allowed that freedom. This claim deserves rethinking, in light of studies of environmental tobacco smoke (ETS) conducted since 1985. These provide further firm and ample proof that second-hand smoke at the relatively dilute concentrations typically found in cigarette smokers' homes, workplaces, and places of entertainment has measurable toxic effects. Added up worldwide, this unintentionally inhaled toxicity exacts a huge price in damaged health of children and nonsmoking adults.

### In Utero

Maternal smoking during pregnancy has been solidly proven to be a common cause of low birthweight babies and premature births. Low birthweight, in turn, is a common intermediary for immature development, congenital anomalies, impaired future intelligence, and infant mortality. In industrial and postindustrial societies, smoking contributes to infant mortality by doubling or tripling the rate of sudden infant death syndrome (SIDS), depending on the duration of the mother's smoking. **(For further information on intrauterine toxicities see the section "In Pregnancy" in Chapter 3.)**

### In Infancy

The damage from parental smoking continues through childhood. A mother or caretaker (such as a babysitter) spends much time in close contact with young children, usually more than a father. As a result, her chemical impact generally is greater than his. Infants raised by a mother who smokes regularly have about double the risk of sudden infant death syndrome (SIDS). For a child whose mother smoked during pregnancy and during its first six months of breathing on its own, the SIDS risk is tripled.

### In Childhood

In the second and subsequent years of childhood, ETS in the home or day care center has been found to be causally associated with an increased risk of lower respiratory infections, such as bronchitis and pneumonia—in the United States alone, between 150,000 and 300,000 additional cases each year in children 1 to 18 months of age are attributed to second-hand tobacco smoke. This results in 7,500 to 15,000 preventable hospitalizations per year in that country. (The wide range of estimated cases is due in part to the changing number of smokers and the differences in smoke concentrations in various homes.)

> *Infants raised by a mother who smokes regularly have about double the risk of sudden infant death syndrome. For a child whose mother smoked during pregnancy and during its first six months of breathing on its own, the risk triples.*

Moreover, since about 1985 a new finding has associated ETS with the prevalence of children having fluid in the middle ear, leading to earache and avoidable medical expenses. Findings regarding the effect of ETS on children's asthma also have been strengthened—among children with asthma, both the severity and frequency of asthma attacks are increased. ETS is estimated to be harmful to about 20% of the 2 to 5 million children with asthma in the United States. The personal suffering and financial costs of an extra one or two million avoidable asthma attacks cannot be calculated. Corresponding data from other nations are not available, but probably correspond to the prevalence of tobacco smoking in children's homes. In addition, ETS might bring on new cases of asthma in children previously free of the disease, but the small number of studies on this point are inconclusive.

Of course, the premature death of a parent from a tobacco disease is socially and emotionally harmful to children and youth.

### In Adults

Consider the following additional facts and estimates regarding ETS effects on nonsmoking adults (EPA, 1993 and WHO, 1997):

- The United States Environmental Protection Agency (EPA) has classified ETS as a Class A carcinogen.

- ETS is the *only* agent rated as Class A by the EPA for which typical environmental exposures (not high-dose laboratory experiments) deliver measurably increased rates of human cancer.

- Evidence from 30 epidemiologic studies conducted in eight countries clearly demonstrates a higher lung cancer risk among nonsmokers exposed to ETS than those living in clean air. There is now such a preponderance of studies showing elevated risks of lung cancer due to ETS, that the statistical chance of them all being wrong is less than 1 in 10 million.

- EPA estimates that ETS is responsible for about 3,000 lung cancers in adult nonsmokers in the United States each year. This is in addition to those lung cancers in non-smokers caused by occupational or smog exposures.

- ETS has subtle but clinically measurable effects on lung function, coughing, and phlegm production.

Two factors operate worldwide to spread the tobacco epidemic—the powerful addictive properties of nicotine and the wealthy tobacco industries that buy their way into developing areas. Tobacco industries market and advertise their products with psychological skill, often targeting young people—even children—by giving away enough free samples to plant an addiction in many.

## THREE PREVENTIVE STRATEGIES

Community and health leaders have three prevention levels available—primordial, primary, and secondary. Tertiary prevention is useless for combating tobacco addiction, because once tobacco diseases are fully present they are not reversible. Stopping tobacco use, however, can halt further disease progress and, over time, allow rates of emergence of full clinical disease to decline.

## Primordial Prevention

This level refers to prevention before the disease agent enters the environment. In another context, for example, this would involve the quarantine of all live animals seeking to enter a given area until they have been proven to be free of rabies. This represents primordial prevention of rabies in those geographic areas. The same principle can be applied to the importation or manufacture of tobacco products, by banning their entry into a given area. This early prevention requires strong political will, as well as the population's support to withstand the enticements of multinational tobacco companies and, sometimes, the pressures of other governments. (Unfortunately, for some decades in the past, the United States Department of Commerce sought to force smaller countries to accept US tobacco products for local marketing.)

If tobacco products cannot be kept out of a country or province, they can be taxed sufficiently to sharply limit their use by children and adults with less money.

A second primordial prevention measure would be to make tobacco products more difficult to obtain. Requiring an expensive license for wholesale distribution will drive up the price of tobacco products. In the United States, for example, there are laws in place that require proof of age (18 years or older) for purchasing tobacco products; they have reduced adolescent usage. Of course, youth can get older friends to purchase cigarettes for them, but it still raises one more barrier. Eliminating machines that sell cigarettes automatically raises another inconvenience. Each trivial barrier increases the effort (the costs) needed, and makes the habit less easy. **(Also see sections "Overlapping Theories of Behavior Change" and "A Sampling of Self-Directed Behavior Change Tactics in Chapter 12.")**

## Primary Prevention

At this level, children are taught how to stay away from tobacco before they even begin experimenting with it. Just trying out cigarettes can start a slippery slide down to addiction. These principles and sentiments should be taught from age 2 years (when children might pick up cigarettes or butts) in homes and child care facilities. This teaching is more effective if the adults involved do not smoke, chew tobacco, or use tobacco products in any way.

Schools, especially primary and secondary schools, hold great potential for primary prevention of tobacco use among children and youth 6 to 18 years old. Governmental and nongovernmental health agencies have developed various curricula. Keep in mind, however, that curricula that simply give out health information alone almost universally fail. Successful curricula include the teaching of attitudes and providing counterarguments to reject invitations to try tobacco. These are reinforced most effectively by discussion and role playing among the participants. School curricula for tobacco prevention are available in most major languages (The problem of childhood smoking, 1996). **(Also see relevant text on tobacco in the section "From Ages 5 through 14 Years" in Chapter 3.)**

### Secondary Prevention

At this level, efforts involve getting tobacco users to quit an existing habit of smoking or chewing tobacco. The United States National Institutes of Health has supported this kind of behavior-change research for about three decades. It has been found that although many intervention programs can get a high percentage of smokers to quit for a while, the critical test of a good program is how many quitters abstain from tobacco for 6 or 12 months after quitting. Skaar, Tsoh, McClure, et al. (1997) offer a comprehensive review of smoking cessation program evaluation and health care policy implications; Fiore, Bailey, Cohen, et al. (1996 or later) have a useful summary of clinical intervention guidelines.

> *Schools, especially primary and secondary schools, hold great potential for primary prevention of tobacco use among children and youth 6 to 18 years old.*

These sources agree that:

1. Smoking cessation programs can be conducted by many kinds of professionals and nonprofessionals, as long as they have had specific training and supervised experience in the kinds of listening, teaching, group process, and problem-solving involved.

2. Nicotine-replacement skin patches or chewing gum, where available and affordable, can be used for a short time to reduce nicotine withdrawal symptoms and facilitate cessation. Patches or gum are relatively ineffective, however, if used without concurrent behavior change group sessions.

3. Teaching the following messages is beneficial: (1) cessation programs do work, even if they do not work the first time, and (2) the program participant has the ability to quit. Success is likely to come by following the program one hour at a time, rather than through vast amounts of willpower.

4. Treatment is more effective when the counselor:

   - **Is perceived as being understanding.** Persons who quit successfully typically report that their counselors were supportive, caring, and enabled them to work out their own solutions. Counselors were not authoritarian, nor did they judge clients negatively. This encouraged discussion and problem-solving.

- **Encourages expressions of feelings and concerns.** Many clients are afraid that stopping smoking will lead to weight gain, for example. Counselors can reassure them that many studies show that some people gain no weight at all, and among those that do, the average gain is less than 10 lbs (4.4 kg). That can be lost later by increasing exercise. Counselors can also relieve clients' embarrassment over brief setbacks in their progress.

- **Helps heavy smokers (more than 20 to 30 cigarettes per day) start a tapering-off program.** This involves smoking on a strict time schedule and lengthening the interval between cigarettes so that one-third fewer cigarettes are smoked each successive week (Cinciripini, Lapitsky, Seay, et al., 1995).

- **Encourages persons smoking fewer than 20 cigarettes per day to set a "quit date."** This is the day that will mark the start of their lives without tobacco. The client will announce to family and friends that he or she will quit on that date, and is getting rid of all tobacco products, cigarette lighters, and ashtrays from home or other places where he or she spends time. The counselor, family, and friends should all give additional social support and encouragement from a few days before the quit date until about 10 days afterward, depending on how well the person is coping with withdrawal.

- **Maintains follow-up to reinforce cessation.** Quitting smoking is easier than staying quit. Some die-hard smokers say, "Quitting smoking is easy! I've done it 10 times." The counselor (or the anti-smoking program) is urged to follow every client, first weekly, then monthly, then quarterly for a year. This enables the program to be evaluated and identifies areas for improvement.

The "stages of change" behavioral model is well suited to the process of smoking cessation (Prochaska, Rossi, et al., 1994). **(Also see Chapter 12 for further discussion and additional resources.)**

Even before the advent of psychologically-based intervention programs, people had been stopping tobacco use on their own. The United States Office of Smoking and Health in 1989 reported that in addition to the 25% of all regular smokers whose deaths are attributable to tobacco, enough living smokers quit smoking to reduce the prevalence of adult smokers in the country from 40% in 1965 to 29% in 1987. At that time, nearly half of all living adults in the United States who had ever smoked had quit. The downward trend appeared to be continuing in the 1990s. As a result of decisions never to start smoking or to quit, an estimated 750,000 smoking deaths were prevented. Similar preventive success

**301**

can be achieved in most nations. Mass media presentations of anti-smoking messages—on television, radio, magazines, and billboards—were deemed effective. Some of these campaigns were paid for by taxes from tobacco sales.

Countries, especially in the developing world, today have a great opportunity to prove wrong the predictions and projections of 8,400,000 tobacco-related deaths in the year 2020. This can be accomplished through aggressive, well-directed primordial and primary prevention targeted to children and young people. If countries can raise a tobacco-free generation until age 25, by then those young adults will be at low risk for starting the tobacco habit. Keeping future generations smoke-free just for their first 25 years would save huge numbers of lives and billions of currency units of unnecessary medical bills. Furthermore, the costs of maintaining such preventive programs would become increasingly cheaper after tobacco advertising is stopped and fewer adults are modeling self-destructive habits.

Teaching materials and intervention program guides may be obtained from WHO in Geneva, Switzerland; PAHO; other WHO Regional Offices; most national ministries of health; and organizations working in health and health-related issues.

## UNSAFE SEX

### DISEASE BURDEN

Sexually transmitted infections (STIs) are estimated to be the third leading cause of disability and the seventh most common cause of death worldwide. Their impact is by far the greatest in economically less developed and transitional areas.

On average, 685,000 people are infected every day with an STI (WHO, 1999). This adds up to about 250 million new infections per year, nearly as many as for malaria. Trichomoniasis, gonorrhea, chlamydia, chancroid, and syphilis are the most prevalent infections. Sampling surveys in gynecology clinics in the United States of America report trichomoniasis prevalence rates as high as 50%. High prevalences occur all over the world. In some places, the rate of gonorrhea infection is as high as 20% in adults coming to general health clinics and up to 50% among commercial sex workers (Cates and Holmes, 1986).

> Every day, an average of 685,000 people are infected with a sexually transmitted infection—which adds up to about 250 million new infections each year.

Human immunodeficiency virus (HIV) infections and clinically apparent acquired immunodeficiency syndrome (AIDS) are sweeping through Sub-Saharan Africa, Southeast Asia, and many other regions. HIV prevalence is difficult to estimate adequately, because many areas lack laboratory facilities to make the diagnosis. In addition, adults infected with HIV can infect others in about four months, yet may remain unaware of their disease until it starts showing signs or symptoms, often as long as three to six years later. Furthermore, full national reporting has political and tourism implications. Without question, AIDS is a worldwide epidemic. One of its more tragic expressions is the tens of thousands of infants with infections acquired in utero, during the birth process, and/or less commonly from breast-feeding. Until now, the AIDS mortality rate has been nearly 100%. Unfortunately, new drugs to delay progression of such retroviruses remain too expensive for use in many countries.

More than 50 different STI syndromes have been recognized; they are traced to more than 20 infectious agents. The field is much more complex than it was thought to be 40 years ago. Yet, by 1995, the teaching about STIs in medical universities in the United States reportedly had dwindled to an annual average of only one hour per student. Health policy leaders may need to correct this deficiency in many nations. However, new advances are continuing to be made with regard to more efficient organization of STI services, more user-friendly delivery of services, less invasive diagnostic tests, improved antibiotic drugs, and better treatment schedules. Finally, in some places modern behavior change methodology is beginning to be used. Perhaps the broadest research program evaluating clinical field trials of state-of-the-art psycho-behavioral theory and practice is that conducted by the Centers for Disease Control and Prevention (U.S.A.) through its Behavioral Interventions and Research Branch in the Division of STD Prevention.

Traditionally, most STI training courses and published guidelines have focused on biological and administrative issues. Inadequate attention to prevention issues and failure to adapt and utilize modern psychological methods has tended to limit STI efforts mainly to getting patients to recognize signs of disease and to self-refer for treatment. Another major problem is that STI services almost everywhere have been understaffed and underfunded.

This Handbook offers the following arguments:

- STIs are social-behavioral in their etiology (cause and spread). They share many of the same psychosocial risk factors as injuries, violence, and alcohol and drug abuse. **(Also see section "Major Health Problems at Ages 15–24" in Chapter 4, and chapters 7 and 11.)**

- STIs express themselves as infectious diseases.

- Primary prevention is better than secondary or tertiary prevention. For HIV/AIDS there is no secondary or tertiary prevention as yet. For chlamydia and gonorrhea that result in pelvic inflammatory disease, recognition is often too late for any restoration of fertility.

## POPULATIONS AT RISK

STIs are sneaky. Most are invisible. They hide among the poor, the rich, the young and old, and among persons of all races, all levels of education, and all occupations—even among nice clean-looking folks. You cannot tell by looking or asking. Therefore, it is important to stress that knowing a prospective partner's group identification is far less important than knowing about their behavior. By far the most common way of contracting STIs is through sexual activity. Ranking second (for viral STIs such as HIV) is by sharing needles or syringes, mainly to inject drugs. Unborn fetuses are at high risk if their mother has an STI; they can be infected during pregnancy, the delivery process, or afterward.

Subgroups that tend to practice unprotected sex, and so are at high risk of carrying STIs, include sexually active youth and young adults, people temporarily living away from home, men and women in the military, long-distance truck drivers, rural migrants to urban areas, commercial sex workers, people using injected illegal drugs, and persons engaging in anal intercourse.

It is important to inform people that ordinary social interactions—shaking hands, hugging, sharing food together, using public toilets—will not transmit STIs, neither will insect nor animal vectors carry them.

## RISK FACTORS

- Failure to follow safer sex practices, especially a person's failure to protect him- or herself with barriers such as condoms every time sexual penetration occurs.

- Having unprotected sex with multiple partners. This is the most dangerous of all, because it multiplies a person's risk, by accumulating the risk each other partner incurred from all previous partners, and then passing it on to the next person involved.

- Having a sex partner who himself/herself has multiple partners. This is how one careful partner can be infected by a careless one.

- Changing one's sex partner from time to time. It adds a new set of contacts.

- Having sex with casual acquaintances whose background and prior sex habits are not known well. These people may be harboring an STI!

- Having sex with commercial sex workers, including prostitutes or their clients.

- Having anal sex.

- Although there is danger in numbers, contact with a single person can be dangerous too, if that person is infected and the contact is not protected by a barrier such as a condom.

## THE MAIN PROTECTIVE FACTOR: THE BRAIN

Contrary to what most STI guidebooks say, the primary protection against these infections, unwanted pregnancies, and all the troubles either can bring, is not the condom, it's the brain. Handing out latex condoms and showing people how to use them is part of primary prevention, but it must not be considered sufficient. Sexual behaviors begin long before the condom is unwrapped, and it is at such beginnings that the brain must be engaged in prevention. By the time the condom begins to be unwrapped—provided this has not been forgotten in the excitement—the brain may no longer be functioning wisely enough.

> *Handing out latex condoms and showing people how to use them is part of primary prevention, but it must not be considered sufficient. Sexual behaviors begin long before the condom is unwrapped, and it is at such beginnings that the brain must be engaged in prevention.*

The teaching of primary STI prevention in children should begin before they begin puberty. Middle childhood is a rational period for children, and many of them talk and act like small, sensible grown-ups. (This may well reveal the bias of an aging author.) Preventive teaching and participatory discussion need not be sex education, which has vocal opposition in many subcultures.

Teaching can simply be oriented around making choices, emphasizing that the choices children and teens make can either build their futures or ruin them. Using street drugs, for example, can damage the body and the brain. Riding a bicycle carelessly on a highway can break arms and legs, or worse. Getting involved with people of either sex in ways that bring fluids or sores near to or in contact with sexual organs—or even with breaks in the skin—can spread serious or even occasionally fatal infectious diseases. These diseases can damage a person's occupational future and his or her prospects for marriage or parenthood. Fortunately, as is the case with other diseases or injuries, sexually transmitted infections can be largely prevented. Children need to learn how to avoid trouble; how to make smart decisions; how to control impulses; how to deal firmly and politely with pressures from friends; and how to continue steering themselves forward to a good life, not damaged by past immature mistakes. Girls especially need to avoid sexual risks, because as a rule they get hurt far more seriously than their male partners. Girls can get pregnant and STIs can linger long and do reproductive damage.

## CAUSES OF SEXUAL BEHAVIOR

Human behavior follows systematically from its "causes." If these causes can be identified and changed, the behaviors will change also. People enter into a new situation or circumstance with predispositions for certain behaviors based on past learning, motives, drives, and intentions or goals. The situation itself holds cues (signals that have meaning), and these cues prompt one of several reactions: to move toward, to move away, to oppose, or to ignore the objects and persons in the new situation.

People differ so widely from one another in culture, past experience, personal needs, and ways of trying to get what they want, that no "cookie cutter" approach will help even half the clients. This is not to say that in a group of 1,000 persons each one has to be treated individually. However, there may be a dozen or so different categories of people in terms of motivations, habits, and approaches to behavior change. To deal with these categories as efficiently as possible warrants the development of flow-charts for behavioral treatment parallel to flow-charts to determine antibiotic treatments for STI syndromes. In the same way that a single shot of penicillin won't cure every STI, a single set of instructions, or one approach such as providing condoms, won't correct all sexual behavior problems.

### Psychosocial Determinants

What are some of the predispositions and needs that might lead adolescents and adults to be too hasty or careless about their sexual activities?

Internal psychological drives:

- Adolescents may want to prove that they are grown up and independent.

- Some may use sexual intimacy to boost low self-regard (often true, but rarely self-reported).

- Sex may be used as a balm for loneliness or to fill an acute hunger for intimacy.

- Youths may want to experience the thrill of sudden passion and sex with a stranger.

- Mature adults may rely on sex as an assurance that they are still attractive and sexually competent.

- Sexual activities that build high excitement and discharge in orgasm deliver great psychological reinforcement that creates a yearning for more. And there are many forms of exciting, fulfilling activities—sexual or other—that are safe.

Social pressures:

- Young people may engage in sex "to be like their friends," "to fit in." In fact, when large groups of high-schoolers are asked how many youth of their own age engage in various presexual and sexual behaviors, they vastly overestimate the percentages for each behavior, as anonymously self-reported by the same group.

- Young people may engage in sexual behavior to get the reputation of being especially "sexy" or popular.

- Adolescents and adults both may want to rebel against their families and childhood value systems.

Pressures to keep or save relationships:

- People may be afraid of losing a current partner unless they move quickly enough to full intimacy, at times including more risk-filled acts.

- Many people use sex activities to enhance and maintain a long-term relationship. This approach to sex is usually safe, unless one partner is infected. If so, safe sex precautions should be used.

- Some people may trade sex for friendship or companionship.

Economic reasons:

- Some people may trade sex for favored treatment or other services such as help with work, quicker promotion, auto repair, or extra groceries. (The author once counseled a divorced woman with two children who came to a prenatal clinic. She explained her third pregnancy by saying, "a mother has to feed her children.")

- Male and female drug abusers may trade sex for more drugs or money to buy drugs. In the desperation of withdrawal symptoms they will do almost anything for a drug fix. Drug addiction often progresses to intravenous drug injection, multiplying the risk of viral infection from shared needles and syringes.

Of course, the prevention counselor should focus on modifying the motives and drives operating in specific individuals, couples, or groups, so that they can fulfill their felt needs, such as those above, by safer and more constructive means than indiscriminant sexual behavior.

Goals in STI prevention counseling include "preparing the brain" to deal wisely and safely with sexual possibilities. For many clients this involves strengthening their sense of self-efficacy ("I can and must guide my own destiny") and level of self-esteem ("I am a worthwhile person who deserves good health and a fulfilling future").

An approach that some counselors and group facilitators use to raise the sense of self-determination and self-value emphasizes that the human race has greater capacities and responsibilities than do all animal species. Animals are prisoners to their instincts and urges, forced to act on impulse because they cannot think reflectively. Animals are hostages of their surroundings. Counselors and facilitators—and their patients, clients, or students—on the other hand, are part of the only species that can work weeks to finish a painting, years to finish a book, and centuries to build a cathedral. Humans can plan their lives and radically reconstruct their environment or move to new ones.

Even those of us who cannot do things on such a grand scale can at least stop and think, manage our behavior, steer clear of danger, and look far enough forward not to swap an hour of (what one hopes will be) fun for years of trouble, regret, or unplanned responsibilities. Only by caring for themselves and their loved ones—constantly and thoughtfully—can humans keep themselves free. Mother Nature does not forgive.

These may seem like unattainable dreams for impulsive teenagers or deprived adults, but we all carry the instinct to move on up a little higher. Counselors can present a client with a personalized vision of where he or she now stands, and calibrate it to fit the client and the social environment. This may also entail re-defining which way is "up"—which is the direction toward which to grow.

For the other personal needs and desires listed above, there are healthier solutions than unsafe sex to meet psychological needs, to make a social statement, to firm up a relationship. Counselors should try to guide clients into better ways to meet their specific needs and resolve their concerns.

> *The STI counselor's job is not to change clients' personalities or world view, nor to solve their deep conflicts. Rather, the counselor should offer better and healthier ways for clients to get what they want.*

The STI counselor's job is not to change clients' personalities or world view, nor to solve their deep conflicts. Rather, the counselor should offer better and healthier ways for clients to get what they want. Ideally, the newly adjusted behaviors will meet the true underlying hungers and needs as well as did the old behaviors (the reward side), but with much less danger of disease, disability, or death as the old behaviors (the cost side of the equation).

## Social Environmental Determinants

So far, this chapter has reviewed some of the predispositions, intentions, needs, and reasons—both true and false—people carry with them as they travel through their environments. Those environments, too, are essential determinants of whether sexual activity will take place or not, and if so, the likelihood that it will be safe.

Throughout history, families and communities have controlled the physical and social environments of fertile females and males so as to minimize the number of pregnancies outside of sanctioned couples. Society also imposed harsh taboos on same-sex partners. As a byproduct of this societal control, the spread of STIs also was kept in check. For example, traditional systems kept youths and young adults living in their families' homes until marriage and, as a rule, the sexes lived in separate quarters in schools, colleges, and even in many factory towns. Moreover, the practice of chaperoning unmarried young women was widespread and accepted as the norm in most Hispanic, Arabic, Asian, and some European cultures. With the rapid worldwide spread of individual and sexual liberation since about the middle of the 20th century, however, the controls began to erode—as the rising birth rate to unwed mothers and the pandemic of STIs amply demonstrates.

The fact is that, with the new sexual and individual freedoms, the responsibility for safer sex has shifted more to the individual, rather than society. Today, more and more individuals "control" the environments they select—and they can select safe or risky ones. STI prevention should work to replace risky circumstances with safer ones. Even if low self-esteem or sexual hunger cannot be counseled away, they won't result in unsafe sex unless the environment provides a partner. Some examples of "environmental safety" that a counselor can share with a client include:

- Avoid frequenting pick-up bars, places where single persons go to drink alcohol and find someone new for intimacy.

- Avoid parts of town where commercial sex workers wait for customers.

- Socialize mainly with groups where sexual activity (regardless of sexual orientation) is unlikely or impossible; for example, groups of monogamous couples, groups sponsored by religious or ethical organizations, or groups so committed to specific purposes and projects that "sexual cruising" is unlikely.

- Avoid circumstances where alcohol or street drugs may numb one's brain so that wise decision-making is hampered.

- Avoid situations where narcotics are being injected.

- Avoid patronizing places where tattooing or body-piercing is done, unless you can determine yourself that needles or lancets have not been used before and are opened from sealed packages, or witness a thorough sterilization process conducted. Don't accept verbal assurances.

- Obtain health care only at first-class medical facilities where strict sanitation is practiced, including boiling and/or chemical disinfection of all instruments that pierce the skin, careful soap scrubbing of workers' hands, or the use of fresh sterile gloves as a worker moves from one patient to another patient (especially when examining body openings).

*With the advent of new sexual and personal freedoms, the responsibility for safe sex has shifted away from society and toward the individual.*

All behavior requires both a predisposition (conscious or unconscious) and an enabling environment (including environments that change intentions). Therefore, keeping people out of sexually enabling environments and circumstances is one effective way to reduce unsafe sexual behaviors.

## AN UNHURRIED DECISION-MAKING PROCESS

Counselors must stress the importance of taking time to make reasoned decisions about sex. Decisions about sexual behavior should not be made in a thoughtless rush. As to "life and death" decisions, a quick "no" just might mean

BUILDING BETTER HEALTH

life, but a quick "yes" just might risk death. Good sex will wait, and mutual anticipation might make it better. The safest of all sexual behaviors, as many religious and ethical systems teach, is abstinence. The only preventive material a person needs is that wonder drug, "self-control." Don't leave home without it.

After the informed, thoughtful, and well-controlled brain is engaged, there may be no need for the "latex reflex." One way to give the brain—and the developing personal relationship—more time is for the client to say something like, "We really don't know each other very well. Let's take a few more occasions to get to know each other better." Clients will then have gained time to change their minds or realize that they may not be ready for sex with the other person. The bottom line: if a person waits, the risk of acquiring an STI or getting pregnant is zero.

If an informed brain that is conscious of the future and in control has postponed for more thought and then still decides to proceed with intimacy, and the social environment enables intimacy to take place, the following measures can be used to considerably reduce risk, but they will not totally eliminate it.

Counselors should encourage clients to:

1. Develop enough mutual openness to discuss the potential partner's STI status. Determine how long ago each party was tested for STIs. Ask about any post-test exposures.

2. Consider engaging in intimacy without penetration. This can be a fully satisfying experience and learning to do it well can, in itself, be fun.

3. Unobtrusively examine the partner around the genital area, looking for any rashes, ulceration, pimples, sores, or warts that may reflect the presence of syphilis, chancroid, herpes (a virus that keeps recurring and is spread by skin-to-skin contact), or genital warts (condylomata acuminata) caused by human papilloma virus (HPV). If some of these skin lesions are not covered by a latex condom and come in contact with uncovered skin they can infect the other partner. This is, of course, a signal that the person so marked has one or more STIs and probably has failed to receive adequate treatment. There is also major risk of oral infection if the mouth contacts such sores. Be aware, however, that a prospective partner already may be seriously infected and yet not show any obvious signs. Chlamydia rarely shows external signs, and most other STIs have extended periods without signs or symptoms including AIDS, syphilis, gonorrhea, human papilloma virus (HPV), and others, including trichomoniasis, which is the most common of all STIs in many areas.

4. Be alert (by looking, touching, asking) for any STI signs that form the basis for the "syndrome approach" to treatment, especially:

  - abnormal discharge from the vagina or penis, especially if it has an atypical color or smell;

  - irritation or pain while urinating (either gender);

  - pain, tenderness, or swelling of the scrotum;

  - lower abdominal tenderness or pain (either gender);

  - tender or swollen lymph glands in the groin; and skin sores or ulcers (as described in the third bullet above).

  If signs and symptoms such as those mentioned in items 3 and 4 are found, the observer should urge the prospective partner to go for diagnosis and treatment, both for his/her own sake and for the sake of others. The person learning about these symptoms should not proceed with intimate contact until antibiotic treatment is completed. Home remedies and folk medicines do not get rid of sexual infections!

5. Use a barrier protection (condom) or avoid contact if he or she has mouth sores or a tendency to bleeding gums, because a person can be infected by having oral contact with a partner's infected skin, sexual organs, or fluids from them.

6. Use latex condoms or similar fluid-tight barriers correctly (health workers can explain this) every time and throughout the exposure. This protects a person from invisible infections and from incubating infections that the partner may not even know about, but which are nevertheless catching. They are the best protection, even if one makes an error in selecting a partner.

7. Before having unprotected/risky sex with anyone, go together to an STI clinic for laboratory testing to make sure you are both free of infection. Both partners' safety will continue as long as they are mutually monogamous.

## PRIMARY PREVENTION

The goal of primary STI prevention is to keep infections from ever happening. Primary prevention must be taught not only to persons already sexually active, but also to those who expect to become sexually active. The public must be reached respectfully, but effectively, with health preserving STI messages. Keep in mind that fear-inducing communications have been shown to be ineffective

312

in preventing STIs. They probably scare as many people away from clinical care as the number scared away from sexual behavior.

Mass media information about STIs sets the agenda for people's conversations. But the mass media in many places send the wrong messages: that sexual urges usually turn into sexual behavior, that "everybody is doing it" casually, without protection, uncontrollably. The media implies a standard for usual behaviors upon which persons "new to the scene" can set their expectations. The first goal is to change the portrayal of sexuality in films, television, and the print media, and to get the mass media to be socially responsible and health-promoting. However, even if this can be achieved, media messages are unlikely to change people already engaging in unsafe habits. That is most effectively achieved in personal discussions among peers, between partners, or with a counselor.

> *The goal of primary prevention of sexually transmitted infections is to keep infections from ever happening. Primary prevention must be taught to persons who are already sexually active, but also to those who expect to become sexually active.*

Primary prevention of STIs has never received adequate attention at the national level, perhaps worldwide. Recently, well-conducted primary prevention efforts have worked wonders in reducing the incidence and prevalence of scores of diseases and disorders. Could the traditional impotence of primary STI prevention programs be responsible for some—maybe even for most—of the 250,000,000 new cases in the world each year?

On the 20th century's medical bookshelf dealing with STIs, most publications do not touch on primary prevention. Most seek only to treat active STIs and teach early self-referral for repeated treatment. Is this public health specialty ready to try out the established strategies using psychological methods for behavior change in clinical trials?

## SECONDARY PREVENTION

Secondary prevention of STIs also is within the scope of this Handbook, because secondary prevention in one partner can (and should) be primary prevention for the other. There are urgent reasons for the prompt identification and effective treatment of STIs:

- If untreated or untreatable (as is the case of sexual viruses), infections easily spread to other persons through sexual contact.

- If untreated or untreatable, the agents can multiply and spread to other organs within the patient, often causing serious damage. *Chlamydia trachomata* has no symptoms in its early stages in more than half of infected men and women. Only later does it produce symptomatic inflammation. It may cause infertility or ectopic pregnancy in women. Syphilis, now becoming epidemic again in some areas, can result in damage to many organs including the brain, and can cause death if not adequately treated.

- Untreated STIs can damage the mucous membranes and the skin near their portals of entry—the genitals, mouth, or anus. This damage opens the system to other infectious agents, particularly HIV. Thus, prompt STI treatment is an important aspect of preventing AIDS, as well as a host of other STIs.

- Gonorrhea infection in pregnancy is often transmitted to the baby's eyes during vaginal birth. This infection can lead to blindness if not treated promptly.

Counseling, advising, and motivating the patient being treated for a current STI has five personal goals. The counselor's task is to enlist the patient in sharing responsibility to achieve them:

1. Get the infection cured;

2. Don't spread this infection, or any other STI;

3. Help your partners get treatment;

4. Come back to the clinic to make sure your infection was cured;

5. Stay cured—prevent another infection—by engaging only in safer sex.

If a woman is pregnant or expecting to become so, she has a sixth goal—protecting her baby.

### SUGGESTIONS FOR STI COUNSELORS

Experienced STI workers will realize that the above goals for changing behaviors represent an overly idealistic scenario for both primary and secondary prevention. Clearly, only parts of the total inquiry and parts of the recommendations can be covered in a single meeting, especially if the client/patient is given adequate time to discuss the problems and become part of their solution. Clients who are not adequately helped the first time will be back again and again, with infections and reinfections. At a return appointment it is better to take more time than is available—more time, in fact, than the counselor can or should—to make that "personal connection," repeat messages, praise progress, or try new approaches. In the long run it is more cost-effective to take an extra hour or two with a reinfected patient, particularly if he or she has new contacts and is infecting others. Remember, the patient's knowledge is not the goal—behavior change is!

Counselors constantly practice the "art of the possible." They negotiate the steps that clients reasonably can do, given their mental, emotional, and circumstantial limitations. For example, a client should not be asked to stop all intercourse. The client will hear only enough of that to decide that you are unrealistic. A reduction in the number of partners could be negotiated, however. Start with the full partner list and negotiate how the client can eliminate some persons and not add new ones. Even commercial sex workers might learn to be more restrictive, by insisting on practicing only safer sex, or by avoiding high risk situations, such as working with belligerent or drugged clients. These are examples of risk behavior negotiations. Follow this by an agreement between client and counselor—a verbal contract—as to what the client promises to do. Then set an appointment in a week or two for him or her to come back, give a progress report, be checked for symptoms, and perhaps get an updated behavioral prescription. Clients should be welcomed to return to the same counselor for support. There must be good reasons to return, especially without a reinfection!

> *In the long run it is more cost-effective to take an extra hour or two with a reinfected patient, particularly if he or she has new contacts and is infecting others. The patient's knowledge is not the goal—behavior change is!*

Behavior change need not be limited to one client at a time. Create opportunities to work with groups, such as military units with above average infection rates, wives who have been infected by husbands who use commercial sex workers, commercial sex workers in a given geographic area, groups of adolescents or students in school dormitories. In all these situations, group interactions, the sharing of problems and solutions, and the support of similar people, can be captured and directed toward self-empowerment, and from that toward behavior change. Several theoretic models of behavior change are now being field tested with encouraging results (Fisher et al., 1996; Kalichman et al., 1999). The group process, guided by a knowledgeable counselor, usually has more enduring persuasive power than a counselor working with individual clients all week long (also see Fishbein, 1998 and Kamb et al., 1998). **(Review the many points in Chapter 12 and see how they can be applied to STI prevention.)**

### RESTRUCTURING STI OUTREACH

New strategies for delivering STI services have been urged over the past decade. Traditionally, STI services have been delivered in separate clinics devoted to this category of disease. Typically, these clinics have been located in old run-down buildings in dangerous parts of the big city. Anyone seeing a patient walking in such an area might suspect where he or she was going and why. The separateness and isolation of STI clinics hints to the insightful observer that at some unconscious level health officials may have suspected that STIs could be spread to other patients with more "acceptable" problems through the waiting room. Perhaps they seek to quarantine the shame they impute to STDs. Such categorical clinics miss seeing the greater majority of persons who need their care, largely because they don't know they are infected.

The new approach recommended by WHO and other health organizations and groups is to incorporate STI screening and treatment into general health services, such as family medicine, obstetrics (for prenatal care), adolescent clinics, occupational health, and hospital admissions routines.

The benefits are clear:

- Sharing clinic and laboratory facilities and staff cuts costs.

- Treating STI patients like all seekers for other health care destigmatizes their plight.

- Treating patients as whole persons, possibly having multiple health care needs, not just as a "case of disease X."

- Reaching people who come to the clinic for other reasons, which presents great opportunities for screening. Prenatal screening for women facilitates primary prevention for neonates.

- And it is convenient, convenient, convenient. **(Also see Chapter 12.)**

### NEWER STRATEGIES FOR EFFICIENT TREATMENT

The same new approaches to diagnosis and treatment of STIs are being promoted by many international agencies. For example, since many STI patients come to a facility only once for diagnosis, never returning for treatment or follow-up, the strategy is to accomplish as much treatment as soon as possible, even in the first visit. This same new approach works well in settings with limited diagnostic capabilities (some clinics may not even have a microscope) and where there is a shortage of STI-trained physicians.

This new clinical system is called the "syndrome approach." Specific combinations of STI symptoms follow infection with one or more pathogens. These easily distinguished combinations are used to identify an appropriate treatment plan, which is provided to the patient immediately. The combinations include the following:

- vaginal discharge in women,

- urethral discharge in men,

- genital ulcer disease in men and women,

- swollen scrotum,

- certain lower abdominal pain in women (for pelvic inflammatory disease), and

- swelling of inguinal lymph nodes (bubos).

The syndrome approach is more efficient for the patient, stops transmission of the pathogen by the patient without waiting an additional week, and is cheaper for the clinic in the longer term. The separate stage of confirming the diagnosis by laboratory results is omitted. This omission results in treating some patients with more drugs than they actually need at that time, but it also eliminates problems of laboratory error and well suits those many patients with multiple concurrent infections. The syndrome approach also permits trained health workers who are not physicians, as well as physicians not trained in STIs, to follow flow charts leading from presenting symptoms, to history of present episode, to physical examination, to administering the most appropriate drugs.

Textbooks and guidebooks for implementing this system are available, and will soon be further translated and more widely distributed. The following were available at the writing of the Handbook, and seem to be comprehensive.

- *WHO STD Case Management Workbook.* Geneva, 1999–2000.

- *Control of Sexually Transmitted Diseases.* Edited by G. Dallabetta, M. Laga, P. Lampty. Arlington, VA (USA): AIDSCAP, Family Health International, Undated (late 1990s).

- *Practical Case Management of Common STD Syndromes.* A.R. Brathwaite for the Primary Health Care Centers. Kingston, Jamaica: Ministry of Health, 1993.

> *Preventing and treating alcohol abuse may go forward more effectively if the condition is not classified either as a moral weakness or a psychiatric problem, but instead as a separate category of concern.*

## ALCOHOL USE

Alcohol use and abuse directly account for a relatively smaller number of deaths than other mega-risk factors. However, many deaths involving alcohol are coded as trauma in the workplace, highway deaths, drownings, liver cirrhosis, homicide, and other outcomes. In addition, alcohol ranks as the second largest cause of disability in industrialized areas, and the fourth largest disabler in the developing world.

Alcohol is a major disabler of local economies because it mostly attacks working age persons. In addition, it destabilizes their families, thus damaging communities. The economic costs of lost production; accidents on the job, on roadways, and at home; medical care for acute episodes and chronic alcohol diseases, all add up to a huge burden.

Alcohol behavior is culturally determined, as is the priority accorded for its prevention and treatment. Ethical and religious issues create conflicts and stigma. Perhaps preventing it and treating it will go forward more effectively if the condition is not classified either as a moral weakness or a psychiatric problem, but instead as a separate category of concern, which the community should begin addressing now for the benefit of the next generation. **(Issues regarding the contributing causes to alcohol abuse, screening for overuse, and possible preventive interventions are presented in the section "Major Problems at Ages 15–24 Years" in Chapter 4 and in the section on "Consumption of Alcohol" in Chapter 5, and the section "Alcohol Abuse and Dependence" in Chapter 7.)**

## HYPERTENSION

Elevated blood pressure is almost always free of unpleasant symptoms. It remains a secret to those who have it. Nevertheless, it causes enough heart disease and cerebrovascular crises to be ranked as the second leading force of death in industrialized nations and third in developing areas (following only hunger and lack of sanitation). See Table 13.1.

Hypertension contributes to several forms of cardiovascular disease, including ischemic, pulmonary, hypertensive, and congestive heart failure. **(The definition of hypertension, its causes, and ways to treat it are discussed more fully in the section "Hypertension and Hypertensive Heart Disease" in Chapter 8.)** Of great potential for developing areas are the five nonpharmacologic behavior changes, each of which can help lower blood pressure to some extent, thus helping to prevent serious disease. Again, the population intervention approach applies. This means that lowering the average blood pressure in a population of adults will usually save more lives than treating all the hypertensives.

## OCCUPATIONAL HEALTH HAZARDS

Occupational health is declining in the world's developing countries. This comes at a time of increasing unemployment and factory closings in many places. Occupational exposures are one remediable cause of disability among 15 to 64 year olds, the economically critical age group.

Attracted by the lure of cash-paying jobs in the big cities and the hopes for a higher standard of living that such cash can buy, men migrate away from subsistence farming to magnet urban centers, only part of the time bringing their families along. The supply of workers is far greater that the supply of jobs, however, which leaves millions unemployed or underemployed. It was estimated that in Central and South America alone there were 10 million unemployed workers in 1990 and 78 million more working only part-time (PAHO, 1994). Furthermore, economic depression and monetary inflation in the 1980s and 1990s have lowered current wages in many nations to equal only 66% of the buying power the same amount of money had in 1980. In effect, wages have gone down for most workers (PAHO, 1994). These occupational problems affect both men and women.

> *In the developing nations of the Americas alone, there are an estimated 95 million workdays lost to occupational injuries and illnesses each year.*

In most countries at early stages of development, workplace health and safety are generally not controlled by the government or by the industries themselves. At first glance this might seem to lead to greater profit for management. But considering the estimated 95 million workdays lost to occupational injuries and illnesses each year in the developing nations of the Americas alone, this may not be true (PAHO, 1994). In addition, mortality rates for work-related accidents—even considering the fact that they are underreported in most developing countries—already slightly exceed the rates in developed countries, which have safety standards.

The leading causes for this damage to people and productivity are:

- **Chemicals.** These include carbon disulfide, vinyl chloride, benzene, arsenic compounds, organophosphates, pesticides, fumes from solvents, fumes from coal and gas refineries, smoke from cigarettes, soot, tars, and many others.

- **Metals.** Metals can be free or in unstable compounds. The most toxic include lead, chromium, mercury, cadmium, beryllium, nickel, and fumes from smelters. Population exposure to lead may be the most widespread of these.

- **Particulates floating in the air.** These can include asbestos, dust from cotton and other fibers, coal, silica, lime, agricultural dusts, particulates in smoke, smog, and chemical spraying.

- **Gases.** These include carbon monoxide from incomplete burning or fumes from industrial processing such as refining, which give off hydrogen sulfide, sulphur dioxide, and fluorocarbons.

319

- **Ionizing radiation.** Such ionizing radiation may come from inadequately shielded nuclear fuels and wastes, and from fabrication of products containing radionuclides. Even inadequately shielded X-ray equipment can be a danger.

- **Machinery.** This is especially true when equipment is operated by unskilled hands, lacks proper protection, or lacks proper maintenance. Of particular danger are trucks; power lifts; road-building equipment; cutting, stamping, drilling machines; farm machinery that cuts or chops; and mining equipment.

- **Acute trauma.** This can be caused by falling objects or when workers fall, especially in construction trades, as well as impacts from moving objects, heat, or steam. Lifting heavy objects without proper training or assistance is another factor.

- **Repetitive motion injuries.** These have emerged from work on assembly-line machinery and at computer terminals. They occur when the same relatively small movements are made thousands of times in a day. Proper ergonomic design for the task and support for affected body parts can relieve much of this.

- **Impact vibration and excessive noise.** Repetitive impact causes musculoskeletal problems; intense noise causes permanent deafness. Working with hand-held mining and highway construction machines or near airplanes and loud machinery are examples. Proper body cushioning and ear protection can help. Child and adolescent workers are more susceptible than adults to all these insults. **(Also see the section "Nurturing the Seeds of a Healthy Future" in Chapter 4.)**

- **Violence**. The workplace is a social setting, and as such, interpersonal and work stresses often are at play. In recent years, the leading cause of death for women while at work in the United States has been homicide. Acts of assault are generally not recorded, but no doubt are a major issue throughout both developed and developing countries. **(Also see the section "Suicide and Violence" in Chapter 11.)**

With such a varied list of dangers, where should initial efforts be focused to improve occupational health? Good spots to consider first are those activities and places that have the highest frequencies of medical care needs and days lost due to injury and illness (per 1,000 person-days of work). Two other ways of setting priorities for initial efforts are to target the hazards to which the greatest number of people are exposed, or to turn first to the hazards that are most easily correctable.

The list of "pathogens" and dangerous work above gives health workers dealing with occupational health and management (including family farmers) a checklist of ways to promote both healthy workers and healthy production. Only a handful of industries are responsible for an alarming share of occupational diseases and mortality. In most countries, the construction, mining, and metal producing industries are the most dangerous. Refining and dust-generating factories and mechanized farms also present dangers that can be lessened.

Workers hardest hit with occupational hazards appear to many to be the first generation exposed to each technological advance, be it mechanical, chemical, physical, ergonomic, or a new kind of process-chain whose side effects are not fully understood. Adequate job training of able and mature trainees, plus safety engineering for handling raw materials, machinery for processing, and end-products should greatly remediate occupational dangers. Regulations alone cannot achieve these goals without full affirmation at all levels of management that the workers are the living building blocks both of this industry and their community. They are not merely raw materials to be used up and replaced.

## PHYSICAL INACTIVITY/SEDENTARY LIFESTYLE

Industrialization and automation take much of the physical labor out of occupational work. This has several advantages—fewer people can accomplish more work in less time; skilled people can have longer careers, not shortened early by diminished strength. Populations in developing areas yearn for these advances to reduce the sweat of their brows.

In post-industrialized areas, however, the dark side of these advances is a growing population who remain sitting most of their waking hours. A person's body—even someone's psychological adjustment—deteriorates relatively quickly under such conditions. As discussed in Chapter 6, "The Older Years: 65 to 100," humans must either use all their capacities or lose them. Physical, mental, and social activity are vital to personal well being at every age.

Sedentary lifestyle ranks third as a risk for mortality and fifth among the precursors of disability in the post-industrialized world. It is much less frequent in countries at earlier stages of economic development. Calculations of the attributable risks for ischemic heart disease (IHD) in the United States in the 1980s found that physical inactivity made the single largest contribution to mortality. Sedentary people have an IHD risk much less than double that of actively working or exercising people (when other risks are controlled), whereas people who smoke or have high LDL cholesterol may each have triple or greater risk. The extremely high prevalence of "sedentarism," however, multiplies the individual relative risk into a community burden that is very large indeed. Thus, prevention at the community level, wherever the diseases fostered by inactivity constitute a problem, should make it a priority to increase daily physical activity. This means that enjoyable (not boring) activities that generate more rapid heart rate, deeper breathing, and muscle movement should be identified. Then, groups, times, and places for exercise should be organized. This may be accomplished without full-time staff and without new facilities, as evidenced by the millions of adults who gather in parks and public places in China's cities to practice Qi-gong each morning that weather permits. Other groups may pursue calisthenics, walking, or vigorous folk dancing. Exercise activities are more likely to be continued regularly if they convey a built-in sense of reward. Shared participation with others is one way to provide this.

---

**A FREQUENTLY PRESCRIBED EXERCISE PROGRAM**

- Participate in physical activities that involve all major muscle groups.
- Exert enough effort to increase the heart rate and the frequency and depth of breathing. Keep the workout at such a level that you are left with enough breath to speak easily. You should not experience pain, pressure, or heaviness in the chest during the workout.
- Make sessions last at least 30 minutes, and do them at least three days each week. The Institute of Medicine in the U.S.A. in 2002 increased its recommendation to one hour per day, five days per week. If this level of exercise represents a major change from a person's usual intensity or kind of exertion, he or she should first check with a health professional to make sure the workout is safe.

---

## LACK OF ESSENTIAL PRIMARY HEALTH SERVICES

The eight overarching risk forces discussed above—each of which causes multiple forms of disease, disability, and death—can be fought at the local and individual levels. But the last two—lack of essential primary health services and chronic endemic poverty—exert their destructive roles on a much larger stage that requires a national response.

The International Conference on Primary Health Care, cosponsored by WHO and UNICEF in 1978 in Alma Ata, USSR, defined essential primary health care to include eight components:

1. Health education on major health problems;

2. Control of local endemic disease;

3. Maternal and child health services, including family planning;

4. Immunizations against infectious diseases;

5. Clean water supply;

6. Sanitary disposal of waste;

7. Food and nutrition services; and

8. Treatment of common ailments, including the use of essential drugs.

Most of these have been dealt with in this Handbook as part of the chapters on specific age groups and the sections on diseases. But they have been discussed piecemeal, and primary health care as a whole is greater than the sum of these eight parts. It deserves fuller treatment.

The establishment and maintenance of primary health care (PHC) services entails the commitment of a nation, state, or province to the health of its population. Staff at PHC centers become health sentinels and advocates scattered throughout the geographic and social environment. The sentinel function involves reporting community needs and health problems upward through the political structure. The advocate function calls for putting people's health high on the priority lists of central decision-makers and citizens.

All eight primary health care components are vital, but two deserve added discussion—immunizations against infectious diseases and maternal and child health services.

## IMMUNIZATIONS AGAINST INFECTIOUS DISEASES

Worldwide, immunization programs have been among the most exciting success stories in public health. The greatly increased survival rates of children can be attributed in large part to the gradual conquest of childhood cluster diseases such as pertussis, poliomyelitis, diphtheria, measles, and tetanus. Recently, however, immunization efforts have become routine in many places, losing some of their past priority. As a result, there are many population pockets where immunization coverage has become frighteningly low. It is glamorous to fight an epidemic, but far wiser to prevent it, and PHC and child health programs must maintain surveillance on immunization coverage. Children in poor families and street children are often left out, for example. Remember, the success of an immunization program can be judged only by the completeness of its coverage.

*The success of an immunization program can be judged only by the completeness of its coverage. Children in poor families and street children, however, often are left out of immunization programs.*

## MATERNAL AND CHILD HEALTH SERVICES

Adequate prenatal care not only reduces infant mortality. More important economically, it reduces the number of mentally and physically impaired infants and children. The GBD Study estimated nearly 33 million healthy years of life lost (DALYs) in infants were due to conditions arising in the perinatal period. Maternal problems during pregnancy and delivery accounted for another 30 million disabled life years among women.

These losses are most concentrated in developing nations, and many causes lie behind such heavy losses. It would seem most appropriate to begin by providing PHC to women and children and allow that experience to identify the more prevalent biomedical causes. Second-stage programs can be designed accordingly. Childhood diarrheas are a major cause of death in children 1–4 years old. The same PHC outreach can teach mothers oral rehydration therapy and other basic skills for identifying and dealing with children's health problems before they become serious.

The focus of PHC should be kept on primary and secondary prevention of common health problems. It should not be allowed to drift into intensive and/or expensive care for terminal or infrequent diseases. Many of the most cost-effective of all health programs take place in PHC work (Bobadilla et al., 1994).

## POVERTY

No matter the level of organization one considers—continent, nation, province, community, or family—wherever there is a rank ordering from rich to middle class to poor, one also will find a parallel ordering from good to fair to poor health. While socioeconomic gradients predict almost every index of health, they manage to explain very few of them. In a nutshell, poverty is a basic force of risk for perhaps 90% of the most common diseases and disabilities in the world.

Much research has been done to see what must be changed to improve the lives of the poor, with solutions ranging from supplementing incomes, providing food, providing free or insured access to health care, and providing health information. All these measures have led to some health improvements in populations thus served. Rich and poor alike tend to improve in areas with comprehensive programs, but counter to expectations, the gaps between rich and poor in disease, disability, and premature death are not shrinking. In fact, they are widening in many places.

Obviously, the ideal solution would be to eliminate poverty. But this is a tall order. Many nations have waged a "War on Poverty" over the centuries. Battles have been won, but not the war. Most people equate poverty with a lack of money or goods, but that is the least toxic of its poisons. The circle of poverty includes poor health, low education, unskilled and insecure jobs, substandard housing, unsafe and disorganized neighborhoods, and social stigma and prejudice. And these lead to a sense of lacking a worthwhile future, lacking hope, and lacking power. Such feelings can become self-fulfilling prophecies.

Poverty is an "agent" for many diseases and can permeate every level of the environment. It invades the "host" by changing the assumptions, attitudes, expectations, behaviors, and lifestyles of communities, families, and individuals. It affects the community's wealthier strata with apathy—the morphine of social structure—generating a numbness to the pain of others. When any thought is given to the sickness and disability of the poor, rationalizations come quickly. "The poor should help themselves." "The plight of the poor is the responsibility of some government agency or a private sector organization." "Poverty has always existed."

> *Most people equate poverty with a lack of money or goods, but that is the least toxic of its poisons. The circle of poverty includes poor health, low education, unskilled and insecure jobs, substandard housing, unsafe and disorganized neighborhoods, and social stigma and prejudice.*

Poverty requires more than money to cure. Community development work can help reverse this spiral. **(Also see the section "Mobilizing the Community" in Chapter 12.)** Other keys include education, available jobs, adequate housing, community safety, health-building, and overcoming helplessness and hopelessness. Upward social mobility has been occurring in industrialized countries throughout the 20th century. It tends to occur selectively, however, leaving behind the people with the worst health status.

In the absence of an ideal solution for eliminating poverty, health planners and epidemiologists may do well to find out which environmental and behavioral elements of poverty are vectors of disease and disability and under which circumstances of poverty health is harmed. Indeed, many of these mechanisms have already been discussed earlier in this Handbook. Simple low-technology behavioral changes that advance biologic and behavioral health are a basic wedge to break the cycle of poverty.

## IS INCOME INEQUALITY AN INDEPENDENT RISK FACTOR?

Social epidemiology research has established that substantial income inequality within a state or nation also is a strong predictor of overall morbidity and mortality. Income inequality can be measured by several indexes. The "Robin Hood Index" arranges households by deciles of income and sums the excess over 10% of income that all "richer" deciles receive. Higher indexes reflect more severe poverty at lower deciles of the population. Another index uses the aggregate income received by the 50% of households with lowest income for each state or unit of study. (These population indexes are relatively easy to estimate, even if only part of the population is enumerated. Details for calculation are presented in the sources cited for this section.)

Several studies report that income inequality is more strongly related to total population death rates than is the absolute level of poverty in the area. Most such studies are based on data from industrialized nations, but the same principles have now been found to apply elsewhere. Income inequality remains a potent predictor of total population mortality, even after adjusted for the percentage of households below a specific poverty level. In the U.S.A., a mere 1% increase in the inequality index was associated with an increase in mortality of 21.7 deaths per 100,000 in the general population. A similar but smaller gradient was reported in England. The effect on those persons actually living in poverty was much greater (Wilkinson, 1996).

In studies conducted in the United States, the correlation of income inequality with mortality was quite similar for African-Americans (r=0.39) and for other, mostly white, citizens (r=0.46). When controlled for level of poverty, the lethal power of income disparity was increased more in African-Americans than in others, however. Another analysis of the same data set by a different team using a wider array of indicators showed a correlation between income inequality and mortality of r=0.62. This broader study also revealed that income disparity correlated with all of the indicators of health and social pathology shown in Table 13.2.

This set of sociomedical correlates sketches an array of environments within industrialized countries, and they hold true anywhere there is a great economic di-

**TABLE 13.2.** Correlation of income disparity with health and social pathology indicators.

| Indicator | r = |
|---|---|
| Low birthweight | 0.65 |
| Homicide rate | 0.74 |
| Violent crime | 0.70 |
| Medical expenditures (log per capita) | 0.67 |
| Police costs (per capita) | 0.38 |
| Education expenditure (as % of government budget) | −0.32 |
| Prisoners (% in population) | 0.44 |
| Current smokers (%) | 0.35 |
| Receiving governmental financial aid (%) | 0.69 |
| Without health insurance (%) | 0.45 |
| Reading ability (4th grade) | −0.58 |
| Math ability | −0.64 |
| No high school education | 0.71 |

*Source:* Selected from Kaplan et al., 1996.

vide between the wealthy and the lowest 30% to 50% of the population. One environment would be where the population is more homogeneous in income and where more babies are born healthy, more people live longer, there is less violent crime, fewer murders, fewer people in prison, fewer families receiving financial assistance, more people having health insurance, more youth continuing into secondary education, and more children with age-appropriate reading and mathematical skills by the ages of 8 and 9 years. An apt definition of a healthy community, indeed!

On the other hand, there are social environments that have similar average levels of financial assets, but a much greater variability around those averages. They have great financial disparities across families, leading many to have great despair. While the cost of shortened life expectancy may be paid only by some people, the costs of medical care, police protection, and early school dropout rates are paid by everyone. Proportionally more money is spent for prisons and less for schools by these governments. The milieu of social pathologies displayed in the prior table automatically accompanies these social environments (Kaplan et al., 1996).

Although mortality data are more available and less debatable than illness data, the same processes work to generate excesses of acute and chronic non-fatal disease and disability. International studies of disability-adjusted life years (DALYs) show a strong gradient, with poorer nations having more disease and disability per 1,000 population. Some of the associations described suggest possible pathways of pathogenesis. Inequality (according to studies conducted in the U.S.A.) has its greatest impact on the following diagnostic categories: homicide, total mortality, infant mortality, ischemic heart disease, tuberculosis, infectious diseases (in total), hypertensive diseases, and some cancers. And all these are preventable and/or curable diseases. In these environments, apparently, the higher per capita expenditures on medical care are not being spent as appropriately as they could be—that is, on prevention. In other climates and cultures other pathologies may head the list.

Further hints as to possible directions for "upstream intervention" have come from linking the concept of "social capital" to income disparity research. Social capital is a property of a community, state, or province (an ecologic variable) that reflects the level of cooperation, cohesion, shared values, behavioral norms, civic participation, concern for mutual benefit, and trust in the community and in outsiders. In a given community, social capital is created, or diminished, as a by-product of social relationships. Everyone in the community shares in the level of social capital. It permeates through the psychosocial, ideological, and even the physical environment.

The hypothesis is that when these levels break down or remain low, people become frustrated, resentful, fearful, more isolated, and take on a siege mentality—they, their family, and their friends come first, everyone else comes last. This mindset manifests itself more acutely at the highest and lowest extremes of the socioeconomic ladder.

Kawachi and colleagues (1997) have linked income inequality with mortality, and both of these to social capital.[1] This team estimated social capital in states in the United States through four indicators: three involved social survey questions about other people's lack of fairness, lack of trustworthiness, and lack of helpfulness; the fourth was the average number of memberships in groups and organizations in the respondent population, as a way to reflect the amount of community engagement. The proportion of people who responded to the three questions stating that other people were unfair, unhelpful, and untrustworthy all correlated very highly with a given state's age-adjusted mortality (r from 0.71 to 0.79). This was greater than the correlations of income inequality and percentage of households below the United States poverty threshold to mortality (r –0.65 and r –0.57, respectively). And when a path model was calculated, it was shown that most of the effect of income inequality on mortality was explained by low social capital. This implies that relative poverty—the display of wealth as viewed by the "have nots"—breaks down morale, erodes the sense that the community is treating people fairly, and dissolves the belief that by hard work one can achieve material success. It sets barriers between groups.

## IMPLICATIONS FOR SOCIAL POLICY

If governments work to increase social participation, fairness, and helpfulness, and help people to increase their trust in others and in the government, will they succeed? If they do, will it improve health? Is reducing income extremes the easiest way to advance health? Or is the solution to reduce social problems associated with striking inequality? These are all unanswered questions. Correlations don't necessarily mean causation. It should be kept in mind that some social experiments have minimal downside risks and just might pay off in more ways than appears on face value.

Governments could certainly respond as follows:

• Increase the proportion of school-age children who attend school regularly.

• Increase the effectiveness of teaching and learning throughout the school system, especially in the first six grades (ages 6–12 years).

---

[1] Again, data from United States states were used. Unfortunately, this is not a replication of findings, but it does expand the range of inferences.

BUILDING BETTER HEALTH

- Increase, on a yearly basis, the number of school years that the majority of children and youth complete, until 90% have advanced literacy, social competence, and job skills adequate for the new century.

- Redistribute health care budgets better to serve the basic needs of the whole population (see Bobadilla, 1994).

- Encourage community members to join associations, civic and religious groups, parent-teacher organizations at schools, and informal mutual support groups. This is especially important in low-income areas as part of community development. Moreover, it has a direct effect on health program participation. **(Also see sections "Mobilizing the Community" and "Spreading New Health Behaviors through the Community" in Chapter 12.)** Besides, most higher income people already belong to multiple organizations and groups.

- Encourage fairness in housing by subsidizing new housing for low-income families, setting health and safety standards for rental housing, and imposing rent ceilings on below-standard units until they are improved.

- Use taxation systems that tend to reduce inequalities, such as progressive rate income taxes, where wealthier persons pay a higher percentage on their earnings than persons at or below the median. Sales taxes on purchases of daily needs should be kept low. They cost low-income people a higher percentage of their earnings than they cost the wealthy. Luxury taxes (such as on jewelry, luxury cars, or imported non-essentials) also serve as a good source of state income. If property taxes provide a "homestead allowance" to shelter lower-price homes and a surtax on high-priced luxury properties, further leveling will be achieved.

- Levy "sin taxes" on alcohol and tobacco. Revenues can help support health programs.

- Provide universal easy access to primary health care and to cost-effective screening and preventive interventions to help break the spiral of poor health and social deprivation.

And what about income redistribution to achieve greater equality? Is it politically possible? Is it necessary? Several of the studies on income disparity and poor health come from the United States, which has a more extreme income disparity than most nations. Nevertheless, the principal findings are supported in multination studies.

Actually, graphs showing the relation of income disparity to excess mortality (among states in the United States) suggest that only limited reductions in the ex-

> *Wherever there are pockets of unusually deep poverty in cities or countryside, health officials can be sure that high sickness and death rates dwell there also. There is an uncanny geographic clustering of biological, psychological, social, and economic pathologies in the same neighborhoods.*

tremity of inequality provide considerable health benefit. All seven of the states with highest age-adjusted mortality had income inequalities such that the poorest 50% of the population received less than 21% of the total household income for the population. Under perfect equality, 50% of the households would receive 50% of the income. Inferences from this single U.S. study are admittedly shaky, and may not apply elsewhere, but temporarily we might proffer the hypothesis that raising the income share of the least well-off half of the population to at least 25% of the population total, would show positive social, psychological, and biological health effects in the whole population, as part of a "preventive package" of services.

More practically stated, wherever traveling about through cities and countryside shows pockets of unusually deep poverty, health officials can be sure that high sickness and death rates dwell there also. There is an uncanny geographic clustering of biological, psychological, social, and economic pathologies in the same neighborhoods. The areas with the highest infant mortality and highest cardiovascular death rates before age 65 years, usually also have high rates of destructive fires, homicide, social service needs, children not attending school, and substandard housing (Jenkins et al., 1977). No fancy studies are needed. The only necessary step is to scan the most recent scientific literature for new proven ways to reduce the health inequities—and to launch the interventions.

# PART V.
# THE AUTHOR'S
# EPILOGUE

# 14. Is Good Health Achievable and Sustainable?

## CONFRONTING BASIC DECISIONS

Every day we live, we come to a crossroad—the crossroad between past and future. The present is only a crowded intersection. Shall we continue onward in our habitual ways of thinking, expecting, and doing? Or, shall we risk making a change? Families, communities, professional groups, and organizations encounter crossroads every day, too. They, like us, are usually too busy keeping on doing what they have always done, and do not look around to see the many possibilities for more rewarding futures.

## CAN THE WORLD, MY COMMUNITY, OR MY FAMILY ACHIEVE BETTER HEALTH?

This Handbook presents many possibilities. In general, these are steps that can advance health without expensive equipment or supplies. Moreover, these steps can be taken by people at all levels of education, at all ages, and in most social circumstances.

Our answer, then, is: "Yes, the world can achieve better health—provided that enough people see the vision." It will happen when enough individuals and groups keep performing the simple tasks required.

## SHOULD WE WAIT FOR NEW DISCOVERIES IN MEDICAL SCIENCES? NEW "MAGIC BULLET" VACCINES?

No. Today we can take many giant steps toward reducing disease, disability, and death based on past discoveries and existing breakthroughs in the health sciences. We already know how to prevent many diseases and injuries and how to drastically reduce the incidence of most others. These preventive technologies already have been proven successful, albeit mostly in economically developed countries. Now, they must be applied on a much broader scale, and adapted to different cultures and geographies.

The history of smallpox control is instructive. Edward Jenner developed the first successful smallpox vaccine in 1796. Improved vaccines were developed in the 19th century, but international epidemics continued. Finally, after hundreds of millions of vaccinations were administered in the 20th century, the vision of possibly eradicating smallpox broke into world thinking. Eradication was achieved in 1977. Remember, however, that smallpox eradication happened only after:

- Enough people believed eradication was possible—they had the "vision."

- Agencies organized surveillance and immunization outreach programs.

- Agencies obtained the required human and financial resources for these programs.

- Agencies diligently executed the programs, readjusting plans and operations to fit "hard to reach" subpopulations, until the job was completed.

We contend that these same four steps are required to conquer other diseases. Poliomyelitis already has been eradicated from the Western Hemisphere. Most health problems, however, are not susceptible to eradication. This limitation holds for infectious diseases whose agents have multiple reservoirs and can survive outside living hosts for long periods. It also applies to chronic degenerative diseases and those caused by common toxins, malnutrition, behavioral and mental disorders, and "external causes."

The time-window of inertia lasted nearly 180 years for smallpox (1796–1977), but it can be as short as a decade for some of the major health problems discussed in this Handbook. The health establishment and community leadership should recognize that the required technology is available—although not yet widely enough known. The same steps listed above are the key to progress now. They can be restated for non-eradicable health problems, as follows:

- Enough people must believe change and progress are possible—and valuable!

- Enough local programs must be conducted and evaluated to learn how to intervene effectively. (This may be as simple as the "Back to Sleep" program in the section "From Birth to 4 Years Old" in Chapter 3.)

- Sufficient human and monetary resources are harnessed to do the job on a larger scale.

- Programs are executed diligently, controlling resources, evaluating progress, and readjusting design and operations to fit the subcultures encountered. **(Also see the section "Spreading New Health Behaviors through the Community" in Chapter 12.)**

Now we must move ahead with the tools that are available. Waiting for new breakthroughs in the biomedical sciences or miracle vaccines will only paralyze progress. The people and nations most in need of such "magic bullets" have rarely been able to afford them, because such high-technology advances cost many millions of dollars to develop. Commercial science laboratories usually focus on those problems whose solution promises high monetary rewards. (*The Economist,* 14 August 1999) cites "Doctors without Borders" ("Médecins Sans Frontières") reporting having counted 1,223 new pharmaceutical compounds placed on the medical market between 1975 and 1997. Only 11 of these were for tropical diseases. The communities and patients suffering from such diseases generally cannot raise enough money to pay for the production of drugs for mass epidemics, nor for the high costs invested in all the unsuccessful compounds that were tested en route to finding the best ones. The trickle-down of expensive high technology is exceedingly slow. And when it arrives, it may not be locally relevant.

## WHAT ARE THE HEALTH GOALS IMPLIED IN THIS HANDBOOK? WHAT MIGHT BE THE HANDBOOK'S MISSION STATEMENT?

Is it to mount as many of the suggested intervention programs that a state or community can? Is it to prevent as many deaths as possible?

No, the goals here are much more modest. The Handbook's basic mission is to inform and stimulate persons who value health and value others, and the organizations with which they are involved, to engage in the following:

- to prevent disease, disability, and premature death as early as possible;

- to do this as inexpensively and effectively as possible;

- to apply techniques and methods that are already proven and sustainable; and

- to select conditions to prevent (and subpopulations to reach) so as to provide the greatest benefit for the greatest proportion of the population as a whole.

As it happens, as we cross into the 21st century, reaching for these health goals will involve generating behavioral and social changes, most of all.

## DECIDING BETWEEN PREVENTION AND ADVANCED TREATMENT

In an ideal world, every nation would be able to find sufficient resources to carry out primary, secondary, and tertiary medical care, as well as all levels of prevention. In the real world, however, most nations have—and others claim to have—a severe shortage of resources for health services. In many Central American and South American nations, expenditures for health care (in inflation-adjusted currency units) actually declined during the economic depression between 1980 and 1990. This may well have happened elsewhere in the world, but data were not available to us from other Regions.

When resources are scarce, difficult decisions must be made. Clinical medicine puts the individual patient's welfare first. But what if that perspective hurts the community as a whole? Community medicine and public health put the health and functioning of the community first. This might include economic considerations, such as giving priority to health protection and promotion for workers and parents of younger children. A healthy workforce can generate the revenues to fund expansion of health care to the entire age range. Parents who are mentally and physically healthy can provide careful (i.e., full of care) common-sense parenting to reduce the frequency and severity of childhood illnesses and injuries, and the costs of their medical care.

In contrast, hospital care of advanced (especially, incurable or terminal) cases spends too much money on too few people, and gives little economic benefit to the community and nation. Of course, it seems to be the only humane thing to do. But, it must be recognized that the resources spent on one advanced case may mean the loss of primary preventive efforts, which might have kept dozens of healthy people from losing their health and becoming economically dependent. Phillips and colleagues estimate that in more affluent countries it costs US $50,000 on average to treat advanced cancer per healthy year of life saved. In contrast, providing pain relief for advanced cancer patients costs between US $100 and US $300 per year. Preventive care contrasts are even greater, with antibiotic treatment of tuberculosis costing US $5 to US $7 per year of healthy life saved (DALY). The Expanded Program on Immunization costs only US $12 to US $30, and treatment of sexually transmitted infections costs US $10 to US $25 per DALY saved. That is a minimum of 2,000 times more cost-effective than intensive cancer treatment, and 480 times more cost-effective than modern anti-viral treatments for AIDS at current prices (Phillips et al., 1992; Murray and Lopez, 1994).

Which, then, is the more humane investment of limited health funding?

## HOW CAN WE DO BOTH: PREVENT AND TREAT?

In theory, if prevention works there will be fewer cases of disease to treat, and medical costs would hopefully decline. But, preventive efforts must reach out to thousands of people because, in most situations, health science cannot predict which few will encounter the "pathogen," be it the measles virus or an automobile that is out of control.

Suppose it costs $1 apiece to reach 1,000 people with a totally effective preventive program. Suppose the disease prevented ordinarily afflicts only 1% of the population (10 people), and each case costs $100 to treat successfully. One could argue that such preventive efforts cost as much as they gain—that they are of neutral value. Such a calculation leaves out the non-cash costs of pain and lost function, as well as the monetary costs of lost work. This can add up to several days or more per worker, resulting in lost productivity to the employers, and perhaps lost wages to the worker. So, even "cash-flow neutral" interventions are likely to be biopsychosocially valuable, once the larger equation is considered.

However, quite many preventive interventions have been demonstrated to create more cash benefits than they cost. Evaluations of many health promotion programs in the workplace show that they typically reduce the amount of illness absences, and both outpatient clinic and hospital costs. A summary of 28 separate studies showed that workplace health promotion usually saves the employers at least three times the money that the program costs. Typically, there is a lag of two to three years between the change in health habits and the reduction in onset of major diseases (reviewed in Fries et al., 1993).

Smoking cessation programs extend life, thus providing more years to accumulate medical costs. Nevertheless, the lifetime medical costs for continuing smokers accumulate so much faster in fewer years, that smoking cessation is cost-effective for the community, as well as for the individual. Therefore, invest in proven smoking prevention efforts.

## REDUCING COSTS OF EACH UNIT OF SERVICE RENDERED

Another way health care programs can reduce costs is by having diagnosis and treatment performed by fully qualified, rather than overqualified, professionals. It does not require a specialty-certified physician to deal with a common respiratory infection or uncomplicated diarrhea, or to do routine monitoring of hypertension or depression. Physicians' assistants, nurses, and other properly trained health workers can provide such care equally effectively.

Of course, brain surgery should be performed only by brain surgeons, often with diagnostic assistance from a certified neurologist. But not everyone with headaches needs to be treated by one of these specialists. There are validated flow diagrams that enable subdoctoral health professionals to screen 1,000 headache patients to identify the 50 to 100 who need further triage by a physician, who then checks thoroughly for possible need for neurological care.

Flow charts and decision-making algorithms have been developed for many symptom patterns, including sexually transmitted infections. **(See the section on "Unsafe Sex" in Chapter 13)**. If they were more widely used, both in industrialized and in developing nations, health professionals could be employed more efficiently, costs would be cut sharply, and more truly sick people could be processed and helped by the health system.

## INCREASING SELF-CARE AND REDUCING DEMAND ON FACILITIES AND PROFESSIONALS

The ultimate step in delegating medical decisions and care to less costly care-givers is to promote care within families and self-care. The general public should know more and do more to promote their own health. Consumer-oriented groups in post-industrialized nations have come forth with sayings such as: "Your health is too important to be left in the hands of others!"

The objective is to teach and motivate the general public:

• to know how to reduce risk factors for many conditions;

• to know how to care for the minor, self-limiting health problems of their families and themselves;

• to recognize, with a margin of safety, when professional evaluation and care is probably required; and

• to ask their health care givers at regular intervals whether any preventive care is timely—e.g., immunization, screening, or assistance with health habits.

The overall goal is to reduce unnecessary or trivial use of health services. Reductions of 7% to 17% have been reported by simple patient education programs (Fries et al., 1993).

## SETTING COST-EFFECTIVE PRIORITIES

In addition to reducing demand for health care, savings (both of healthy function and medical costs) can be achieved by wider use of some true preventive health bargains (see Bobadilla et al., 1994). Popular thinking says that a surgeon who charges US$ 2,000 for a given operation must do twice as good a job as one who charges US$ 1,000, or that the more a health program costs, the better it must be. In fact, the per capita costs of prevention programs have little relation to their economic and social benefits.

The ten following interventions are among the most cost-effective in developing and transitional countries per healthy-life-year preserved:

1. expanded programs of immunization for children (the six vaccines, plus hepatitis B vaccine and vitamin A);

2. iodine supplementation (only in iodine-deficient areas);

3. removal of intestinal parasites (by sanitation and drugs);

4. effective antibiotic treatment of tuberculosis and Hanson's disease;

5. prevention and control of HIV and other STIs;

6. effective tobacco control;

7. effective alcohol control;

8. family planning;

9. prenatal and delivery care; and

10. school health programs (including providing a nutritious meal where under-nutrition is common).

Other preventive programs may also deliver large local health bonuses at low costs, depending on the environment and prevalence of specific conditions, and ease of program delivery.

The "bottom line" is not to spend money on cost-ineffective prevention or treatment programs until more cost-effective interventions have been carried out. Note that the 10 most effective programs (in most places) are all low in technology and high in personal contact by caring health workers. Issues of equity also should enter into setting priorities (more comprehensive evaluations of more than 40 kinds of interventions are presented in the World Bank publication by Jamison and colleagues (1993).

## WHAT MIGHT THE FUTURE HOLD?

Long-range planning for advancing health must, of course, look to the future. Economists, health statisticians, and specialists in specific diseases have published many predictions for the first portion of the 21st century. The predictions come from mathematical models that combine different assumptions about future population growth, economic development, and national health programming. Inasmuch as there are multiple scenarios for each of these domains, the total of all likely combinations is overwhelming. Some scenarios assume past trends will continue into the future; others assume governments will be converted to pro-health policies. Longer predictions have more time for cumulative error than do short predictions.

## POPULATION AND INCOME PROJECTIONS

Table 14.1 presents world population growth by Regions, based on 1990 data and projected to the year 2020. For the first 20 years of the 21st century, population is expected to grow overall by 27.3%. Of particular concern are the expected growth rates in Sub-Saharan Africa of almost 70% and in the Middle Eastern Crescent of 53%; the latter also includes the southern and eastern former Soviet republics, which are primarily of Islamic culture. Such explosive population growth will overwhelm the capacity of the Regional economic systems to feed and house such masses, and the health system to care for the sick. Even the 27% increases in Latin America and the Caribbean and in Southeast Asia and Islands are beyond what the nations in those Regions can adequately care for, given their present health circumstances and health service infrastructure.

Although such rapid growth raises fears about future health worldwide, it is those Regions themselves that will experience greater starvation and more diseases of poverty, disabilities, and premature deaths. The rapid increase in the

**TABLE 14.1.** World population growth, by Region, 1990 data and projections to 2020.

| Regions | Population (in millions) | | | | Population increase (%) | Projected per capita GDP[a] | |
|---|---|---|---|---|---|---|---|
| | 1990 | 2000 | 2010 | 2020 | 2000–2020 | 2000 | 2020 |
| Established market economies | 798 | 839 | 874 | 905 | 7.9 | 18 | 32 |
| Former socialist economies of Europe | 346 | 358 | 363 | 365 | 2.0 | 5 | 8 |
| India | 850 | 995 | 1,124 | 1,127 | 13.3 | 2 | 3 |
| China | 1,134 | 1,280 | 1,378 | 1,469 | 14.8 | 4 | 9 |
| Southeast Asia and Islands | 683 | 808 | 922 | 1,024 | 26.7 | 4 | 6 |
| Sub-Saharan Africa | 510 | 691 | 912 | 1,172 | 69.6 | 1 | 2 |
| Latin America and the Caribbean | 444 | 533 | 607 | 678 | 27.2 | 4 | 8 |
| Middle Eastern Crescent[b] | 503 | 656 | 821 | 1,003 | 52.9 | 2 | 3 |
| World total | 5,267 | 6,160 | 7,000 | 7,844 | 27.3 | — | — |

**Source:** Abstracted from Murray and Lopez, 1996, Annex Table II and Figure 7.1.

[a] GDP enumerated in internationally adjusted, inflation-adjusted US$ (in thousands per average household).
[b] Includes seven former Soviet republics in Southeast, of largely Islamic culture.

BUILDING BETTER HEALTH

proportion of the child population that is dependent on others, combined with constricted economic resources, which are not expected to grow by much (see the GDP data in Table 14.1), might well open these Regions to even greater deprivation and civil unrest.

Programs to provide family planning are not designed to reduce the size of ethnic or geographic groups, but rather to enable families and populations to grow at modest enough levels so that children can be adequately fed, kept healthy, and educated sufficiently to prepare them for full lives. These are the goals of national family planning programs that should be emphasized. More importantly, they are goals that almost all families share. But, where future thinking extends only to the next day's food, the next harvest, and to "who will help us," dreams or fears about the next decade—even for one's family and for oneself—are not allowed to intrude upon dealing with daily crisis.

The huge differences in per capita income between wealthy and poor nations will actually widen between 2000 and 2020. Established market economies will capture 45% of the total world product in both these years, but by 2020 the established market economies will comprise only 11.5% of the world population vs. 13.6% in 2000.

An additional demographic force that will change the face of world health in the next 20 years is the aging of the population expected in all countries. The population will have proportionally more people over age 50, and hence an increase in chronic disease prevalence and in proportional mortality due to diseases of older adults. Economically, the cost to care for frail, dependent elders will multiply.

**HEALTH PROJECTIONS**

Table 14.2 presents comparisons of the relative importance of selected causes of years of healthy life lost (DALYs) between estimates for 1990 (based on partial data) and projections for 2010 (based on extrapolation of trends and anticipated medical progress). We have chosen 2010 rather than more distant projections because the margin of error should be smaller.

Projections for changes in world DALYs from 1990 to 2010 point to improved health for women (10% fewer DALYs) and worse health for men (5% more DALYs). This happens despite similar population increases for both genders. (We present total DALYs rather than DALYs per million population, because the former better represents the overall need for health services.)

The burden of all infectious and parasitic diseases is expected to decline about 27%, with HIV/AIDS being the only exception—its burden quadruples. Dis-

**TABLE 14.2.** Burden of disability and years lost to death (combined as DALYs), selected major categories and all causes, by sex, projected for 2010.[a]

| Ranking | | | DALYs (in millions) | |
|---|---|---|---|---|
| Men | Women | Selected major categories | Men | Women |
| 1 | 1 | Infectious and parasitic diseases | 125 | 106 |
| 4 | 2 | Neuropsychiatric disorders | 91 | 95 |
| 3 | 3 | All cardiovascular diseases | 105 | 71 |
| 2 | 4 | Unintentional injuries | 113 | 57 |
| 5 | 5 | Malignant neoplasms (cancers) | 67 | 44 |
| 6 | 6 | Chronic respiratory diseases | 46 | 37 |
| | | **All causes** | **757** | **592** |

*Source:* Murray and Lopez, 1996.

[a] World population is expected to grow to 7 billion by 2010.

abling and fatal respiratory infections in children are expected to drop by nearly half, as are nutritional deficiencies and the pathologies of the perinatal period. In general, the greatest improvements are projected for the aggregate of "Communicable, Maternal, Perinatal, and Nutritional Conditions," referred to as Category 1 in *World Health Statistics*. This apparently assumes a spread of preventive health programs from wealthier nations in temperate climates to economically deprived nations in tropical regions. Despite these expected sharp declines, this category will remain the single greatest health burden for the foreseeable future.

Increases—often large—in the burden of chronic and degenerative diseases also are anticipated. The projected total burden (not population prevalence) for malignant neoplasms is expected to increase 71% for men and 42% for women by the year 2010. For all cardiovascular disorders, the corresponding increases are 49% and 13%, respectively; increases for chronic respiratory disorders are 39% for men and 32% for women. The already substantial margin by which men die younger than women will increase sharply in the next decade.

Neuropsychiatric disability will continue to rise in both men (26%) and women (30%). All the major conditions are expected to increase in number. Cases of major depression may increase by 38%, causing the overall loss of more than 70 million healthy life years in 2010. Women are more affected than men, bearing 65% of this burden.

Injuries are expected to increase overall, again with men more stricken than women. The most alarming increase will occur for road traffic disability and death, rising by 65% for men and 79% for women in just the 20 years between 1990 and 2010!

The offsetting effects of anticipated major incidence reductions and population increases will result in infectious and parasitic diseases remaining the causes of the greatest health loss. Diarrheal diseases, HIV/AIDS, tuberculosis, and vaccine-preventable diseases of childhood will be the top four subcategories for both sexes. The reversed sequences of the 2nd, 3rd, and 4th sources of disablement for men and women are of interest, and warrant special attention when planning preventive outreach (see Table 14.2).

The overall priority issues for 2010 are similar to those in 1990. Respiratory infections in children will become less serious, but chronic obstructive pulmonary diseases of adults will increase sharply.

The large projected increases in malignancies have their roots in the past. Many cancers do not appear clinically until 20 to 30 years after carcinogenic exposures have begun. Similarly, stopping exposures to cancerous chemicals this year and subsequently will start showing benefits only after a similar delay. The same kinds of malignancies that caused most death and disability in 1990 will do so in 2010, but in greater volume. The expected increases (both genders combined) are as follows:

| | |
|---|---|
| Stomach cancer | up 66% |
| Liver cancer | up 80% |
| Trachea, bronchus, lung | up 109% |
| Women's breast cancer | up 31% |

The doubling of lung cancer burden in just 20 years is part of the worldwide pandemic of tobacco-related diseases. Its roots are already planted so deeply as to be fatal for about one-third of heavy users of tobacco who are now alive. There is no need for this pandemic to continue. It will stop, but only when the community of nations and peoples has the will to make it happen.

On the other hand, consider the positive predictions of drastic reductions in disease burden from infectious, parasitic, and perinatal conditions. The 2010 outcomes may fall short of the goals unless more effective outreach is made to the many high mortality areas. Again, the key is collective will—the will of the populations affected, the will of their leaders, and the will of those organizations (read: decision-makers) who control the resources needed to make it happen.

The future is not foreordained. It is malleable and it is in our hands.

## PROTECTIVE FORCES TO ADVANCE HEALTH

Chapter 13 reviewed ten of the major forces that diminish life to the end-points of disability and death. It also suggested ways to combat those damaging forces.

Built into the core of the human species is a life force to survive, to function, to be fruitful, and to raise descendants who will do the same. For uncounted millennia, the life force has prevailed over the "bad stuff," even though more and more of the latter is of human making. I will now discuss a number of proven protective forces that can be used to augment humans' inborn drive to survive and, even, to realize a newer desire to thrive.

Many simple, protective, and health-promoting steps are ready to be taken. They are assembled in outline form here, since most have been explained more completely earlier in this Handbook. The steps will be sorted by whether the primary responsibility for them is likely to rest with the community (or state), the family or primary group, or the individual.

### COMMUNITY AND STATE RESPONSIBILITIES

1. Work to have an adequate food supply—enough to prevent both general and specific malnutrition. Ensure that essential foods get to all young children.

2. Provide a safe drinking water supply. One clean well protected from drainage is a good start. Build onward from there.

3. Provide and maintain a safe waste and sewage disposal system.

4. Maintain purity standards for foods sold commercially.

5. Teach and facilitate personal and domestic hygiene.

6. Provide basic primary health care available for all, including prenatal and infant care, family planning, immunizations, school health, sexual disease prevention and treatment, tuberculosis treatment. and health promotion. Prenatal and infant clinics can teach good parenting.

7. Encourage disease prevention through community policies and teaching to prevent: tobacco use, alcohol and drug abuse, unsafe sex, carelessness with vehicles, and risk-taking. Cooperate with schools and other channels of influence. **(Also see the section on "Motor Vehicle Injuries" in Chapter 11.)**

8. Encourage health promotion, through community policies and teaching, to improve parenting and to promote anger management skills from childhood onward.

9. Teach and enforce traffic laws for motor vehicles, bicycles, and pedestrians.

10. Prevent and control community health hazards, which might otherwise be generated by factories, large farms, mines, etc.

11. Restrict the flow of lethal weapons, especially those that can quickly kill multiple persons.

12. Encourage local organizations to build social cohesion, to create foundations for fair behavior and social trust, thereby to repair faults and schisms in the social structure. This will advance everyone's health. **(Also see the section on "Poverty" in Chapter 13.)**

13. Encourage and facilitate groups, families, and individuals to respond healthfully to concerns at their levels.

Communities stand poised in the middle of a "high-wire balancing act." There is a delicate balance involved in properly allocating responsibilities to nations and provinces, to communities, or to organizations, families, or individuals. The political system has much to do with whether responsibilities tend to get pushed upward or downward. A general rule is that each level prefers having the benefits rather than the responsibilities. One strategy is to keep both at the same level, so that those who carry on the responsibility successfully reap the rewards. This keeps up the good work. When a given level of the social structure does not have the resources or the degree of control necessary to fulfill a responsibility, however, that work needs to be reassigned upward to a higher level.

## GROUP AND FAMILY RESPONSIBILITIES

Group here refers to neighborhoods, extended families, coworkers, students in a classroom, and any other assemblage of people that has ongoing close interactions.

1. Set standards for personal interaction that are fair, caring, trustworthy, helpful, and dependable. This could start anywhere, but should certainly include marital partners and extend to infants, children, families, schools, workplaces, and neighborhoods. This is a prime component of "social capital," which underlies the physical, mental, and social health of a community. It creates a social fabric that encourages persons, families, and communities to flourish.

2. Encourage and facilitate domestic hygiene, at least sufficiently to prevent transmission of disease. Reward personal hygiene for all in the group.

3. Teach and practice healthy lifestyles—build that into the group or family culture. This includes eating a healthy diet, regularly engaging in exercise, getting adequate sleep, avoiding personal toxins (alcohol, tobacco, illicit drugs), avoiding unsafe sex, and steering clear of risk taking that could be self-destructive or destructive to others.

4. Teach and facilitate timely use of preventive health services, as well as use of primary medical care when required.

5. Collectively keep the immediate environment free of health hazards, including those leading to trauma, falls, burns, poisons, insects, parasites, toxins, and infectious exposures.

6. Work collectively to encourage local schools, the community, city, and state to address their health responsibilities effectively.

7. Teach and strengthen coping abilities to reduce distress, fears, depression, and especially to manage anger. Teach problem solving so that no one loses.

8. Build and maintain social support networks that provide information, practical assistance, emotional sharing, and a sense of belonging to everyone in the group or family, especially those who might otherwise be isolated. Social support is a potent force for physical and mental health. It hastens recovery from illness and extends healthy years of life.

9. Encourage and facilitate individuals to respond healthfully to concerns at their levels both for their personal benefit and for the well being of the group.

## INDIVIDUAL RESPONSIBILITIES

1. Respond positively to the health initiatives of the state and community.

2. Follow the positive health teaching and practice of families and other groups, and urge others to do the same.

3. Practice a healthy lifestyle, as described in public health or preventive medicine textbooks and in this Handbook.

4. Use one's roles in the family, workplace, and as a citizen to encourage one's family, social groups, community, and state to fully meet their responsibilities to advance health.

5. Be informed and take responsibility for one's own well being and health.

## STEPS ALONG THE ROAD

This Handbook has emphasized using low technology for preventive interventions and primary health care. This relates to the "hardware" involved. In contrast, we have called for changes in knowledge, attitudes, expectations, behaviors, and social values. Doesn't achieving these require an even higher technology? Probably so. But the "high technology" for behavioral and social change resides in the "software"—the way we prepare ourselves, our collaborators, and our health programs to excite people, to enlist them in health goals and activities, and to participate in those opportunities offered to advance health. Health psychologists are still working on the software: writing new programs and debugging old ones. Different cultures and climates run on different operating systems, so programming may continue for years. Nevertheless, we stress again, we can begin now, right where we are. **(Review "the toolbox" of ideas for facilitating changes shown in Chapter 12.)**

## TAKE ONE STEP AT A TIME

Large system-wide changes are dramatic, but they are not always fully successful and may not be sustainable. Professor B.F. Skinner, a founder of behavior modification, could teach pigeons to do remarkable tricks, such as pushing a ping-pong ball back and forth to each other. Such skills, however, were learned one small step at a time, starting by paying attention to the ball, then touching it, and onward over many days and weeks.

Many personal and community changes are best approached in the same way, gradually—one cluster of services at a time or in one demonstration neighborhood only, until the program can be "fine tuned." That way, problems can be identified and corrected by the team when they are small, and at a small cost. For big programs, the critics will covet the money spent and be quick to raise an outcry about every shortcoming, hoping to get the whole effort cancelled.

Critics may also sabotage a proposed program (of any kind) by overenthusiasm. Years ago, I was a junior member of a health team trying to convince a corporation to field-test a small preventive medicine program in one of their factories. We met around the table with an occupational physician from the factory and with corporate officers. After criticism of the idea and efforts to find gaps in the proposal failed, the tide turned. Former critics became staunch supporters. They now said they had underestimated the program's value, and really it should be expanded to reach more workers than originally proposed, and to include most of the corporations' factories. Our health team agreed, and the corporate conferees took the proposal to top management. Top management shot it down immediately, pointing out it was too big a program; it lacked field-testing; and no data on the cost-benefit balance were available.

Hey! Let's set up a committee!

This cry, like bad television, is spreading like a plague from developed to developing countries. Yes, much important work is decided upon and organized by committees, but often sharp ideas come to a committee and get filed down to dullness—or just get filed.

An epidemiologist working in a state in the United States discovered specific poverty areas where age-sex adjusted mortality was 30% higher than in the state as a whole and 60% higher than that in more affluent areas. These findings were published in a prestigious medical journal, and reported dramatically by newspapers and television in a dozen states. Reporters came to the state governor and the mayor of the largest city asking what they would do to resolve the problem. Certainly time was needed for further review and planning. The governor and mayor both exclaimed, "Hey! Let's set up a committee."

Setting up the committee went slowly, as did its work. By the time the official report and plan of action were delivered, three months had passed. The public and the reporters were chasing new headlines. The pressure was off health issues. Nothing ever was done. Government officials were honestly busy with other pressing issues. (Perhaps referring them to other committees.) Momentum, timing, and insights into the sources of power are vital. Many a national or provincial health official has stumbled over the complexities of local politics and competing personalities, or waited until the fickle wave of momentum had passed.

Working incrementally has other advantages, too. Since facing changes is threatening, smaller changes should cause less anxiety. A helpful approach is to link the new effort to activities and purposes that are already familiar and accepted, so that the public will recognize that the new elements will fit in comfortably. Furthermore, after new changes become connected to the ongoing flow of community life, and prove to generate benefits greater than their costs, they will require less program energy to be maintained. That energy can then be shifted to advance the next innovation. In localities where sanitation and universally available child health clinics, for example, become accepted as parts of "what makes our community such a good one," there will be few barriers to their sustainability.

Automobile manufacturers offer new improvements and conveniences as options each new model year. Those that are perceived as making a positive addition to the autos after a few years, soon become an intrinsic part of the "standard model." Community health programs that prove valuable follow the same natural history. Existing competition between neighborhoods or cities can provide the motivation to get additional public health services started and maintained. **(Also see the section "Mobilizing the Community" in Chapter 12.)**

## ENLISTING NEW KINDS OF HEALTH WORKERS

Health needs are so intense in so many places that the available human resources cannot meet the demand. What can be done? Let's consider these possibilities:

1. Train a new category of community health facilitators. Select candidates carefully for keen minds and caring hearts. Add perhaps one year of practical training at first, with continuing opportunities for learning and improving skills each year thereafter. No nation has a shortage of intelligent people. Only the training system, the career path, and the resource "set aside" to fund the network are missing. These facilitators would learn the basis of preventive medicine, the rationale and techniques to render the simplest of primary health care, and the psychosocial skills to facilitate behavioral changes that build health.

2. Once health facilitators are available in a state or province, more intensively trained and credentialed health workers can supervise and sharpen their skills in tasks that can be safely delegated. In effect, this would multiply the services delivered, without increasing the number of physicians and nurse practitioners. Further it would cut costs considerably per unit of service delivered.

3. Augment the training of health educators by having them participate in clinical health behavior change and community development work. Participatory learning is powerful. In most places, health educators' skills in providing information, packaging messages, and leading groups, exceed their familiarity with issues of psychological processes, motivation, and behavior change. That can be remedied.

4. Health facilitators and health educators/promoters together can enlist and prepare a majority of the public to participate more actively in health promotion, disease prevention, and basic minor care for themselves and their families. This has two outcomes: it lowers health care costs and it builds a health-conscious constituency. The latter will support health-related initiatives politically in the community, state, and nation.

5. Different kinds of environmental scientists are needed—ones trained to work with the social and cultural environments. There are shortages of scientists who work with problems in the physical and biological environments, but the most acute shortage—and the one to fix first—is the virtual absence in health agencies of scientists who work with the social, cultural, and ideological environments. We need such scientists whose first commitment is to building health. The contributions of health economists, political scientists, and successful practicing politicians should also be enlisted. These profes-

sionals can help move good ideas into good programs, good programs into effective public actions, and effective actions into rewarding health outcomes.

6. Find ways to develop more "salutogenic people." The late Professor Aaron Antonovsky popularized the term "salutogenesis," derived from the Latin "salus" (health) and the Greek "genesis" (originating or giving birth). Simply put, the word means "giving birth to health." In reviewing the pages of this Handbook, we will recall many conditions in life that are salutogenic: good nutrition, a safe environment, loving parenting, social encouragement and support.

Are there ways to add a great throng of ordinary citizens to the ranks of "salutogenic people"?

Yes, the world has hundreds of thousands of doctors and perhaps millions of nurses, hospital personnel, and allied health workers. At a less institutionalized level, there are the "barefoot doctors of China," the community health aids in Yemen, and traditional birth-attendants almost everywhere. The world's current health status—better than ever in all of history—attests to the dedication, skills, and labor of all of them.

Yet, the journey toward world health has a long distance to go, and more helpers are needed than the nations can afford to train and to hire. Could mass training of people to promote health and prevent disease for themselves and their families be the most powerful and cost-effective step the world health community can now take?

Could these community participants in personal and family health extend their outreach, perhaps only in times of special need or when requested, to their neighbors? To a local school? To a community group? With the guidance of professionals, self-help groups might be started. In communities where many persons have diabetes, groups of such persons could inform and support each other in all the aspects of managing this disease, with occasional guidance from a physician, nurse, nutritionist, and a physical education teacher. For tuberculosis patients, groups could meet to assist in Directly Observed Treatment Short-course (DOTS). DOTS is the most effective way to assure medication adherence. Successfully treated patients could return to help current patients, under the supervision of a health professional, if needed. The ranks of "salutogenic people" could be increased with such approaches at very low costs. Such volunteers would need educational supplies, a place to meet, and encouraging visits from professionals to keep activities going.

In every community there are already unpaid "salutogenic people"—the grandmother to whom neighborhood children run to be comforted, the respected wise man to whom people come for advice, the schoolteacher with whom students share personal and family concerns. And health workers, too, give valuable informal services outside their professional roles.

How can any of us "give birth to health"? There are many ways; here are some:

- Offer accurate information about health promotion, how to reduce risk factors, how to increase protective factors, and about family and self-care. Do this simply and clearly.

- Find ways to motivate the desire for better health, and to believe it is attainable.

- Listen to people, and help them find their own solutions to the problems they face. Do not push behavioral prescriptions to people who are not ready for them.

- Help identify barriers to people's good health or health behavior change. Cooperatively discuss possible ways to overcome them.

- Model a healthy lifestyle yourself—no self-destructive habits. Be healthy. Look healthy. (Sumo wrestlers do not make convincing dietitians.)

- Encourage reduction or resolution of conflicts, particularly if they affect health behavior, the safety of the immediate environment, or entail chronic psychoemotional or interpersonal turmoil. These can lead to physiological, psychological, and/or behavioral ill health in those involved. Often, the "salutogenic person" will let the person "pour out the problem," which in itself is helpful. Depending on the nature of the conflicts, the "salutogenic person" may urge one or more of the people involved to seek appropriate help—from a family friend, a friend of both parties, a social or religious advisor. The "salutogenic person" should ordinarily refer the problem and not get involved personally, lest it diminish her or his other health efforts.

- Let people know you care about them and their family's health and well being. You cannot respond to all kinds of problems, and you cannot always resolve the ones you do respond to. You are not a physician, a psychiatrist, a lawyer, or a rescuer. But you can be a coach and help people consider some alternatives. And, most of all, convey that you care about their well being and wellness, and will do what you are able.

- Link people who can help each other. It may be as simple as finding a babysitter while a mother goes to clinic. This is like "making referrals," but it is usually non-professional and quite informal. It is best to discuss the matter first with the person to whom the referral will be made to see if the idea is acceptable. Self-help groups usually welcome new people. This process increases community engagement and builds "social capital." **(Also see the section "Poverty" in Chapter 13.)**

- Help people who feel or act socially isolated to connect with others. Follow up to see if the connection continues.

- Try to keep relationships reciprocal. If you are able to help someone, allow them to help you in some way also. You and they will feel more comfortable if there is a two-way give and take, but do steer clear of keeping a tally. Don't try to keep things even or remember who owes one more assist to the other. Remember that over the long-term, it will all even out—if it doesn't, that's OK, too, among friends.

- As the community program develops over several years, perhaps from among the throng of community participants newly educated to nurture health, some 5% or 10% will emerge who have the gifts to become especially salutogenic. Would it be possible to give them the community recognition that would motivate them to continue sharing their gifts? Could they get additional training and materials to upgrade their health work?

The burden of disease, disability, and premature death in many places is as big as a mountain. No one approach, no package of programs will take it away. But we hope some of the ideas in this Handbook will enable you, and those with you, to chip off chunks of the problem, a few at a time. And perhaps, people like you on the other side of the mountain will be doing the same. You can be a mover among the "salutogenic people."

## SAVING LIVES IS MORE THAN REDUCING MORTALITY

This Handbook has talked about elementary medical procedures (e.g., how to mix oral rehydration solution), about counseling on sensitive matters (e.g., the mixed motives of sexually transmitted illness patients), about community development, about earthy politics (e.g., name the new water treatment plant after the community leader who obtained the funds), about how gross income inequalities appear to increase a nation's mortality, and about changing cultures on a worldwide scale. Quite a bookful!

Why? To what end? To give officials, epidemiologists, and health professionals at all levels the thrill of sharply lowering disability and mortality rates? Yes, there is a deep sense of reward for saving lives. But saving lives consists of far more than reducing mortality. Yes, that must be done first, and preventing disability is the next great challenge.

But whole strata of people in the world today are not motivated to work for future health, even their own. They spend their life energies to survive, to grasp some pleasure, to make a splash so others will know they existed. Even in youth, their vision of the future may be clouded over by people they know who have died, run away, lost jobs, failed their families for reasons beyond their control.

Too commonly, such people believe that they are castaways in social environments and economic straits against which they are helpless. They then become hopeless, alienated. For some, the consequent anger leads to destructiveness and crime. For others, it leads to living in the moment, because the future is painful at worst and formless at best. For all of these persons and groups, future health is too uncertain, too unlikely, to work toward.

The basic point is that life must seem worth surviving for, or people will not make the effort to do so. People's efforts must have a reasonable chance of achieving their goals, or they will be redirected to other rewards, perceived as more likely, more immediate, or more pleasurable.

So, saving lives reaches beyond reducing mortality, disability, and morbidity. The good healthy life means growing, learning, developing, living with people who are loving and helpful, and reflecting those behaviors to others. It means being productive in some way, to add a positive touch to the human journey. This expresses incompletely some widely affirmed visions of what humanity can become. It goes beyond what the health professions can ever do. It will take all sectors of society and all people of goodwill to make this happen.

Healthy people can travel this road more successfully than sick or troubled ones.

So, let us begin.

# References and Additional Resources

## 1. GENERAL PRINCIPLES OF HEALTH PROMOTION AND DISEASE PREVENTION

Last JM. *Public Health and Human Ecology*. Norwalk: Appleton & Lange; 1987.

McGinnis JM, Foege WH. Actual causes of death in the United States. *JAMA* 1993; 270:2207–2212.

Rose G. *The Strategy of Preventive Medicine*. Oxford: Oxford University Press; 1992.

## 2. PRINCIPLES OF COMMUNITY HEALTH INTERVENTION

Barnes ST, Jenkins CD. Changing personal and social behavior: Experiences of health workers in a tribal society. *Soc Sci Med*. 1972; 6:1–5.

Last JM. *Public Health and Human Ecology*. Norwalk: Appleton & Lange; 1987.

Mrazek PH, Haggerty RJ, eds. *Reducing risks for mental disorders: Frontiers for preventive intervention research*. Washington, DC: National Academy Press; 1994.

Murray CJL, Lopez AD, eds. Vol 1: *The Global Burden of Disease*. Cambridge: Harvard University Press; 1996.

Rose G. *The Strategy of Preventive Medicine*. Oxford: Oxford University Press; 1992.

## 3. INFANTS AND CHILDREN UP TO 14 YEARS OLD

American Academy of Pediatrics, Committee on Child Abuse and Neglect. Shaken baby syndrome: Inflicted cerebral trauma. *Pediatrics* 1993; 92:872–875.

American Academy of Pediatrics, Task Force on Infant Positioning and SIDS. Positioning and Sudden Infant Death Syndrome (SIDS): Update. *Pediatrics* 1996; 98: 1216–1218.

Baildam EM, Hillier VF, Ward BS, et al. Duration and pattern of crying in the first year of life. *Devel Med Child Neurol* 1995; 37:345–353.

Bass JL, Christoffel KK, Windome M, et al. Child injury prevention counseling in primary care settings: A critical review of the literature. *Pediatrics* 1993; 92:544–550. (42 references).

Bobadilla JL, Cowley P, Musgrove P, et al. Design, content and financing of an essential national package of health services. *Bull WHO* 1994; 72: 653–662.

Botash AS, Fuller PG, Blatt SD, et al. Child abuse, sudden infant death syndrome and psychosocial development. *Curr Opin Pediatr* 1996; 8: 195–200.

Cates W Jr., Holmes KK. Sexually transmitted diseases. In Last JM, ed. *Public Health and Preventive Medicine* 12th ed. Norwalk: Appleton-Century Crofts; 1986.

Centers for Disease Control and Prevention. Postnatal causes of developmental disabilities in children aged 3–10 years. *MMWR* 1991; 45 (6): 130–134.

Centers for Disease Control and Prevention. Certification of poliomyelitis eradication—the Americas, 1994. *MMWR* 1994;43:720–722. [Also see *JAMA* 1994;272:1319–1320.]

Centers for Disease Control and Prevention. MMWR 1996; 45(10) (15 March) 211–215.

Chin J. *Control of Communicable Diseases Manual.* 17th edition. Washington DC: American Public Health Association; 2000.

Coreil J, Mull JD, eds. Anthropological studies of diarrheal illness. *Soc Sci Med* 1998; 27 (1)(Suppl).

Creighton SJ. The incidence of child abuse and neglect. In Brown K, Davies C, Stratton P, eds. *Early Prediction and Prevention of Child Abuse*. Chichester: Wiley, 1988.

Feachem RGA, Kjellstrom T, Murray CJL, et al., eds. *The Health of Adults in the Developing World.* Oxford: Oxford University Press; 1992.

Feindler EL. Adolescent anger control: Review and Critique. *Prog Behav Modif.* 1990; 26: 11–59 (Review 120 refs.).

Fleming PJ. Understanding and Preventing SIDS. *Curr Opin Pediatr* 1994; 6:158–162.

Frank DA, Bresnaham K, Zuckerman BS. Maternal cocaine use: Impact on child health and development *Curr Prob Pediatr* 1996; 26:57–70. (Review of 159 refs.)

Gibson E, Cullen JA, Spinner S, et al. Infant sleep position following new AAP guidelines. *Pediatr* 1995; 96: 6–72.

Gortmaker SL, Sappenfield W. Chronic childhood disorders: prevalence and impact. *Pediatr Clin North Am* 1984; 31:3–18. (Review 113 refs.)

Grossman DC, Rivara FP. Injury control in childhood. *Pediatr Clin North Am* 1992; 39: 471–485.

Guerrant RL. Diarrheal diseases: New challenges and merging opportunities. In Walker DH, ed. *Global Infectious Diseases*. New York: Springer-Verlag Wien; 1992: 87–102.

Guerrant RL, McAuliffe JF. Special problems in developing countries. In Gorbach SL, ed. *Infectious Diarrhea*. Boston: Blackwell Scientific; 1986: 287–307.

Hartunian NS, Smart CN, Thompson MS. The incidence and economic cost of cancer, motor vehicle injuries, coronary heart disease and stroke: A comparative analysis. *Amer J Public Health*. 1980; 7:1249–1260.

Henderson-Smart DJ, Ponsonby AL, Murphy E. Reducing the risk of sudden infant death syndrome: A review of the scietfic literature. *J Paediatr Child Health* 1998; 34:213–219.

Hijazi SS, Abulaban A, Waterlow JC. The duration for which exclusive breastfeeding is adequate: A study in Jordan. *Acta Paediatr Scand* 1989; 78:23–28.

Hirschhorn N, Greenough WB. Progress in oral rehydration therapy. *Sci Am* 1991; 264(5):16–22.

Horwood LJ, Ferbusson DM. Breastfeeding and later cognitive and academic outcomes. *Pediatr* 1998; 101(1):E9.

Hutchinson MK, Sandall SR. Congenital TORCH infections in infants and young children. *Top Early Child Spec Educ* 1995; 15:65–82.

Huttly SR, Morris SS, Pisani V. Prevention of diarrhea in young children in developing countries. *Bull WHO* 1997; 75 (2):163–174. (Review 111 refs.)

Jakobsen MS, Sodeman M, Molbak K, et al. Promoting breast feeding through health education at the time of immunizations: a randomized trial from Guinea-Bisau. *Acta Paediatr* 1999;88:741–747.

Kendrick D. Role of the primary health care team in preventing accidents to children. *Brit J Gen Pract* 1994; 44: 372–375.

Kerfoot M. Guidance to health workers and parents where child abuse is suspected. Geneva: WHO, Division of Mental Health; 1992. Behavioral Science Learning Module.

Last JM, ed. *Public Health and Preventive Medicine*.12th ed. New York: Appleton-Century-Crofts; 1986.

Lederman RP. Relationship of anxiety, stress and psychosocial development to reproductive health. *Behav Med*. 1995(a); 21:101–112. (Review 110 refs.)

Lederman RP. Treatment strategies for anxiety, stress and developmental confict during reproduction. *Behav Med*. 1995(b); 21:113–132. (Review 69 refs.)

Lipkin PH. Epidemiology of developmental disabilities. In Caputo AJ, Accardo PJ, eds. *Developmental Disabilities in Infancy and Childhood*. Baltimore: Brookes; 1991: 43–67.

MacMillan HL, MacMillan JH, Offord DR. Periodic health examination, 1993 update: 1. Primary prevention of child maltreatment. *Can Med Assoc J* 1993;148:151–163. (126 refs.)

Milerad J, Sundall H. Nicotine exposure and the risk of SIDS. *Acta Paediatr*. 1993; 389(Suppl): 70–72. (Review.)

Monte CM, Ashworth A, Nations MK, etal. Designing educational messages to improve weaning food hygiene practices of families living in poverty. *Soc Sci Med*. 1997; 44: 1453–1464.

Mrazek PJ, Haggerty RJ, eds. *Reducing Risks for Mental Disorders: Frontiers for Preventive Intervention Research*. Washington DC: National Academy Press; 1994.

Murray CJL, Lopez AD, eds.*The Global Burden of Disease*. Cambridge: Harvard University Press; 1996.

Murray CJL, Lopez AD. Mortality by cause for eight regions of the world: Global Burden of Disease Study. *Lancet*. 1997(a) May 3; 349: 1269–1276.

Murray CJL, Lopez AD. Regional patterns of disability-free life expectancy and disability-adjusted life expectancy: Global Burden of Disease Study. *Lancet*. 1997(b) May 10; 349: 1347–1352.

Murray CJL, Lopez AD.Global mortality, disability, and the contribution of risk factors: Global Burden of Disease Study. *Lancet*. 1997(c) May 17; 349: 1436–1442.

Murray CJL, Lopez AD.Alternative projections of mortality and disability by cause 1990–2020: Global Burden of Disease Study. *Lancet*. 1997(d) May 24; 349: 1498–1504.

Norvenius SG, Milerad J, Rammer L. Epidemiological change of SIDS in Sweden since 1979. *Acta Paedr*. 1993; 389(Suppl): 40–41.

Olweus D. Bully/victim problems among schoolchildren: Basic facts and effects of a school-based intervention program. In Pepler DJ, Rubin KH, eds. *The Development and Treatment of Childhood Aggression*. Hillsdale: Erlbaum; 1991.

Pan American Health Organization *Health Conditions in the Americas*. 1994 ed. Washington DC: PAHO; 1994 (Scientific Publication 549; 2 vols).

Pan American Health Organization *Health Conditions in the Americas*. 1998 ed. Washington DC: PAHO; 1998 (Scientific Publication 569; 2 vols).

Pan American Health Organization *Health Conditions in the Americas* 2002 ed. Washington DC: PAHO; 2002 (Scientific Publication 587; 2 vols).

Perez-Escamilla R, Pollitt E. Causes and consequences of intrauterine growth retardation in Latin America. *Bull PAHO*. 1992; 26:128–147.

Reeb KG, Graham AV, Zyzanski SJ, et al. Predicting low-birth weight and complicated labor in urban black women: A biopsychosocial perspective. *Soc Sci Med* 1987; 25: 1321–1327.

Rutter DR, Quine L. Inequalities in pregnancy outcome: A review of psychosocial and behavioral mediators. *Soc Sci Med*. 1990;30: 553–568.

Schoendorf KC, Kiely JL. Relationship of sudden infant death syndrome to maternal smoking during and after pregnancy. *Pediatr* 1992;90: 905–908.

Scrimshaw NS. Nutrition and preventive medicine. In Last JM, ed. *Public Health and Preventive Medicine*. 12th ed. Norwalk: Appleton-Century Crofts;1986: 1515–1542.

Smedby B, Irgens L, Norvenius G. Consensus statement on epidemiology (of SIDS). *Acta Paedriatr* 1993;389 (Suppl): 42–43.

St. James-Roberts I. Persistent infant crying. *Arch Diseases Child* 1991; 66: 653–655.

Straus MA, Gelles RJ. Societal change and change in family violence from 1975 to 1985 as revealed by two national surveys. *J Marriage Fam* 1986;48: 465–479.

Texas Department of Health. *Dis Prev News* 56(8), 15 April, 1996.

Thielman NM, Guerrant RL. From Rwanda to Wisconsin: the global relevance of diarrheal diseases [editorial]. *J Med Microbiol* 1996;44: 155–156.

Torres-Pereyra J. Emphasis on preventive perinatology: A suitable alternative for developing countries. *Semin Perinatol* 1988;12: 381–388.

Trichopoulos D, Willett WC, eds. Nutrition and Cancer. *Cancer Causes Control* 1996; 7(1)(Special Issue): 3-180, 1996.

Tulloch J, Richards L. Childhood diarrhea and acute respiratory infections in developing countries. *Med J Aust* 1993;159: 46–51.

United States Environmental Protection Agency. Respiratory health effects of passive smoking: Lung cancer and other disorders. Report of the US Environmental Protection Agency. Washington DC: Department of Health and Human Services and Environmental Protection Agency; 1993. (NIH Publication No. 93-3605.)

United States Preventive Services Task Force. *Guide to Clinical Preventive Services*. 2nd ed. Baltimore: Williams and Wilkins; 1996.

Victoria CG, Vaughan JP, Smith PG, et al. Evidence for protection by breastfeeding against infant deaths from infectious diseases in Brazil. *Lancet* 1987; (2): 319–3222.

Werner SB. Food Poisoning. In Last JM, ed. *Public Health and Preventive Medicine* 12th ed. Norwalk: Appleton-Century Crofts; 1986: Chapter 7.

Widom CS. The cycle of violence. *Science* 1989;244:160–166.

Williams RB, Williams V. *Anger Kills*. New York: Times Books; 1993. (Later paperback editions by New York: Harper Perennial.)

Willis WO, Fullerton JT. Prevention of infant mortality: An agenda for nurse-midwifery. *J Nurse Midwifery* 1991;36: 343–350.

World Health Organization. *World Health Statistics Quarterly* 1980;33: 197–224.

## 4. ADOLESCENTS AND YOUNG ADULTS 15–24 YEARS OLD

Acierno R, Resnick HG, Kilpatrick DG. Health impact of interpersonal violence *Behav Med* 1997; 23: 53–84. (Three reviews.)

Bradburn NM. *The Structure of Psychological Well-Being*. Chicago: Aldine; 1969. (NORC Monograph.)

Elster A, Panzarine S, Holt K, eds. American Medical Association State of the Art Conference on Adolescent Healthy Promotion: Proceedings. Arlington: National Center for Education in Maternal and Child Health; 1993.

Ewing JA. The CAGE questionnaire. *JAMA* 1984; 252: 1905–1907.

Hsu LKG. Epidemiology of the eating disorders. *Psychiatr Clin North Am* 1996;19: 681–699.

Marmot MG, Shipley MJ, Rose G. Inequalities in death. *Lancet*. 1984;1:1003–1006. [Also see data in Chapter 13.]

Mrazek PJ, Haggerty RJ, eds. *Reducing Risks for Mental Disorders: Frontiers for Preventive Intervention Research*. Washington, DC: National Academy Press; 1994.

Murray CJL, Lopez AD, eds. *The Global Burden of Disease*. Cambridge: Harvard University Press; 1996.

Pan American Health Organization *Health Conditions in the Americas*. 1994 ed. Washington DC: PAHO; 1994 (Scientific Publication 549; 2 vols).

UNICEF. *State of the World's Children: 1991*. New York: Oxford; 1992.

United States Bureau of Census. National Hospital Discharge Survey. Wahington DC: US Bureau of Census; 1990.

United States Preventive Services Task Force. *Guide to Clinical Preventive Services*. 2nd ed. Baltimore: Williams and Wilkins; 1996.

Ware JE, Jr, Johnston SA, Davies-Avery A, et al. Vol III: *Conceptualization and Measurement of Health for Adults in the Health Insurance Study*. Santa Monica: Rand Corp; 1979.

Williamson DF. Prevalence of obesity. In Brownell KD, Fairburn CG, eds. *Eating Disorders and Obesity*. New York: Guilford; 1995: Chapter 68.

World Health Organization. *Tobacco or Health: A Global Status Report*. Geneva: WHO; 1997.

World Health Organization. *World Health Statistics Annual*, 1994.


## 5. PRIME OF LIFE AGES 25 TO 64 YEARS

Acierno R, et al. Health impact of interpersonal violence. *Behav Med* 1997; 23: 53–64.

*American Psychologist*. January 1999;54(1)(Special issue on family violence).

Comstock GW. Tuberculosis. In Last JM. *Public Health and Preventive Medicine*. 12th ed. Norwalk: Appleton-Century Crofts; 1986..

Evans L. *Traffic Safety and the Driver*. New York: Van Nostrand Reinhold; 1991.

Feachem RGA, Kjellstrom T, Over M, Phillips MA, eds. *The Health of Adults in the Developing World*. Oxford: Oxford University Press; 1992.

Murray CJL, Lopez AD, eds. *The Global Burden of Disease*. Cambridge: Harvard University Press; 1996.

Murray CJL, Lopez AD. Regional patterns of disability-free life expectancy and disability-adjusted life expectancy: Global Burden of Disease Study. *Lancet*. 1997 May 10; 349: 1347–1352.

Paluska SA, Schwenk TL. Physical activity and mental health current concepts. *Sports Med* 2000;29:167–180. (Review 110 refs.)

Pan American Health Organization. Vol I: *Health Conditions in the Americas*. 1994 ed. Washington DC: PAHO; 1994 (Scientific Publication 549).

Reiss AJ Jr, Roth JA, eds. *Understanding and Preventing Violence*. Washington: National Academy Press; 1993.

Resnick, HS, et al. *Behav Med* 1997; 23:65–78.

Schofield A. The CAGE questionnaire and psychological health. *Brit J Addict* 1998;83: 761–764.

Sudman S, Bradburn NM. *Asking Questions*. San Francisco: Jossey-Bass; 1982 and later editions.

United States Preventive Services Task Force. *Guide to Clinical Preventive Services*. 2nd ed. Baltimore: Williams and Wilkins; 1996.


## 6. THE OLDER YEARS: 65 TO 100

Carlson JE, Ostin GV, Black SA, et al. Physical activity as prevention. *Behav Med* 1999;24: 157–168.

Disability in Older Adults: Special issue. *Behav Med* 1999;24(4) Winter 1999.

Haber D. *Health Promotion and Aging*. New York: Springer; 1994 and later editions.

Lillie JM, Arie T, Chilvers CED. Accidents involving older people: A review of the literature. *Age and Aging* 24: 346–365, 1995.

Murray CJL, Lopez AD, eds. *The Global Burden of Disease*. Cambridge: Harvard University Press; 1996.

Rowe JW, Kahn RL. *Successful Aging*. New York: Random House (Pantheon); 1998.

Lorig KR, Sobel DS, Stewart AL, et al. Evidence suggesting that a chronic disease self-management program can improve health status while reducing hospitaliation: a randomized trial. *Med Care* 1999;37:5–14.

## 7. BRAIN AND BEHAVIORAL DISORDERS

Barrish HH, Saunders M, Wolf MM. The Good Behavior Game. *J Appl Behav Anal* 1969;2:119–124.

Beck AT, Rusk AJ, Shaw BF, et al. *Cognitive Therapy of Depression: A Treatment Manual*. New York: Guilford; 1979.

Bennetts MP. Depression and suicide. In Matzen RN, Lang RS, eds. *Clinical preventive medicine*. St. Louis: Mosby; 1993.

Center for Mental Health Services. Estimation methodology for children with serious emotional disturbance. *U.S. Fed Register* 6 October 1997; 62(193).

Clarke GN, Hawkins W, Murphy M, et al. Targeted prevention of unipolar depressive disorders in an at-risk sample of high school adolescents. *J Am Acad Child Adolesc Psychiatry* 1995;34:312–321.

Dolan LJ, Turkkan J, Wertheimer-Lawson L, et al. *The Good Behavior Game Training Manual*. Baltimore: Johns Hopkins Prevention Research Center; 1989.

Feindler EL. Adolescent anger control: Review and critique. (120 refs) *Prog Behav Modif* 1990;26:11–59.

Gloaguen V, Cottraux J, Cucherat M, et al. A meta-analysis of the effects of congitive therapy in depressed patients. *J Affect Disord* 1998;49:59–72.

Hansen WB, Graham JW. Preventing alcohol, marijuana and cigarette use among adolescents. *Preventive Med* 1991;20: 414–430.

Hansen WB. School-based substance abuse prevention. *Health Educ Res* 1992;7:403–430.

Hersen M, et al., eds. Vol. 25 and later vols: *Progress in Behavior Modification*. Newbury Park: Sage; 1996.

Hosking G, Murphy G, eds. *Prevention of Mental Handicap: A World View*. London: Royal Society of Medicine Services; 1987 (International Congress and Symposium Series No. 112).

Kellam SG, Anthony JC. Targeting early antecedents to prevent tobacco smoking: Findings from an epidemiologically based randomized field trial. *Am J Public Health* 1998; 88: 1490–1495.

Kendall PC, ed. *Child and Adolescent Therapy*. New York: Guilford; 1991: especially chapters by Feindler EL and Lochman JE).

Kolko DJ, Brent DA, Baugher M, et al. Cognitive and family therapies for adolescent depression: Treatment specificity, mediation, and moderation. *J Consult Clin Psychol* 2000; 68:603–614.

Last JM. *Public Health and Human Ecology*. Norwalk: Appleton & Lange; 1987.

Levav I, Restrepo R, Guerra de Macedo C. The restructuring of psychiatric care in Latin America. *J Pub Health Policy* 1994;15: 71–84.

Manning D, Francis A, eds. *Combination Drug and Psychotherapy in Depression*. Washington DC: American Psychiatric Press; 1990.

Matzen RN, Lang RS, eds. *Clinical preventive medicine*. St. Louis: Mosby; 1993.

Murray CJL, Lopez AD. Quantifying disability. *Bull WHO* 1994;72: 481–494.

Murray CJL, Lopez AD, eds. *The Global Burden of Disease*. Cambridge: Harvard University Press; 1996.

Murray CJL, Lopez AD.Global mortality, disability, and the contribution of risk factors: Global Burden of Disease Study. *Lancet*. 1997(a) May 17; 349: 1436–1442.

Murray CJL, Lopez AD.Alternative projections of mortality and disability by cause 1990–2020: Global Burden of Disease Study. *Lancet*. 1997(b) May 24; 349: 1498–1504.

Mrazek PJ, Haggerty RJ, eds. *Reducing Risks for Mental Disorders: Frontiers for Preventive Intervention Research*. Washington, DC: National Academy Press; 1994.

Pearson JL, Ialongo NS, Hunter AG, Kellam SG. Family structure and aggressive behavior in a population of urban elementary school children. *J Am Acad Child Adolesc Psychiatry* 1994; 33: 540–548; 1994.

Roeleveld N, Zielkuis GA, Gabreels F. The prevalence of mental retardation: A critical review of recent literature (71 refs). *Devel Med Child Neurol* 1997;39: 125–132.

Rowland N, Bower P, Mellor C, et al. Counseling for depression in primary care. Cochrane Database of Systematic Reviews (1:CD001025;2001).

Rutter M. Resilience in the face of adversity: Protective factors and resistance to psychiatric disorder. *Br J Psychiatry* 1985;147: 598–611.

Seligman MEP. *Learned Optimism*. New York: Knopf; 1991.

Substance Abuse and Mental Health Services Administration. Estimation methodology for adults with serious mental illness. *U.S. Fed Register* 24 June 1999; 64(121).

Suomi S. Attachment in rhesus monkeys. In Cassidy J, Shaver P, eds. *Handbook of Attachment: Theory, Research and Clinical Applications*. New York: Guilford; 1999.

## 8. DISEASES OF THE HEART AND BLOOD VESSELS

Blaufox MD, Langford HG. *Nonpharmacologic Therapy of Hypertension*. Basel: Karger; 1987.

Chaithiraphan S, Tanphaichitr V. Nutritional heart disease. In Cheng TO, ed. *The International Textbook of Cardiology*. New York: Pergamon; 1986.

Cheng TO, ed. *The International Textbook of Cardiology*. New York: Pergamon, 1986.

Datta BN. Heart disease in the tropics and parasitic heart diseases. In Cheng TO, ed. *The International Textbook of Cardiology*. New York: Pergamon, 1986.

Gorelick PB. Stroke prevention. *Arch Neurol* 1995;52: 347–355. (Review 126 refs.)

Last JM, ed. *Public Health and Preventive Medicine* 12th ed. Norwalk: Appleton-Century Crofts; 1986:372–374.

Lenfant C. Pulmonary heart disease (cor pulmonale). In Cheng TO, ed. *The International Textbook of Cardiology*. New York: Pergamon, 1986.

MacMahon S, Neal B, Rodgers A. Blood pressure lowering for the primary and secondary prevention of coronary and cerebrovascular disease. *J Suisse Med* 1995;125: 2479–2486. (Review 28 refs.)

MacMahon S. Blood pressure and the prevention of stroke. (Rev. 33 refs.) *J Hypertension* 1996;(Suppl14):S 39–S 46.

Murray CJL, Lopez AD, eds. *The Global Burden of Disease*. Cambridge: Harvard University Press; 1996.

Ostfeld AM, Shekelle R. Psychological variables and blood pressure. In Stamler J, ed, *Epidemiology of Hypertension*. New York: Grune & Stratton; 1967.

Pan American Health Organization. *Health Statistics from the Americas*. Washington, DC: PAHO; 1995.

Rose RM, Jenkins CD, Hurst M. Air-traffic controller health change study. Washington: Federal Aviation Administration; 1978.

Sila C. Stroke. In Cheng TO, ed. *The International Textbook of Cardiology*. New York: Pergamon; 1986.

Simonsick EM, Wallace RB, Blazer DG, et al. Depressive symptomatology and hypertension-associated morbidity and mortality in older adults. *Psychosom Med* 1995;57: 427–435.

World Health Organization. World Health Statistics Manual. Geneva: WHO; issued annually.

Yusuf S, Lessem J, Jha P, et al. Primary and secondary prevention of myocardial infarction and stroke: An update of randomly allocated, controlled trials. *J Hypertension* 1993;11(Suppl 4):S61–S73.

## 9. CANCERS

Aoki M, et al, eds. *Smoking and Health, 1987*. Amsterdam: Elservier, Excerpta Medica; 1988.

Belinson JL. Cancers of the female genital tract. In Matzen RN, Lang RS, eds. *Clinical preventive medicine*. St. Louis: Mosby; 1993: 618–629.

Biesalski HK, de Mesquita BB, Chesson H, et al. European consensus statement on lung cancer: Risk factors and prevention. Lung Cancer Panel *Eur J Cancer Prev* 1997;6: 316–322; 1997. (Review 38 refs.)

Blot WJ, Fraumeni JF, Jr. Cancers of the lung and pluera. In Schottenfeld D, Fraumeni JF, Jr., eds. *Cancer Epidemiology and Prevention*. 2nd ed. New York: Oxford University; 1996.

Budd GT, Bhatia A. Breast cancer. In Matzen RN, Lang RS, eds. *Clinical preventive medicine*. St. Louis: Mosby; 1993: 618–629.

Chin J. *Control of Communicable Diseases Manual*. 17th edition. Washington DC: American Public Health Association; 2000.

Clark NM, Becker MH. Health education ahd health promotion in cancer prevention. In Schottenfeld D, Fraumeni JF, Jr., eds. *Cancer Epidemiology and Prevention*. 2nd ed. New York: Oxford University; 1996.

Colditz GA, Cannuscio CC, Frazier AL. Physical activity and reduced risk for colon cancer. (Rev. 110 refs). *Cancer Causes Control* 1997;8: 647–667. (Rev. 110 refs.)

Denis L, Morton MS, Griffiths K. Diet and its preventive role in prostatic disease. (Rev. 87 ref). *Eur Urol* 1999;35: 377–387. (Rev. 87 refs.)

Fletcher SW, Black W, Harris R, et al. Report of the international workshop on screening for breast cancer. *J Natl Cancer Inst*. 1993; 85:1644–1656.

Friedman RJ, Rigel DS, Silverman MK, et al. Malignant melanoma in the 1990's. *CA-Cancer J Clinicians* 1991;41: 201–226. (Rev. 84 refs.)

Gallagher RP, Fleshner N. Prostate cancer. 3 Individual risk factors. *CMAJ* 1998;159: 807–813. (Rev. 79 refs.)

Hansluwka H. Cancer mortality in developing countries. In Khogali M, et al, eds. *Cancer Prevention in Developing Countries*. Oxford: Pergamon; 1986: 85–92.

Higginson J. Proportion of cancers due occupation. *Prev Med* 1980; 9:180–188.

Hirayama T. Guidelines for cancer prevention in developing countries. In Khogali M, et al, eds. *Cancer Prevention in Developing Countries*. Oxford: Pergamon; 1986:327–334.

Hirayama T. Health effects of active and passive smoking. In Aoki M, et al, eds. *Smoking and Health, 1987*. Amsterdam: Elservier, Excerpta Medica; 1988. [Conference proceedings.]

Khogali M, Omar YT, Gjorgov A, Ismail AS, eds. *Cancer Prevention in Developing Countries*. Oxford: Pergamon; 1986.

London WT, McGlynn KA. Liver cancer. In Schottenfeld D, Fraumeni JF, Jr., eds. *Cancer Epidemiology and Prevention*. 2nd ed. New York: Oxford University; 1996.

Madan NC, Dhawan IK, Sahn D. Epidemiology and risk factors in oral cancer. In Khogali M, et al, eds. *Cancer Prevention in Developing Countries*. Oxford: Pergamon; 1986: 115–118.

Matzen RN, Lang RS, eds. *Clinical preventive medicine*. St. Louis: Mosby; 1993.

McGinnis JM, Foege WH. Actual causes of death in the United States. *JAMA* 1993;270: 2207–2212.

Murray CJL, Lopez AD, eds. Vol.1: *The Global Burden of Disease*. Cambridge: Harvard University Press; 1996.

Pan American Health Organization. *Health Statistics from the Americas*. 1992 ed. Washington, DC: PAHO; 1992 [Scientific publication 542].

Pan American Health Organization. *Health Statistics from the Americas*. 1995 ed. Washington, DC: PAHO; 1995 [Scientific publication 556].

Parkin DM, Whelan SL, Ferlay J, et al. Vol VII: Cancer Incidence in Five Continents. Lyon: International Agency for Research on Cancer; 1997 [Scientific Publication No. 143].

Peters RK, Bear MB, Thomas D. Barriers to screening for cancer of the cervix. *Prev Med* 1989;18: 133–146.

Peters RK, et al. Risk factors for invasive and non-invasive cervical cancer among Latinas and non-Latinas in Los Angeles County. *J Natl Cancer Inst* 1986; 77:106–77.

Potter JD. Nutrition and colorectal cancer. In Trichopoulos D, Willett WC, eds. Nutrition and Cancer. *Cancer Causes Control* 1996;7(1)(Special Issue): 3–180, 1996: 127–146.

E Riboli. Nutrition and cancer of the respiratory and digestive tract: results from observation and chemoprevention studies. *Eur J Cancer Prev* 1996; 5(Suppl.2):9–17.

Schottenfeld D, Fraumeni JF, Jr., eds. *Cancer Epidemiology and Prevention*. 2nd ed. New York: Oxford University; 1996.

Thomas DB. Cancer. In Last JM, ed. *Public Health and Preventive Medicine* 12th ed. Norwalk: Appleton-Century Crofts; 1986.

Thorisdottir K, Dijkstra J, Tomecki K. Skin cancer and protection of the skin. In Matzen RN, Lang RS, eds. *Clinical preventive medicine*. St. Louis: Mosby; 1993.

Thun MJ. NSAID use and decreased risk of gastrointestinal cancers. *Gastroenterol Clin North Am*. 1996;25: 333–348. (Review 71 refs.)

Trichopoulos D, Willett WC, eds. Nutrition and Cancer. *Cancer Causes Control* 1996;7(1) (Special Issue): 3–180, 1996.

Ursin G, Pike MC, Preston-Martin S, et al. Sexual, reproductive and other risk factors for adenocarcinoma of the cervix: Results from a population-based case-control study (California, US) *Cancer Causes and Control* 1996;7:391–401.

World Health Organization. *Tobacco or Health*. Geneva: WHO; 1997.

## 10. CHRONIC LUNG DISORDERS

Chin J. *Control of Communicable Diseases Manual*. 17th edition. Washington DC: American Public Health Association; 2000.

Doll R. Foreword. In Hirsch A, Goldberg M, Martin JP, Masse R. *Prevention of Respiratory Disease*. New York: Dekker; 1993.

Last JM, ed. *Public Health and Preventive Medicine*. 12th ed. New York: Appleton-Century-Crofts; 1986.

McKeown T. *The Role of Medicine: Dream, Mirage, or Nemesis*. London: Nuffield Provincial Hospital Trust; 1976.

Mur JM. Epidemiology of occupational respiratory hazards: recent advances. In Hirsch A, Goldberg M, Martin JP, Masse R. *Prevention of Respiratory Disease*. New York: Dekker; 1993.

Murray CJL, Lopez AD, eds. *The Global Burden of Disease*. Cambridge: Harvard University Press; 1996.

Petty TL. Chronic obstructive lung disease and other disorders of the chest. In Matzen RN, Lang RS, eds. *Clinical preventive medicine*. St. Louis: Mosby; 1993.

Samet JM, Spengler JD. Prevention of respiratory diseases from indoor and outdoor air pollution. In Hirsch A, Goldberg M, Martin JP, Masse R. *Prevention of Respiratory Disease*. New York: Dekker; 1993.

World Health Organization. *Tobacco or Health*. Geneva: WHO; 1997.

## 11. INJURIES AND VIOLENCE

Bennets MP. Chapter 10. In Matzen RN, Lang RS, eds. *Clinical preventive medicine*. St. Louis: Mosby; 1993.

Campbell BJ. Former Director, North Carolina Highway Safety Research Center. Personal communication.

Ellsberg MC, Pena R, Herrera A, et al. Wife abuse among women of childbearing age in Nicaragua. *Am. J Public Health* 1999;89:241–242.

Evans L. *Traffic Safety and the Driver*. New York: Van Nostrand Reinhold; 1991.

Guze SB, Robins E. Suicide and primary affective disorders. *Br J Psychiatry* 1970;117: 437–438.

Killias M. International correlations between gun ownership and rates of homicide and suicide. *Can Med Assoc J* 1993;148:1721–1725.

Murray CJL, Lopez AD, eds. Vol.1: *The Global Burden of Disease*. Cambridge: Harvard University Press; 1996.

## 12. PRINCIPLES AND METHODS OF BEHAVIOR CHANGE

Becker MH, Maiman LA. Strategies for enhancing patient compliance. *J Community Health* 1980;6:113–135.

Campbell MK, DeVelis RF, Strecher VJ, et al. Improving dietary behavior: The effectiveness of tailored messages in primary care settings. *Am J Public Health* 1994;84: 783–787.

Coyne CA, Hohman K, Levinson A. Reaching special populations with breast and cervical cancer public education. *J Cancer Educ* 1992;7(4):293–303.

Glanz K, Lewis FM, Rimer BK. *Health Behavior and Health Education*, 2nd ed. San Francisco: Jossey-Bass; 1997.

Jenkins CD, Tuthill RW, Tannenbaum SI, Kirby CR. Zones of excess mortality in Massachusetts. *New Engl J Med* 1977;296:1354–1356.

Jenkins CD, Hewitt LO. A two-dimensional intervention plan to reduce risk factors for ischemic heart disease. *Ann Acad Med Singapore* 1992;21:84–91.

Johnson AL, Jenkins CD, Patrick R, Northcutt TJ. *Epidemiology of Polio Vaccine Acceptance*. Jacksonville: Florida State Board of Health; 1962. (Monograph No.3).

Maiman LA, Becker MH, Liptak GS, et al. Improving pediatricians compliance-enhancing practices. A randomized trial. *Am J Dis Child* 1988;142: 773–779.

Montano DE, Taplin SH. A test of an expanded theory or reasoned action to predict mammography participation. *Soc Sci Med* 1991;32:733–741.

Morgan LM. *Community Participation in Health: The Politics of Primary Care in Costa Rica*. Cambridge: University of Cambridge; 1993.

Northcutt TJ, Johnson AL, etal. Factors influencing vaccine acceptance. In Neill JS, Bond JO, eds. *Hillsborough County Oral Polio Vaccine Program*. Jacksonville: Florida State Board of Health; 1964. (Monograph No. 6).

Oldenburg B, Hardcastle DM, Kok G. Diffusion of innovations. In Glanz K, Lewis FM, Rimer BK. *Health Behavior and Health Education*, 2nd ed. San Francisco: Jossey-Bass; 1997.

Prochaska JO, Diclemente CC, Velicer WF, et al. Standardized, individualized, interactive and personalized self-help programs for smoking cessation. *Health Psychol* 1993;12: 399–405.

Prochaska JO, Diclemente CC, Norcross JC. In search of how people change. Applications to addictive behaviors. *Amer Psychol* 1992;47:1102–1114.

Rifkin SB. *Community Participation in Maternal and Child Health/family Planning Programmes*. Geneva: WHO; 1990.

Rogers E. *Diffusion of Innovations*. 4th ed. New York: Free Press; 1995.

Rojas Aleta I. *Imperatives for community participation in health development: Processes, strategies, and issues*. Kingston: University of the West Indies for the Caribbean Community Secretariat. Univ. Of the West Indies; April 1984.

Stebbins KR. Clearing the air: Challenges to introducing smoking restrictions in West Virginia. *Soc Sci Med* 1997;44:1393–1401.

Ugalde A Ideological dimensions of community participation in Latin American health programs. *Soc Sci Med* 1985;21:41–53.

Urban N, Taplin SH, Taylor VM, et al. Community organization to promote breast cancer screening among women ages 50–75. (Randomized Clinical Trial) *Prev Med* 1995;24: 477–484, 1995.

Whyte AV. Guidelines for planning community participation activities in water supply and sanitation projects. Geneva: WHO; 1986. (WHO Offset Publication No. 96).

## 13. GETTING SPECIFIC: ACTIONS TO REVERSE THE MOST DESTRUCTIVE RISK FORCES

Bobadilla JL, Cowley P, Musgrove P, et al. Design, content and financing of an essential national package of health services. *Bull WHO* 1994;72: 653–662.

Brathwaite AR. Practical case management of common STD syndromes. Kingston: Ministry of Health; 1993.

Cates W, Holmes KK. Sexually-transmitted diseases. In Last JM, ed. *Public Health and Preventive Medicine*. 12th ed. Norwalk: Appleton-Century;1986: 257–281.

Cinciripini PM, Lapitsky L, Seay S, et al. The effects of smoking schedules on cessation outcome: Can we improve on common methods of gradual and abrupt nicotine withdrawal? *J Consult Clin Psychol* 1995;63: 388–399.

Dallabetta G, Laga M, Lamptey P. *Control of Sexually-transmitted Diseases: A Handbook for the Design and Management of Programs*. Arlington: Family Health International, undated.

Fiore MC, Bailey WC, Cohen SJ, et al. *Smoking Cessation. Clinical Practice Guideline No. 18* [or later edition]. AHCPR Publication No. 96-0692. Rockville: United States Department of Health and Human Services, Agency for Health Care Policy and Research; 1996.

Fishbein M. Changing behavior to prevent STD/AIDS. *Int J Gynecol Obstet* 1998;63 (Suppl):S175–S81, 1998.

Fisher JD, Fisher WA, Misovich SJ, et al. Changing AIDS risk behavior: Effects of an intervention *Health Psychol* 1996;15:114–123.

Hirsch A, Goldberg M, Martin JP, Masse R. *Prevention of Respiratory Disease.* New York: Dekker; 1993.

Hunger Project. *Ending Hunger: An Idea Whose Time Has Come.* New York: Praeger; 1985.

Jenkins CD, Tuthill RW, Tannenbaum SI, Kirby CR. Zones of excess mortality in Massachusetts. *New Engl J Med* 1977;296:1354–1356.

Kalichman SC, Williams E, Nachimson D. Brief behavioral skills building intervention for female controlled methods of STD-HIV prevention: Outcomes of a randomized clinical field trial. *Int J STD AIDS* 1999;10:174–181.

Kamb ML, Fishbein M, Douglas JM, et al. Efficacy of risk reduction counselling to prevent HIV and STD: A randomized control trial. *JAMA* 1998;280:1161–1167.

Kaplan GA, Pamuk ER, Lynch JW, et al. Inequality in income and mortality in the United States: Analysis of mortality and potential pathways. *Br Med J* 1996;312: 999–1003.

Kawachi I, Kennedy BP, Lochner K, et al. Social capital, income inequality and morality. *Am J Public Health* 1997;87:1491–1498.

Kennedy BP, Kawachi I, Prothrow-Stith D. Income distribution and mortality: Cross-sectional ecological study of the Robin Hood index in the United States. *Br Med J* 1996; 312:1004–1007. (Also see series of related papers in the same issue.)

Lynch JW, Kaplan GA, Pamuk ER, et al. Income inequality and mortality in metropolitan areas of the United States. *Am J Public Health* 1998;88:1074–1080. (Covers 282 areas.)

Murray CJL, Lopez AD, eds. *The Global Burden of Disease.* Cambridge: Harvard University Press; 1996.

Pan American Health Organization. *Smoking and Health in the Americas.* Washington, DC: PAHO; 1992.

Pan American Health Organization. Vol 1: *Health conditions in the Americas.* Washington DC: PAHO, 1994 (Scientific publication 569).

Prochaska JO, Velicer WF, Rossi JS, et al. Stages of change and decisional balance for 12 problem behaviors. *Health Psychol* 1994;13: 39–46.

The problem of childhood smoking [editorial]. *Eur J Cancer Prev* 1996;5:3–4.

Skaar KL, Tsoh JY, McClure JB, et al. *Behav Med* 23: 5-34, 1997. (Three review papers on stopping smoking.)

United States Environmental Protection Agency. Respiratory health effects of passive smoking: Lung cancer and other disorders. Report of the US Environmental Protection Agency. Washington DC: Department of Health and Human Services and Environmental Protection Agency; 1993. (NIH Publication No. 93-3605.)

Whyte AV. Guidelines for planning community participation activities in water supply and sanitation projects. Geneva: WHO; 1986. (WHO Offset Publication No. 96).

Wilkinson RG. *Unhealthy Societies: The Affliction of Inequality.* London: Routledge; 1996.

World Health Organization. *Tobacco or Health*. Geneva: WHO; 1997.

World Health Organization. *STD Case Management Workbook*. Geneva: WHO. In press.


## 14. IS GOOD HEALTH ACHIEVABLE
## AND SUSTAINABLE?

Bobadilla JL, Cowley P, Musgrove P, et al. Design content and financing of an essential national package of health services. In Murray CJL, Lopez AD, eds. *Global Comparative Assessments in the Health Sector: Disease Burden, Expenditures and Intervention Packages*. Geneva: WHO, 1994. (This article was reprinted in *Bull WHO* 1994;72(4):653–662.

*The Economist* [London]. 1999; 14 August:17–20, 63–65.

Fries JF, Koop CE, Beadle CE, et al. Reducing health care costs by reducing need and demand for medical services. *New Engl J Med* 1993;329: 321–325.

Jamison D, et al, eds. *Disease Control Principles for Developing Countries*. New York: Oxford, 1993.

Murray CJL, Lopez AD, eds. Vol.1: *The Global Burden of Disease*. Cambridge: Harvard University Press; 1996.

Murray CJL, Lopez AD, eds. *Global Comparative Assessments in the Health Sector: Disease Burden Expenditures and Intervention Packages*. Geneva: WHO; 1994.

Phillips MA, et al. The emerging agenda for adult health. In Feachem RGA, Kjellstrom T, Murray CJL, et al. *The Health of Adults in the Developing World*. Oxford: Oxford University; 1992.

# Index

BUILDING BETTER HEALTH

# Notes

# Notes